Multiple Sclerosis

Multiple Sclerosis

Diagnosis and Therapy

EDITED BY

Howard L. Weiner, MD

Robert L. Kroc Professor of Neurology
Harvard Medical School
Director, Partners Multiple Sclerosis Center
Co-Director, Center for Neurologic Diseases
Brigham and Women's Hospital
Boston, MA, USA

James M. Stankiewicz, MD

Assistant Professor of Neurology
Harvard Medical School
Director of Education, Partners Multiple Sclerosis Center
Neurology Clerkship Director
Brigham and Women's Hospital
Boston, MA, USA

WILEY-BLACKWELL

A John Wiley & Sons, Ltd., Publication

Library of Congress Cataloging-in-Publication Data

Multiple sclerosis : diagnosis and therapy / edited by Howard L. Weiner, James M. Stankiewicz.
    p. ; cm.
  Includes bibliographical references and index.
  ISBN-13: 978-0-470-65463-7 (hardcover : alk. paper)
  ISBN-10: 0-470-65463-5
  I. Weiner, Howard L. II. Stankiewicz, James M.
  [DNLM: 1. Multiple Sclerosis–etiology. 2. Multiple Sclerosis–therapy. WL 360]
  LC classification not assigned
  616.8'34–dc23   2011031415

A catalogue record for this book is available from the British Library.

Wiley also publishes its books in a variety of electronic formats. Some content that appears in print may not be available in electronic books.

Set in 9.5/13pt Meridien by Thomson Digital, Noida, India
Printed and bound in Singapore by Markono Print Media Pte Ltd

1   2012

Contents

List of Contributors

Rohit Bakshi, MD FAAN
Laboratory for Neuroimaging Research
Partners Multiple Sclerosis Center
Brigham and Women's Hospital,
Department of Neurology
Harvard Medical School
Boston, MA, USA

Brandon Brown, PharmD
Novartis Pharmaceuticals
West Roxbury, MA, USA

Guy J. Buckle, MD MPH
Partners Multiple Sclerosis Center
Brigham and Women's Hospital
Department of Neurology
Harvard Medical School
Boston, MA, USA

Antonia Ceccarelli, MD
Laboratory for Neuroimaging Research
Partners Multiple Sclerosis Center
Brigham and Women's Hospital,
Department of Neurology
Harvard Medical School
Boston, MA, USA

Varun Chaubal, MD
Partners Multiple Sclerosis Center
Brigham and Women's Hospital
Department of Neurology
Harvard Medical School
Boston, MA, USA

Tanuja Chitnis, MD
Assistant Professor of Neurology
Harvard Medical School;
Director, Partners Pediatric Multiple
Sclerosis Center
Department of Pediatric Neurology
Massachusetts General Hospital for Children
Boston, MA, USA

Manuel Comabella, MD
Centre d'Esclerosi Múltiple de Catalunya,
CEM-Cat
Unitat de Neuroimmunologia Clinica
Hospital Universitari Vall d'Hebron (HUVH)
Barcelona, Spain

Philip L. De Jager, MD, PhD
Program in Translational NeuroPsychiatric
Genomics
Institute for the Neurosciences
Department of Neurology
Brigham and Women's Hospital
and Harvard Medical School, Boston
Program in Medical & Population Genetics
Broad Institute of Harvard University
and Massachusetts Institute of Technology
Cambridge, MA, USA

Laura Edwards, PhD
Partners Multiple Sclerosis Center
Brigham and Women's Hospital
Department of Neurology
Harvard Medical School
Boston, MA, USA

Roopali Gandhi, PhD
Partners Multiple Sclerosis Center
Brigham and Women's Hospital
Department of Neurology
Harvard Medical School
Boston, MA, USA

Bonnie I. Glanz, PhD
Partners Multiple Sclerosis Center
Brigham and Women's Hospital
Department of Neurology
Harvard Medical School
Boston, MA, USA

Brian Healy, PhD
Partners Multiple Sclerosis Center
Brigham and Women's Hospital
Department of Neurology
Harvard Medical School
Boston, MA, USA

Maria K. Houtchens, MD, Msci
Director, Women's Health Program
Partners Multiple Sclerosis Center
Brigham and Women's Hospital
Department of Neurology
Harvard Medical School
Boston, MA, USA

Jonathan S. Jackson, PhD
Laboratory for Neuroimaging Research
Partners Multiple Sclerosis Center
Brigham and Women's Hospital,
Department of Neurology
Harvard Medical School
Boston, MA, USA

Samia J. Khoury, MD, FAAN
Jack, Sadie and David Breakstone Professor of
Neurology
Harvard Medical School
Co-Director, Partners Multiple Sclerosis Center
Brigham and Women's Hospital
Boston, MA, USA

Maria Liguori, MD, PhD
National Research Council
Institute of Neurological Sciences
Mangone, Italy
Laboratory for Neuroimaging Research
Partners Multiple Sclerosis Center
Brigham and Women's Hospital, and
Department of Neurology
Harvard Medical School
Boston, MA, USA

Mohit Neema, MD
Laboratory for Neuroimaging Research
Partners Multiple Sclerosis Center
Brigham and Women's Hospital
Department of Neurology
Harvard Medical School
Boston, MA, USA

David J. Rintell, EdD
Clinical Instructor in Psychiatry
Partners Multiple Sclerosis Center
Brigham and Women's Hospital
Boston, MA, USA

Lynn Stazzone, RN, MSN, NP
Partners Multiple Sclerosis Center
Brigham and Women's Hospital
Department of Neurology
Harvard Medical School
Boston, MA, USA

Preface

Until it was shown that immunosuppressive therapy could affect the course of multiple sclerosis (MS) in the early 1980s, the disease was considered to be untreatable. Today a patient receiving a diagnosis of MS has reason to hope. Great strides have been made in our understandings of MS in the last three decades and several drugs have now been approved by the FDA for the treatment of this disease. Because we now have treatments to offer, a diagnosis of MS can be made more frequently and often at earlier stages of the disease. A number of genetic loci involved in susceptibility to the disease have been identified. Immunologic discoveries continue, sometimes driven by treatments that are shown to confer protection from the disease. Although the T cell remains at center stage, the B cell now shares some of the limelight with other components of the immune system, such as dendritic cells and microglia. We are now able to profile the immune system for signatures that are characteristic of different stages of the disease. This ability will ultimately help us to administer a more individualized treatment, and increase our chances of success. We now have the first orally approved medication with others on the way.

Despite these advances, many challenges remain. MS is still the most common non-traumatic cause of disability in the young. More sophisticated imaging techniques have revealed that injury occurs early in the disease and that even tissue with a normal appearance can be damaged. MS can affect not only white matter, but gray matter. We now better appreciate how MS affects children, often causing cognitive and psychiatric challenges. Sometimes, notwithstanding our best efforts, the symptoms of MS remain and we have no medicine that can halt the progressive phase of the disease.

This book endeavors to define our current understanding of MS in terms of diagnosis and treatment, as well as its underlying pathophysiology. We continue to be deluged with clinical and research findings that expand our conception of the disease, and have done our best to provide an up-to-date, informative, and as engaging as possible view of MS in the current era. We hope it will also serve as a practical guide that can be used to help clinicians to provide the best possible care to patients.

PART I
Pathology and Diagnosis

CHAPTER 1

Disease Pathogenesis

Roopali Gandhi and Howard L. Weiner
Partners Multiple Sclerosis Center, Center for Neurologic Diseases, Brigham and Women's Hospital and Department of Neurology, Harvard Medical School, Boston, MA, USA

Introduction

Multiple sclerosis (MS) is a chronic inflammatory disease of the central nervous system (CNS) that primarily affects young adults [1]. The role of immune system in MS is indisputable. The primary function of the immune system is to protect the body against myriad ever-evolving pathogens and it broadly falls into two categories the "innate immune system" and "adaptive immune system." The important difference in the innate and adaptive arms of immunity is that the adaptive immune system is highly specific toward an antigen. The immune-mediated inflammation of MS was initially recognized in 1948 by Elvin Kabat who observed the presence of oligoclonal immunoglobulins in the cerebrospinal fluid from MS patients. In following years, great strides have been made in understanding the role of both adaptive and innate immune system in Experimental Autoimmune Encephalomyelitis (EAE, an animal model of MS) MS but it is not known the degree to which the adaptive and innate immune systems interact in MS.

In most instances, MS begins as a relapsing remitting disease that in many patients becomes secondary progressive. Approximately 10% of patients begin with a primary progressive form of the disease. Although primary progressive MS differs clinically and in treatment response from relapsing MS [2], it is somehow related as there are families in which one member has relapsing MS and another the primary progressive form. Not all patients enter the secondary progressive stage and, in addition to these, there are benign and malignant forms of MS. This heterogeneity of the clinical course may relate to changes that occur in the adaptive and innate immune system over the course of the illness (Figure 1.1). The progressive forms of the disease are the most disabling and are likely similar in terms of pathogenic mechanisms. Epidemiologic studies have raised the question

Multiple Sclerosis: Diagnosis and Therapy, First Edition. Edited by Howard L. Weiner and James M. Stankiewicz. © 2012 John Wiley & Sons, Ltd. Published 2012 by John Wiley and Sons, Ltd.

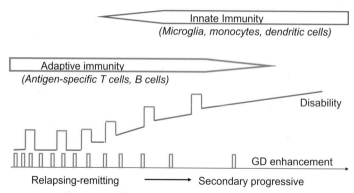

Figure 1.1 Immune status and disease course in multiple sclerosis. MS involves a relapsing-remitting phase followed by a secondary progressive phase. The relapsing-remitting phase is characterized by clinical attacks, gadolinium enhancement on MRI, minimal disability, and is driven by the adaptive immune response. The secondary progressive phase is characterized by the progressive accumulation of disability in the absence of clinical attacks and is driven by the innate immune system. (Reproduced from Weiner [147] with permission from Wiley–Blackwell.)

whether relapses are related to or are independent from the development of progressive MS [3]. This raises the central question: will current therapy that is effective in reducing relapses also delay or prevent the onset of progression? The understanding of MS pathology and immune system helped us to design various treatment strategies for MS and, given this progress, we must now ask: "What would it mean to cure MS?" and "What is needed to achieve this goal?" [4]. When one examines these questions, it becomes clear that there are three definitions of "cure" as it relates to MS: (1) halt progression of the disease; (2) reverse neurologic deficits; and (3) develop a strategy to prevent MS. We are making progress in halting or slowing the progression of MS, have approaches that may help to reverse neurologic deficits, and, for the first time, are beginning to develop strategies to prevent MS.

Clinical and pathologic heterogeneity of MS

Multiple sclerosis is a nondescript term that refers to "multiple scars" that accumulate in the brain and spinal cord. MS is more a syndrome than a single disease entity and the MS syndrome has both clinical and pathologic heterogeneity [5–6]. The clinical heterogeneity is reflected in the different types and stages of the disease. An important question in MS is the relationship of the progressive to relapsing forms. Devic disease appears to be an MS variant associated with antibodies to the aquaporin receptor [7–8]. There are rare malignant forms including Marburg's variant, tumefactive MS and Balo's concentric sclerosis. An unanswered question relates to why benign forms of MS exist [9–10]. Although some cases of MS are defined as benign, and progress with prolonged follow up [11] there are clearly benign forms of the disease. By definition patients with benign MS do not enter the progressive phase. The ability to identify benign or malignant MS early in the course of the illness is very important for treatment strategies. We compared brain parenchymal fraction (BPF) over a 2-year period in benign vs early relapsing-remitting MS matched for age and the EDSS and found that patients with benign MS had a smaller loss of BPF [12]. As it impinges on the EDSS, the majority of disability in MS relates to spinal cord dysfunction. The relationship between spinal cord changes and brain MRI changes is not well known, but changes in the medulla oblongata which reflect spinal cord can be visualized on brain MRI and may correlate with entering the progressive phase [13]. In addition, an HLA-DR2 dose effect may be associated with a more severe form of the disease [14].

What triggers MS?

The etiology of MS is still debatable but the current data suggests that environmental factors in genetically susceptible background can predispose an individual to MS. Family studies assessing the risk of relatives suggests that first-degree relatives are 10–25 times at greater risk of developing MS than the general population[15–17]. The strongest genetic effect is correlated with HLA haplotypes. For instance HLA*1501, *HLA-DRB1*0301, HLA-DRB1*0405, HLA-DRB1*1303, HLA-DRB1*03, HLA-DRB1*01, HLA-DRB1*10, HLA-DRB1*11, HLA-DRB1*14* and *HLA-DRB1*08* have been shown to have either positive or negative association with MS [15]. Ethnicity and sex are other contributors in susceptibility to MS. The white population is more susceptible to disease than the African American population and women are at higher risk of developing MS than men [18], which is not associated with any MS-related gene present on the X chromosome but is more correlated with female physiology and hormones [19]. Other potential environmental risk factors are infections, vaccination, climate, and diet. Infections are considered the most common risk factor for MS as many infections and antibodies generated in response to these infections are present in sera or the cerebrospinal fluid (CSF) of MS patients at higher titers than controls. Epstein–Barr virus (EBV) is of great interest as >99% of MS patients and approximately 94% of age-matched controls are infected with EBV and increased antibody titers to EBV nuclear antigen 1 (EBNA-1) antigen are reported in MS [20–21]. Other infectious agents linked to MS etiology are herpes virus 6, retroviruses and *Chlamydia pneumonia* [22]. Evidence for association of *Chlamydia pneumonia* with MS is debatable, as contradictory presence of this virus has been reported by different groups [23–26]. Decreased sunlight exposure, vitamin D level, and vitamin intake are also associated with MS incidence or protection [27–28]. In addition, studies using different cohorts of MS patients have shown a strong association between smoking and MS [29–30]. The etiology of MS is discussed in detail in the Chapter 3.

TOP TIPS 1.1: Risk factors for MS

- HLA susceptible genes
- Ethnicity
- Infections
- Vaccinations
- Climate
- Gender
- Smoking
- Diet

Pathology of MS

The pathology of MS lesion is defined by the presence of large, multifocal, demyelinated plaques, oligodendrocyte loss, and axonal degeneration. During the early development of MS lesions, the integrity of the blood–brain barrier is compromised, permitting the invasion of monocytes and T cells to the brain parenchyma. Mononuclear cells including activated microglia and peripheral monocytes are the primary cells involved in the demyelination of MS lesions. According to Trapp's classification, MS lesions are categorized into three groups, active (acute), chronic active, and chronic inactive. Active and chronic active lesions are characterized by the presence of evenly distributed MHC class II positive cells [31]. Chronic active plaques are characterized by the presence of MHC class II and myelin lipid positive cells that are distributed perivascularly [31], whereas, chronic inactive lesion have few MHC class II positive cells [31] (Figure 1.2). Microarray results of autopsies from acute/active vs chronic silent lesions revealed a number of differentially expressed genes present only in active lesions [32]. These differentially expressed genes are mostly related to cytokines and their associated downstream pathways [32]. According to another classification based upon a broad spectrum of immunological and neurological markers on a large set of MS pathological samples, MS lesions were characterized into four different patterns. Patterns I and II are defined by the T cell and macrophage-mediated inflammation where pattern II exclusively showed antibody and complement dependent demyelination [33]. Pattern III lesions also contained T cells and macrophages and are defined by distal oligodendrogliopathy [33]. Pattern IV is characterized by the complete loss

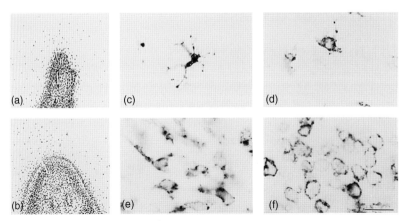

Figure 1.2 Schematic illustration (artistic rendition) of the distribution of MHC class II positive cells in active and chronic active MS lesions (A and B). Each dot represents an MHC class II positive cell. In active demyelinating lesions (A), MHC class II positive cells are evenly distributed throughout the lesion. In chronic active lesions (B), MHC class II positive cells are more concentrated at the lesion edge than within the lesion. Free-floating sections (30 μm thick) from MS brains stained with MHC class II antibody (C–F) demonstrate the morphological changes of parenchymal MHC class II positive cells that are located outside the lesion (C), near the edge of (D), at the edge of (E), and in the center of the demyelinated region (F). MHC class II positive cells closer to the lesion sites are rounder, larger than cells that are further away from the lesion site and extend fewer and shorter processes. Scale bar = 30 μm. (Reproduced from Trapp et al. [31] with permission from Elsevier.)

of oligodendrocyte in addition to the presence of inflammatory infiltrates mostly dominated by T cells and macrophages [33] (Plate 1.1).

We have identified a unique pattern of antibody reactivities to the CNS and lipid antigens in these pathological subtypes of MS patients [34]. In addition to these lesions in white matter, gray matter can be involved with evidence of brain cortical lesions or spinal cord gray matter involvement [35]. These lesions are characterized by less inflammatory infiltrates, microglial cell activation, and astrogliosis than white matter lesions and are independent of white matter lesions [36–38]. Regarding the role of B cells in MS pathology, postmortem analysis of brain tissue from secondary progressive patients, in which the initial relapsing-remitting phase was followed by a progressive phase, showed the formation of secondary B cell follicles containing germinal centers in the inflamed cerebral meninges [39] and the authors suggest that follicular positive SPMS patients have more severe disease [40], although this has yet to be confirmed. Investigation of MS pathology has provided targets for disease therapy, which are primarily directed at reduction of inflammatory cells invading the CNS.

Initiation of disease

(Th1/Th17) T cells

Cd4+ Pathogenic T cells: Upon antigenic stimulation, naïve CD4$^+$ T cells activate, expand and differentiate into distinct subsets of T cells which are characterized by the production of different cytokines upon activation [41]. It is generally believed that acute MS lesions are initiated by a myelin reactive CD4$^+$ T cell that is stimulated in the periphery and enters the brain and spinal cord (Figure 1.3). These CD4$^+$ T cells have previously been felt to be IFN-γ secreting Th1 cells as IFN-γ was found to be present at the site of inflammation [42–45] and adoptive transfer of Th1 cells were able to transfer the disease [46]. However, it was found later that IFN-γ deficient mice are not resistant but highly susceptible to organ-specific autoimmune diseases [47]. It is now recognized that Th17 cells play a crucial role in autoimmunity in the experimental allergic encephalomyelitis (EAE) model [48] and increased numbers of Th17 cells have also been identified in MS [49]. Both types of pathogenic cell (Th1 and Th17] most probably play a role in MS and could account for the immunologic and clinical hetero-geneity of the disease [50]. Immunohistochemical examinations of the brain demonstrate Th1/Th17 immune responses [51]. Th1 vs Th17 responses have been associated with different types of EAE [50]. TGF-β, a central cytokine in the induction of regulatory T cells, induces Th17 cells when combined with IL-6 [52]. Anti-IL-6 therapy is being investigated for the treatment of autoimmunity.

Cd8+ Pathogenic T cells: These cells are another subset of T cells that mostly provide defense against viral infections using cytotoxic weapons. Although CD8$^+$ T cells have not been at the forefront of thinking in MS, CD8$^+$ T cells are found in MS lesions at a higher frequency and CD8$^+$ T cells reactive to myelin antigens have been reported in MS. It is likely that CD8$^+$ T cells play a role in MS and also contribute to disease heterogeneity [53–54]. CD8$^+$ T cells are also well poised to contribute directly to demyelination and axonal loss during inflammation by expression of various cytotoxic molecules (e.g. perforin and granzyme B) as well as death receptor ligands (e.g. FasL, TNF-α, TNF-related molecules). CD8$^+$ T cells isolated from brain lesions show evidence of antigen-driven clonal expansion [55]. T cell lines generated from CD8$^+$ T cell clones isolated from MS patients and healthy controls could mediate MHC class I restricted lysis of oligodendrocytes [56]. CD8$^+$ T cells could also target other CNS resident cells including microglia, astrocytes, and neurons [57] suggesting a pathogenic potential of these cells in MS biology. The same group also observed the close proximity of granzyme B expressing CD8$^+$ T cells to injured axons in MS lesions, which furthermore emphasizes their role in the direct cytotoxicity of axons [57]. The importance of CD4$^+$ and CD8$^+$ T cells in EAE was compared in CD4 and CD8 knockout mice in a MOG-DBA/1 model. CD8$^{-/-}$ mice had reduced demyelination and CNS inflammation compared to wild type animals. CD4$^{-/-}$ animals, however, were refractory to EAE induction, suggesting a pathogenic role for CD8$^+$ T cells [58]. Furthermore, CD8$^+$ T cells are also able to contribute toward the secretion of IL-17 [59] and IFN-γ [57], which, as discussed above, are the important cytokines involved in disease pathology. These observations suggest that both CD4$^+$ and CD8$^+$ T cells are capable of playing pathogenic roles and their relative contribution might be responsible for disease heterogeneity.

B cells and antibodies

B cells are another essential component of an adaptive immune system, which mediates immunity against pathogens by the secretion of antigen-specific antibodies and by acting as an antigen presenting the cells required for T cell differentiation. Like T cells, B cells are also efficient in the production of various cytokines including IL-1, IL-4, IL-6, IL-10, IL-12, IL-23 and IL-16 [60–61]. Antibodies secreted by B cells or immune complexes can also activate other antigen-presenting cells like dendritic cells (DCs) and macrophages through the Fc receptor (Figure 1.3). Although autoantibodies (antibodies against self-antigens) have been reported in MS, there is no evidence that there are high affinity pathogenic antibodies in MS as in other antibody mediated autoimmune diseases such as myasthenia gravis [62]. Antibodies to myelin components, however, may participate in myelin loss [63]. A classic finding in MS is increased locally produced IgG and oligoclonal bands in the CSF, the pathogenic significance of which remains unknown. Treatment with rituximab, a monoclonal antibody that deletes B cells, dramatically reduces inflammatory disease activity as measured by MRI without affecting immunoglobulin levels, demonstrating a clear role for B cells in relapsing forms of MS [64]. The almost immediate response to rituximab suggests that B cells are either affecting T cell regulation via their antigen presentation function or by directly participating in lesion formation. B cells may have both anti-inflammatory and pro-inflammatory functions [60–65].

Regulation/remission of disease

Regulatory cells

Cd4$^+$ and CD8$^+$ regulatory T cells: It is now clear that the adaptive immune system consists of a network of regulatory T cells (Tregs) [66]. Regulatory

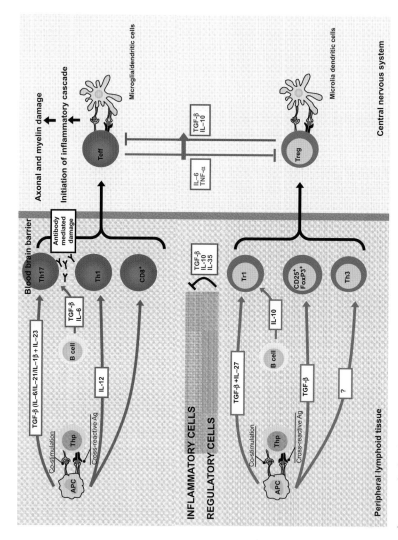

Figure 1.3 Immune pathways and adaptive immunity in the initiation of MS. MS is initiated by myelin reactive inflammatory T cells that cross the blood brain barrier and initiate an inflammatory cascade in the CNS. These inflammatory T cells are modulated by regulatory T cells both inside and outside the CNS. B cells may influence both inflammatory and regulatory T cells. (Reproduced from Weiner [147] with permission from Wiley–Blackwell.)

T cells mediate active suppression of self-antigen specific T cell responses and in the maintenance of peripheral tolerance [67–68]. Regulatory T cells can broadly be classified as natural Tregs and induced Tregs. Foxp3 is the major transcription factor for Tregs. CD25 marks natural Tregs and TGF-β induces Treg differentiation. Th3 cells are induced Tregs that secrete TGF-β [69] and Tr1 cells are induced Treg cells that secrete IL–10 [70]. Defects in regulatory T cell percentages[71–72] and function have been described in MS [73–75] and a major goal of MS immunotherapy is to induce regulatory cells in a physiologic and nontoxic fashion [76–77]. Th2 cells which are recognized by secretion of IL-4, IL-5, and IL-13, may also have regulatory T cell function as patients with parasitic infections that induce Th2 type responses have a milder form of MS [78]. Experimental data suggests that regulatory cells may not be effective if there is ongoing CNS inflammation [79]. We have taken the approach of using the mucosal immune system to induce regulatory cells and have found that oral anti-CD3 monoclonal antibody [80], and ligands that bind the aryl hydrocarbon receptor induce TGF-β dependent regulatory T cells that suppress EAE and provide a novel avenue for treating MS [81–82]. The regulatory function of $CD8^+$ T cells is mostly ascribed to a population of T cells lacking expression of CD28 on their cell surface. These cells induce regulatory effect in a MOG-induced EAE model via induction of tolerogenic dendritic cells which in turn induces $CD4^+$ and $CD8^+$ regulatory T cell subpopulations [83–85]. Another interesting regulatory population in $CD8^+$ T cell subset is $CD8^+CD122^+$ T cells which mediate suppressive effects via IL-10 [85–86]. The human counterpart of this population is recognized as $CD8^+CXCR3^+$ [87]. Depletion of $CD8^+CD122^+$ T cells increased the duration of disease symptoms. Conversely, transfer of this population ameliorated the disease in the MOG EAE model on a C57BL/6 background, suggesting a protective role of this population [88]. In addition, we have described the existence of a novel LAP^+CD8^+ T cell population that exhibited regulatory properties in EAE mice in a TGF-β and IFN-γ dependent manner [89].

Disease relapses

Disease relapses/exacerbation are the defining feature of the relapsing-remitting form of MS and reflect focal inflammatory events in the CNS. Relapse events occur on average 1.1 times per year during the early course of disease and decrease as the disease advances with increasing neurologic symptoms and age [90]. Disease relapse could last for a week to months or even more. Thus it's important to identify the conditions that could trigger relapse to determine if preventative measures could be taken to avoid relapse. A strong correlation was found between upper respiratory tract infections and MS relapses [91–92]. This study confirmed that two-thirds of the attacks occur during a period of risk (the interval 1 week before and 5 weeks after the initiation of URI symptoms) and attack rates were 2.92 per year at risk compared to 1.16 per year when not at risk [92]. Another longitudinal study with 73 patients also confirmed these results, showing an increased attacks rate (rate ratio 2.1) during the period of risk that was associated with an increase in the number of gadolinium-enhancing regions suggesting that systemic infections result in more sustained damage than other disease exacerbations [93]. No specific virus was identified among these studies. Viral infection is associated with activation of autoreactive T cells through molecular mimicry (T cell reactive to viral antigen cross-react with self-antigen) [94], epitope spreading (release of sequestered antigen secondary to tissue destruction

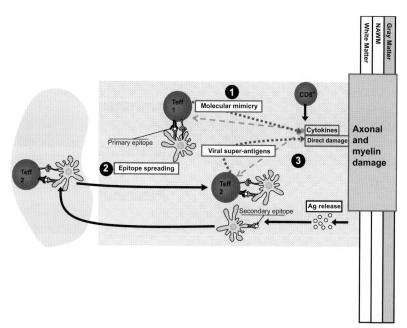

Figure 1.4 Disease relapse. (1) Cells reactive to a viral antigen can cross react to myelin self-antigen (molecular mimicry) and initiate a self-reactive immune response. (2) Inflammatory T cells that enter the CNS initiate a complex immunologic cascade consisting of epitope spreading which triggers new attacks through activation of more self-reactive T cells (epitope spreading). (3) Nonspecific activation of autoreactive T cells through cytokines released during an immune response against viral infection (viral super antigens). Dashed arrows indicate activation of T cells and dotted arrows suggest inflammation mediated by T cells through cytokine secretion and by direct damage of myelin sheath. (Reproduced from Weiner [147] with permission from Wiley–Blackwell.)

mediated by viral antigen) [95–96], and viral superantigens (nonspecific stimulation of autoreactive T cells) (Figure 1.4) [97]. Similarly, inflammatory cytokines like TNF-α and IFN-γ also increase during disease relapses [98]. Thus treatments targeting or controlling these cytokine responses should help to reduce relapse rates. Blocking TNF-α using antibodies or soluble receptors could decrease disease severity in murine EAE but has a worsening effect in MS patients [99–101]. Other factors that contribute toward disease relapse include a stressful life event [102–103], pregnancy [104], and high-dose cranial radiation [105–106]. Based upon studies describing important factors in the initiation, relapse, and progression of the disease it appears that lifestyle changes (including stress management, diet, exercise, smoking, alcohol consumption) in combination with anti-inflammatory therapy can modify the disease activity and should be suggested to MS patients.

Disease progression

Activation of the innate immune system

The innate immune system consists of dendritic cells, monocytes, microglia, natural killer (NK), and mast cells. It is increasingly recognized that the innate immune system plays an important role in the immunopathogenesis of MS. Although the secondary progressive phase of MS may be related to neuorodegenerative changes in the CNS, it is now clear that the peripheral innate immune system changes when patients transition from the relapsing-remitting to the progressive stage. We found increased expression of osteopontin and costimulatory (CD40) [107] molecules and decreased expression of IL-27 (unpublished) in dendritic cells isolated from relapsing MS. Coversely, we observed abnormalities in the expression of CD80 and secretion of IL-12 and IL-18 in the dendritic cells from progressive patients [108–110]. Chronic microglial activation also occurs in MS [111] and this activation contributes to MS and EAE pathology via secretion of various proinflammatory cytokines and through antigen presentation [112]. Persistent activation of microglial cells has also been observed in the chronic phase of relapsing-remitting EAE and a correlation has been found between activated microglia and the loss of neuronal synapses [113]. Natural killer (NK) cells, another component of innate immune cells, are present in demyelinating lesions of patients with MS [114] and are thought to play a protective role through the production of various neurotrophic factors [115] and cytokines. An increase in IL-5 and IL-13 secreting "NK2" subpopulation was observed in MS patients in remission compared to patients in relapse, suggesting that the NK2 subpopulation

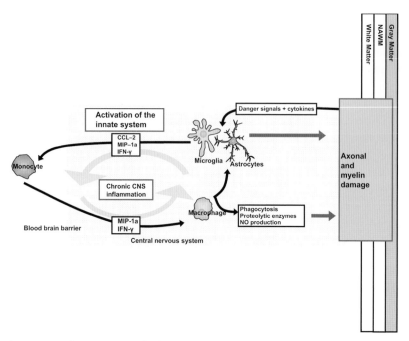

Figure 1.5 Inflammatory T cells that enter the CNS initiate a complex immunologic cascade consisting of cytokine secretion and exposure of new self-antigens that could triggers new attacks through activation of the innate immune system (microglia, dendritic cells, astrocytes, B cells), which leads to chronic CNS inflammation. (Reproduced from Weiner [147] with permission from Wiley–Blackwell.)

may have a beneficial role in maintaining the remission phase [116]. The same subset of NK cells seemed to negatively regulate the activation of antigen-specific autoreactive T cells [117]. In addition, a decreased cytotoxic activity of circulating NK cells has been described in patients with MS in their clinical relapses [118–119]. We have recently described a reduction of another subpopulation of NK cells, characterized as $CD8^{dim}CD56^{+}CD3^{-}CD4^{-}$, in untreated subjects with MS as well as clinical isolated syndrome (CIS) [120]. Treatment with immunomodulatory and immunosuppressant therapies, like daclizumab [121], interferon-β [122], and cyclophosphamide [123] show a beneficial effect through their action on a $CD56^{bright}$ NK cell subset in MS. Mast cells contain cytoplasmic granules rich in histamine and are known for their role in allergic and anaphylactic response. These cells can interact with the innate and acquired immune systems, including dendritric cells, neutrophils, and T and B lymphocytes [124–126]. In MS, histopathological analysis showed an accumulation of mast cells in MS plaques and normal appearing white matter [127–128]. In addition, the mast cell specific enzyme tryptase is elevated in the CSF of MS patients [129] along with other mast-cell-specific genes in MS plaques.

In summary, the immunopathogenesis of MS integrates both limbs of the immune system and links them to different disease stages and processes. Thus, the adaptive immune system drives acute inflammatory events (attacks, gadolinium enhancement on MRI) whereas innate immunity drives progressive aspects of MS. A major question is whether aggressive and early anti-inflammatory treatment will prevent the secondary progressive form of the disease. There is some evidence that this is occurring; studies are beginning to show that treatment with interferons delays the onset of the progressive stage [130]. Of note, there is a form of EAE driven by the innate, rather than the adaptive, immune system [131]. There are no specific therapies designed to affect the innate immune system in MS, and efforts to investigate the innate immune system in MS and characterize it are now being explored to determine how the innate immune system relates to the disease stage and response to therapy. Furthermore, like the adaptive immune system, there are different classes of innate immune responses, e.g. protective and tolerogenic vs pathogenic and pro-inflammatory.

TOP TIPS 1.2: Immune cell involvement in MS pathogenesis

- Decreased percentages of CD4+ regulatory T cells
- Increased frequency of Th1 and Th17 CD4+ T cells
- CD8+ T cells
- B cells
- Activated dendritic cells
- Natural killer cells
- Microglial cells and monocytes

Neurodegeneration in MS

Axonal and myelin loss are prominent pathologic features of MS [132] and can be directly caused by immune cells (e.g. cytotoxic CD8 cells damaging neurons or macrophages stripping myelin from the axon [133]); or can result from release of toxic intermediates (e.g. glutamate, nitric oxide). These intermediates can trigger immune cascades that further enhance inflammatory-mediated CNS damage. Thus, glutamate and nitric oxide can lead to enhanced expression of CCL2 on astrocytes which, in turn, leads to infiltration of CD11b cells and additional tissue damage [134]. AMPA antagonists have been shown to have an ameliorating affect in acute EAE models [135–136] and we have found that a carbon-based fullerene linked to an NMDA receptor with anti-excitotoxic properties slows progression and prevents axonal damage in the spinal cord in a model of chronic progressive EAE [134]. Although the compound is not an immune compound, it reduces the infiltration of CD11b cells into the CNS. Another important component of neurodegeneration relates to changes in sodium channels, suggesting that these could be potential therapeutic targets [137].

TOP TIPS 1.3: Potential therapeutic pathways for the treatment of MS

- Decease Th1/Th17 cells
- Induce regulatory T cells
- Prevent lymphocyte trafficking
- Deplete B cells
- Affect innate immunity
- Provide neuroprotection
- Promote remyelin

Conclusion

In summary, MS represents an immune cell mediated neurologic syndrome rather than a single disease entity that has both clinical and pathologic heterogeneity [5–6]. A major tool to address the pathological heterogeneity of MS and devise appropriate treatment strategies is to develop reliable biomarkers. MRI has served as the primary biomarker for MS [138] and although conventional imaging does not link strongly to clinical outcomes, every FDA-approved MS drug has shown efficacy on MRI outcomes. Advances in magnetic resonance imaging are beginning to better define MS and its heterogeneity. We have also developed a Magnetic Resonance Disease Severity Scale (MRDSS) which combines multiple measures to provide an index of disease severity and progression as measured by MRI [139]. The addition of spinal cord imaging and gray matter involvement to the MRDSS should enhance its value as a biomarker. In addition, we and others have shown immune measures that are associated with disease activity and MRI activity [140–142]. RNA profiling is beginning to identify gene expression patterns associated with different forms of MS and disease progression [143–144]. In addition, we have demonstrated unique serum immune signatures linked to different stages and pathologic processes in MS that could provide a new avenue to understand disease heterogeneity, to monitor MS, and to characterize immunopathogenic mechanisms and therapeutic targets in the disease.

A complex disease such as MS will require treatment(s) that can affect multiple pathways, including (1) suppression of Th1/Th17 responses, (2) induction of Tregs, (3) altering the traffic of cells into the CNS, (4) protecting axons and myelin from degeneration initiated by inflammation that affects the innate immune system. If multiple drugs are required to achieve this effect, we must be certain that one treatment does not interfere with another. For example, it has been reported that statins may interfere with the action of interferons [145]. Because of disease heterogeneity, there will be responders and nonresponders to each "effective" therapy and the earlier that treatment is initiated, the more likely it is to be effective. Inherent in the concept of curing MS by halting progression is the ability to demonstrate that progression has been halted in a group of patients and to identify those factors associated with preventing the onset of progressive disease. We have thus initiated the CLIMB natural history study in which more than 2000 patients with MS will be followed over a period of time with clinical evaluation, MRI studies, and immune and genetic markers, to identify the factors that are associated with the various stages of the disease and disease progression [146]. We believe that the identification of such factors may lead to the stratification of MS patients into smaller subclinical groups with defined common mechanisms of initiation of disease, inflammation, and demyelination during the disease progression that could help in designing/selecting subtype-specific treatment.

References

1 McFarland HF, Martin R. Multiple sclerosis: a complicated picture of autoimmunity. Nat Immunol 2007 Sep; 8(9): 913–19.
2 Miller DH, Leary SM. Primary-progressive multiple sclerosis. Lancet Neurol 2007 Oct; 6(10): 903–12.
3 Confavreux C, Vukusic S, Moreau T, et al. Relapses and progression of disability in multiple sclerosis. N Engl J Med 2000 Nov; 343(20): 1430–8.
4 Weiner H. Curing MS How Science is Solving the Mysteries of Multiple Sclerosis. New York: Crown Publishers; 2004.
5 Lassmann H, Bruck W, Lucchinetti CF. The immunopathology of multiple sclerosis: an overview. Brain Pathol 2007 Apr; 17(2): 210–18.
6 Breij EC, Brink BP, Veerhuis R, et al. Homogeneity of active demyelinating lesions in established multiple sclerosis. Ann Neurol 2008 Jan; 63(1): 16–25.
7 Hinson SR, Roemer SF, Lucchinetti CF, et al. Aquaporin-4-binding autoantibodies in patients with neuromyelitis optica impair glutamate transport by down-regulating EAAT2. J Exp Med 2008 Oct; 205(11): 2473–81.
8 Misu T, Fujihara K, Kakita A, et al. Loss of aquaporin 4 in lesions of neuromyelitis optica: distinction from multiple sclerosis. Brain 2007 May; 130(Pt 5): 1224–34.
9 Ramsaransing GS, De Keyser J. Benign course in multiple sclerosis: a review. Acta Neurol Scand 2006 Jun; 113(6): 359–69.
10 Pittock SJ, McClelland RL, Mayr WT, et al. Clinical implications of benign multiple sclerosis: a 20-year population-based follow-up study. Ann Neurol 2004 Aug; 56(2): 303–6.
11 Hawkins SA, McDonnell GV. Benign multiple sclerosis? Clinical course, long term follow up, and assessment of prognostic factors. J Neurol Neurosurg Psychiat 1999 Aug; 67(2): 148–52.
12 Gauthier S, Berger AM, Liptak Z, et al. Benign MS is characterized by a lower rate of brain atrophy as compared to early MS. Arch Neurol 2008.

13 Liptak Z, Berger AM, Sampat MP, et al. Medulla oblongata volume: a biomarker of spinal cord damage and disability in multiple sclerosis. Am J Neuroradiol 2008 Sep; 29(8): 1465–70.

14 Barcellos LF, Oksenberg JR, Begovich AB, et al. HLA-DR2 dose effect on susceptibility to multiple sclerosis and influence on disease course. Am J Hum Genet 2003 Mar; 72(3): 710–6.

15 Trapp BD, Nave KA. Multiple sclerosis: an immune or neurodegenerative disorder? Annu Rev Neurosci 2008; 31: 247–69.

16 Sadovnick AD, Baird PA, Ward RH. Multiple sclerosis: updated risks for relatives. Am J Med Genet 1988 Mar; 29(3): 533–41.

17 Ebers GC, Sadovnick AD, Dyment DA, Yee IM, Willer CJ, Risch N. Parent-of-origin effect in multiple sclerosis: observations in half-siblings. Lancet 2004 May; 363(9423): 1773–4.

18 Wallin MT, Page WF, Kurtzke JF. Multiple sclerosis in US veterans of the Vietnam era and later military service: race, sex, and geography. Ann Neurol 2004 Jan; 55(1): 65–71.

19 Whitacre CC. Sex differences in autoimmune disease. Nat Immunol 2001 Sep; 2(9): 777–80.

20 Sundstrom P, Juto P, Wadell G, Hallmans G, Svenningsson A, Nystrom L, et al. An altered immune response to Epstein-Barr virus in multiple sclerosis: a prospective study. Neurology 2004 Jun; 62(12): 2277–82.

21 Levin LI, Munger KL, Rubertone MV, Peck CA, Lennette ET, Spiegelman D, et al. Temporal relationship between elevation of epstein-barr virus antibody titers and initial onset of neurological symptoms in multiple sclerosis. JAMA 2005 May; 293(20): 2496–500.

22 Marrie RA. Environmental risk factors in multiple sclerosis aetiology. Lancet Neurol 2004 Dec; 3(12): 709–18.

23 Layh-Schmitt G, Bendl C, Hildt U, Dong-Si T, Juttler E, Schnitzler P, et al. Evidence for infection with Chlamydia pneumoniae in a subgroup of patients with multiple sclerosis. Ann Neurol 2000 May; 47(5): 652–5.

24 Munger KL, Peeling RW, Hernan MA, Chasan-Taber L, Olek MJ, Hankinson SE, et al. Infection with Chlamydia pneumoniae and risk of multiple sclerosis. Epidemiology 2003 Mar; 14(2): 141–7.

25 Sriram S, Stratton CW, Yao S, Tharp A, Ding L, Bannan JD, et al. Chlamydia pneumoniae infection of the central nervous system in multiple sclerosis. Ann Neurol 1999 Jul; 46(1): 6–14.

26 Numazaki K, Chibar S. Failure to detect Chlamydia pneumoniae in the central nervous system of patients with MS. Neurology 2001 Aug; 57(4): 746.

27 Munger KL, Zhang SM, O'Reilly E, Hernan MA, Olek MJ, Willett WC, et al. Vitamin D intake and incidence of multiple sclerosis. Neurology 2004 Jan; 62(1): 60–5.

28 Munger KL, Levin LI, Hollis BW, Howard NS, Ascherio A. Serum 25-hydroxyvitamin D levels and risk of multiple sclerosis. JAMA 2006 Dec; 296(23): 2832–8.

29 Riise T, Nortvedt MW, Ascherio A. Smoking is a risk factor for multiple sclerosis. Neurology 2003 Oct; 61(8): 1122–4.

30 Hedstrom AK, Sundqvist E, Baarnhielm M, Nordin N, Hillert J, Kockum I, et al. Smoking and two human leukocyte antigen genes interact to increase the risk for multiple sclerosis. Brain 2011 Mar; 134(Pt 3): 653–64.

31 Trapp BD, Bo L, Mork S, Chang A. Pathogenesis of tissue injury in MS lesions. J Neuroimmunol 1999 Jul; 98(1): 49–56.

32 Lock C, Hermans G, Pedotti R, Brendolan A, Schadt E, Garren H, et al. Gene-microarray analysis of multiple sclerosis lesions yields new targets validated in autoimmune encephalomyelitis. Nat Med 2002 May; 8(5): 500–8.

33 Lucchinetti C, Bruck W, Parisi J, Scheithauer B, Rodriguez M, Lassmann H. Heterogeneity of multiple sclerosis lesions: implications for the pathogenesis of demyelination. Ann Neurol 2000 Jun; 47(6): 707–17.

34 Quintana FJ, Farez MF, Viglietta V, Iglesias AH, Merbl Y, Izquierdo G, et al. Antigen microarrays identify unique serum autoantibody signatures in clinical and pathologic subtypes of multiple sclerosis. Proc Natl Acad Sci U S A 2008 Dec; 105(48): 18889–94.

35 Wegner C, Stadelmann C. Gray matter pathology and multiple sclerosis. Curr Neurol Neurosci Rep 2009 Sep; 9(5): 399–404.

36 Pirko I, Lucchinetti CF, Sriram S, Bakshi R. Gray matter involvement in multiple sclerosis. Neurology 2007 Feb; 68(9): 634–42.

37 Brink BP, Veerhuis R, Breij EC, van der Valk P, Dijkstra CD, Bo L. The pathology of multiple sclerosis is location-dependent: no significant complement activation is detected in purely cortical lesions. J Neuropathol Exp Neurol 2005 Feb; 64(2): 147–55.

38 van Horssen J, Brink BP, de Vries HE, van der Valk P, Bo L. The blood--brain barrier in cortical multiple sclerosis lesions. J Neuropathol Exp Neurol 2007 Apr; 66(4): 321–8.

39 Serafini B, Rosicarelli B, Magliozzi R, Stigliano E, Aloisi F. Detection of ectopic B-cell follicles with germinal centers in the meninges of patients with secondary progressive multiple sclerosis. Brain Pathol 2004 Apr; 14(2): 164–74.

40 Magliozzi R, Howell O, Vora A, Serafini B, Nicholas R, Puopolo M, et al. Meningeal B-cell follicles in secondary progressive multiple sclerosis associate with early onset of disease and severe cortical pathology. Brain 2007 Apr; 130(Pt 4): 1089–104.

41 Mosmann TR, Cherwinski H, Bond MW, Giedlin MA, Coffman RL. Two types of murine helper T cell clone. I. Definition according to profiles of lymphokine activities and secreted proteins. J Immunol 1986 Apr; 136(7): 2348–57.

42 Merrill JE, Kono DH, Clayton J, Ando DG, Hinton DR, Hofman FM. Inflammatory leukocytes and cytokines in the peptide-induced disease of experimental allergic encephalomyelitis in SJL and B10. PL mice. Proc Natl Acad Sci USA 1992 Jan; 89(2): 574–8.

43 Ando DG, Clayton J, Kono D, Urban JL, Sercarz EE. Encephalitogenic T cells in the B10. PL model of experimental allergic encephalomyelitis (EAE) are of the Th1 lymphokine subtype. Cell Immunol 1989 Nov; 124(1): 132–43.

44 Traugott U, Lebon P. Multiple sclerosis: involvement of interferons in lesion pathogenesis. Ann Neurol 1988 Aug; 24(2): 243–51.

45 Traugott U, Lebon P. Interferon-gamma and Ia antigen are present on astrocytes in active chronic multiple sclerosis lesions. J Neurol Sci 1988 Apr; 84(2–3): 257–64.

46 Pettinelli CB, McFarlin DE. Adoptive transfer of experimental allergic encephalomyelitis in SJL/J mice after in vitro activation of lymph node cells by myelin basic protein: requirement for Lyt 1+ 2-T lymphocytes. J Immunol 1981 Oct; 127(4): 1420–3.

47 Ferber IA, Brocke S, Taylor-Edwards C, Ridgway W, Dinisco C, Steinman L, et al. Mice with a disrupted IFN-gamma gene are susceptible to the induction of experimental autoimmune encephalomyelitis (EAE). J Immunol 1996 Jan; 156(1): 5–7.

48 Bettelli E, Korn T, Oukka M, et al. Induction and effector functions of T(H)17 cells. Nature 2008 Jun; 453(7198): 1051–7.

49 Kebir H, Kreymborg K, Ifergan I, et al. Human TH17 lymphocytes promote blood-brain barrier disruption and central nervous system inflammation. Nat Med 2007 Oct; 13(10): 1173–5.

50 Stromnes IM, Cerretti LM, Liggitt D, et al. Differential regulation of central nervous system autoimmunity by T(H)1 and T(H)17 cells. Nat Med 2008 Mar; 14(3): 337–42.

51 Montes M, Zhang X, Berthelot L, et al. Oligoclonal myelin-reactive T-cell infiltrates derived from multiple sclerosis lesions are enriched in Th17 cells. Clin Immunol 2009; 130(2): 133-44.

52 Bettelli E, Carrier Y, Gao W, et al. Reciprocal developmental pathways for the generation of pathogenic effector TH17 and regulatory T cells. Nature 2006 May; 441(7090): 235–8.

53 Crawford MP, Yan SX, Ortega SB, et al. High prevalence of autoreactive, neuroantigen-specific CD8+ T cells in multiple sclerosis revealed by novel flow cytometric assay. Blood 2004 Jun; 103(11): 4222–31.

54 Saxena A, Bauer J, Scheikl T, et al. Cutting edge: multiple sclerosis-like lesions induced by effector CD8 T cells recognizing a sequestered antigen on oligodendrocytes. J Immunol 2008 Aug; 181(3): 1617–21.

55 Babbe H, Roers A, Waisman A, Lassmann H, Goebels N, Hohlfeld R, et al. Clonal expansions of CD8(+) T cells dominate the T cell infiltrate in active multiple sclerosis lesions as shown by micromanipulation and single cell polymerase chain reaction. J Exp Med 2000 Aug; 192(3): 393–404.

56 Jurewicz A, Biddison WE, Antel JP. MHC class I-restricted lysis of human oligodendrocytes by myelin basic protein peptide-specific CD8 T lymphocytes. J Immunol 1998 Mar; 160(6): 3056–9.

57 Neumann H, Medana IM, Bauer J, Lassmann H. Cytotoxic T lymphocytes in auto-immune and degenerative CNS diseases. Trends Neurosci 2002 Jun; 25(6): 313–19.

58 Abdul-Majid KB, Wefer J, Stadelmann C, Stefferl A, Lassmann H, Olsson T, et al. Comparing the pathogenesis of experimental autoimmune encephalomyelitis in CD4-/- and CD8-/- DBA/1 mice defines qualitative roles of different T cell subsets. J Neuroimmunol 2003 Aug; 141(1-2): 10–19.

59 Kolls JK, Linden A. Interleukin-17 family members and inflammation. Immunity 2004 Oct; 21(4): 467–76.

60 Duddy M, Niino M, Adatia F, et al. Distinct effector cytokine profiles of memory and naive human B cell subsets and implication in multiple sclerosis. J Immunol 2007 May; 178(10): 6092–9.

61 Lund FE, Garvy BA, Randall TD, Harris DP. Regulatory roles for cytokine-producing B cells in infection and autoimmune disease. Curr Dir Autoimmun 2005; 8: 25–54.

62 O'Connor KC, McLaughlin KA, De Jager PL, et al. Self-antigen tetramers discriminate between myelin autoantibodies to native or denatured protein. Nat Med 2007 Feb; 13(2): 211–17.

63 Genain CP, Cannella B, et al. Identification of autoantibodies associated with myelin damage in multiple sclerosis. Nat Med 1999 Feb; 5(2): 170–5.

64 Hauser SL, Waubant E, Arnold DL, et al. B-cell depletion with rituximab in relapsing-remitting multiple sclerosis. N Engl J Med 2008 Feb; 358(7): 676–88.

65 Mizoguchi A, Bhan AK. A case for regulatory B cells. J Immunol 2006 Jan; 176(2): 705–10.

66 Sakaguchi S, Yamaguchi T, Nomura T, et al. Regulatory T cells and immune tolerance. Cell 2008 May; 133(5): 775–87.

67 Sakaguchi S. Regulatory T cells: key controllers of immunologic self-tolerance. Cell 2000 May; 101(5): 455–8.

68 Shevach EM, McHugh RS, Piccirillo CA, Thornton AM. Control of T-cell activation by CD4+ CD25+ suppressor T cells. Immunol Rev 2001 Aug; 182: 58–67.

69 Weiner HL. Induction and mechanism of action of transforming growth factor-beta-secreting Th3 regulatory cells. Immunol Rev 2001 Aug; 182: 207–14.

70 Roncarolo MG, Gregori S, Battaglia M, et al. Interleukin–10-secreting type 1 regulatory T cells in rodents and humans. Immunol Rev 2006 Aug; 212: 28–50.

71 Borsellino G, Kleinewietfeld M, Di Mitri D, Sternjak A, Diamantini A, Giometto R, et al. Expression of ectonucleotidase CD39 by Foxp3+ Treg cells: hydrolysis of extracellular ATP and immune suppression. Blood 2007 Aug; 110(4): 1225–32.

72 Venken K, Hellings N, Hensen K, Rummens JL, Medaer R, D'Hooghe MB, et al. Secondary progressive in contrast to relapsing-remitting multiple sclerosis patients show a normal CD4+CD25+ regulatory T-cell function and FOXP3 expression. J Neurosci Res 2006 Jun; 83(8): 1432–46.

73 Viglietta V, Baecher-Allan C, Weiner HL, et al. Loss of functional suppression by CD4+CD25+ regulatory T cells in patients with multiple sclerosis. J Exp Med 2004 Apr; 199(7): 971–9.

74 Martinez-Forero I, Garcia-Munoz R, Martinez-Pasamar S, et al. IL-10 suppressor activity and ex vivo Tr1 cell function are impaired in multiple sclerosis. Eur J Immunol 2008 Feb; 38(2): 576–86.

75 Astier AL, Meiffren G, Freeman S, et al. Alterations in CD46-mediated Tr1 regulatory T cells in patients with multiple sclerosis. J Clin Invest 2006 Dec; 116(12): 3252–7.

76 Haas J, Korporal M, Balint B, Fritzsching B, Schwarz A, Wildemann B. Glatiramer acetate improves regulatory T-cell function by expansion of naive CD4(+) CD25(+) FOXP3(+) CD31(+) T-cells in patients with multiple sclerosis. J Neuroimmunol 2009 Nov; 216(1–2): 113–17.

77 Korporal M, Haas J, Balint B, Fritzsching B, Schwarz A, Moeller S, et al. Interferon beta-induced restoration of regulatory T-cell function in multiple sclerosis is prompted by an increase in newly generated naive regulatory T cells. Arch Neurol 2008 Nov; 65(11): 1434–9.

78 Correale J, Farez M. Association between parasite infection and immune responses in multiple sclerosis. Ann Neurol 2007 Feb; 61(2): 97–108.

79 Korn T, Reddy J, Gao W, et al. Myelin-specific regulatory T cells accumulate in the CNS but fail to control autoimmune inflammation. Nat Med 2007 Apr; 13(4): 423–31.

80 Ochi H, Abraham M, Ishikawa H, et al. Oral CD3-specific antibody suppresses autoimmune encephalomyelitis by inducing CD4+ CD25- LAP+ T cells. Nat Med 2006 Jun; 12(6): 627–35.

81 Quintana FJ, Basso AS, Iglesias AH, et al. Control of T(reg) and T(H)17 cell differentiation by the aryl hydrocarbon receptor. Nature 2008 May; 453(7191): 65–71.

82 Gandhi R, Kumar D, Burns EJ, Nadeau M, Dake B, Laroni A, et al. Activation of the aryl hydrocarbon receptor induces human type 1 regulatory T cell-like and Foxp3(+) regulatory T cells. Nat Immunol 2010 Sep; 11(9): 846–53.

83 Najafian N, Chitnis T, Salama AD, Zhu B, Benou C, Yuan X, et al. Regulatory functions of CD8+CD28- T cells in an autoimmune disease model. J Clin Invest 2003 Oct; 112(7): 1037–48.

84 Chang CC, Ciubotariu R, Manavalan JS, Yuan J, Colovai AI, Piazza F, et al. Tolerization of dendritic cells by T(S) cells: the crucial role of inhibitory receptors ILT3 and ILT4. Nat Immunol 2002 Mar; 3(3): 237–43.

85 Suciu-Foca N, Manavalan JS, Scotto L, Kim-Schulze S, Galluzzo S, Naiyer AJ, et al. Molecular characterization of allospecific T suppressor and tolerogenic dendritic cells: review. Int Immunopharmacol 2005 Jan; 5(1): 7–11.

86 Endharti AT, Rifa IM, Shi Z, Fukuoka Y, Nakahara Y, Kawamoto Y, et al. Cutting edge: CD8+CD122+ regulatory T cells produce IL-10 to suppress IFN-gamma production and proliferation of CD8+ T cells. J Immunol 2005 Dec; 175(11): 7093–7.

87 Suzuki H, Shi Z, Okuno Y, Isobe K. Are CD8+CD122+ cells regulatory T cells or memory T cells? Hum Immunol 2008 Nov; 69(11): 751–4.

88 Lee YH, Ishida Y, Rifa'i M, Shi Z, Isobe K, Suzuki H. Essential role of CD8+CD122+ regulatory T cells in the recovery from experimental autoimmune encephalomyelitis. J Immunol 2008 Jan; 180(2): 825–32.

89 Chen ML, Yan BS, Kozoriz D, Weiner HL. Novel CD8+ Treg suppress EAE by TGF-beta- and IFN-gamma-dependent mechanisms. Eur J Immunol 2009 Dec; 39(12): 3423–35.

90 Patzold U, Pocklington PR. Course of multiple sclerosis. First results of a prospective study carried out of 102 MS patients from 1976 to 1980. Acta Neurol Scand 1982 Apr; 65(4): 248–66.

91 Edwards S, Zvartau M, Clarke H, Irving W, Blumhardt LD. Clinical relapses and disease activity on magnetic resonance imaging associated with viral upper respiratory tract infections in multiple sclerosis. J Neurol Neurosurg Psychiat 1998 Jun; 64(6): 736–41.

92 Panitch HS. Influence of infection on exacerbations of multiple sclerosis. Ann Neurol 1994; 36Suppl: S25–8.

93 Buljevac D, Flach HZ, Hop WC, Hijdra D, Laman JD, Savelkoul HF, et al. Prospective study on the relationship between infections and multiple sclerosis exacerbations. Brain 2002 May; 125(Pt 5): 952–60.

94 Fujinami RS, Oldstone MB. Amino acid homology between the encephalitogenic site of myelin basic protein and virus: mechanism for autoimmunity. Science 1985 Nov; 230(4729): 1043–5.

95 Vanderlugt CL, Begolka WS, Neville KL, Katz-Levy Y, Howard LM, Eagar TN, et al. The functional significance of epitope spreading and its regulation by co-stimulatory molecules. Immunol Rev 1998 Aug; 164: 63–72.

96 Miller SD, Karpus WJ. The immunopathogenesis and regulation of T-cell-mediated demyelinating diseases. Immunol Today 1994 Aug; 15(8): 356–61.

97 Scherer MT, Ignatowicz L, Winslow GM, Kappler JW, Marrack P. Superantigens: bacterial and viral proteins that manipulate the immune system. Annu Rev Cell Biol 1993; 9: 101–28.

98 Caggiula M, Batocchi AP, Frisullo G, Angelucci F, Patanella AK, Sancricca C, et al. Neurotrophic factors and clinical recovery in relapsing-remitting multiple sclerosis. Scand J Immunol 2005 Aug; 62(2): 176–82.

99 Selmaj KW, Raine CS. Experimental autoimmune encephalomyelitis: immunotherapy with anti-tumor necrosis factor antibodies and soluble tumor necrosis factor receptors. Neurology 1995 Jun; 45 (6 Suppl 6): S44–9.

100 van Oosten BW, Barkhof F, Truyen L, Boringa JB, Bertelsmann FW, von Blomberg BM, et al. Increased MRI activity and immune activation in two multiple sclerosis patients treated with the monoclonal anti-tumor necrosis factor antibody cA2. Neurology 1996 Dec; 47(6): 1531–4.

101 TNF neutralization in MS: results of a randomized, placebo-controlled multicenter study. The Lenercept Multiple Sclerosis Study Group and The University of British Columbia MS/MRI Analysis Group. Neurology 1999 Aug; 53(3): 457–65.

102 Mohr DC, Hart SL, Julian L, Cox D, Pelletier D. Association between stressful life events and exacerbation in multiple sclerosis: a meta-analysis. BMJ 2004 Mar; 328(7442): 731.

103 Rabins PV, Brooks BR, O'Donnell P, Pearlson GD, Moberg P, Jubelt B, et al. Structural brain correlates of emotional disorder in multiple sclerosis. Brain 1986 Aug; 109(Pt 4): 585–97.

104 Confavreux C, Hutchinson M, Hours MM, Cortinovis-Tourniaire P, Moreau T. Rate of pregnancy-related relapse in multiple sclerosis. Pregnancy in Multiple Sclerosis Group. N Engl J Med 1998 Jul; 339(5): 285–91.

105 Peterson K, Rosenblum MK, Powers JM, Alvord E, Walker RW, Posner JB. Effect of brain irradiation on demyelinating lesions. Neurology 1993 Oct; 43(10): 2105–12.

106 Murphy CB, Hashimoto SA, Graeb D, Thiessen BA. Clinical exacerbation of multiple sclerosis following radiotherapy. Arch Neurol 2003 Feb; 60(2): 273–5.

107 Gopal M, Mittal A, Weiner H. Increased osteopontin expression in dendritic cells amplifies IL–17 production by CD4+ T cells in experimental autoimmune encephalomyelitis and in multiple sclerosis. JI 2008.

108 Karni A, Abraham M, Monsonego A, et al. Innate immunity in multiple sclerosis: myeloid dendritic cells in secondary progressive multiple sclerosis are activated and drive a proinflammatory immune response. J Immunol 2006 Sep; 177(6): 4196–202.

109 Balashov KE, Smith DR, Khoury SJ, et al. Increased interleukin 12 production in progressive multiple sclerosis: induction by activated CD4+ T cells via CD40 ligand. Proc Natl Acad Sci U S A 1997 Jan; 94(2): 599–603.

110 Karni A, Koldzic DN, Bharanidharan P, et al. IL–18 is linked to raised IFN-gamma in multiple sclerosis and is induced by activated CD4(+) T cells via CD40-CD40 ligand interactions. J Neuroimmunol 2002 Apr; 125(1–2): 134–40.

111 Kutzelnigg A, Lucchinetti CF, Stadelmann C, et al. Cortical demyelination and diffuse white matter injury in multiple sclerosis. Brain 2005 Nov; 128(Pt 11): 2705–12.

112 Benveniste EN. Cytokines: influence on glial cell gene expression and function. Chem Immunol 1997; 69: 31–75.

113 Rasmussen S, Wang Y, Kivisakk P, Bronson RT, Meyer M, Imitola J, et al. Persistent activation of microglia is associated with neuronal dysfunction of callosal projecting pathways and multiple sclerosis-like lesions in relapsing–remitting experimental autoimmune encephalomyelitis. Brain 2007 Nov; 130(Pt 11): 2816–29.

114 Traugott U. Characterization and distribution of lymphocyte subpopulations in multiple sclerosis plaques versus autoimmune demyelinating lesions. Springer Semin Immunopathol 1985; 8(1–2): 71–95.

115 Hammarberg H, Lidman O, Lundberg C, Eltayeb SY, Gielen AW, Muhallab S, et al. Neuroprotection by encephalomyelitis: rescue of mechanically injured neurons and neurotrophin production by CNS-infiltrating T and natural killer cells. J Neurosci 2000 Jul; 20(14): 5283–91.

116 Takahashi K, Miyake S, Kondo T, Terao K, Hatakenaka M, Hashimoto S, et al. Natural killer type 2 bias in remission of multiple sclerosis. J Clin Invest 2001 Mar; 107(5): R23–9.

117 Takahashi K, Aranami T, Endoh M, Miyake S, Yamamura T. The regulatory role of natural killer cells in multiple sclerosis. Brain 2004 Sep; 127(Pt 9): 1917–27.

118 Kastrukoff LF, Morgan NG, Zecchini D, White R, Petkau AJ, Satoh J, et al. A role for natural killer cells in the immunopathogenesis of multiple sclerosis. J Neuroimmunol 1998 Jun; 86(2): 123–33.

119 Kastrukoff LF, Lau A, Wee R, Zecchini D, White R, Paty DW. Clinical relapses of multiple sclerosis are associated with 'novel' valleys in natural killer cell functional activity. J Neuroimmunol 2003 Dec; 145(1–2): 103–14.

120 De Jager PL, Rossin E, Pyne S, Tamayo P, Ottoboni L, Viglietta V, et al. Cytometric profiling in multiple sclerosis uncovers patient population structure and a reduction of CD8low cells. Brain 2008 Jul; 131 I (Pt 7): 1701–11.

121 Bielekova B, Catalfamo M, Reichert-Scrivner S, Packer A, Cerna M, Waldmann TA, et al. Regulatory CD56(bright) natural killer cells mediate immunomodulatory effects of IL–2Ralpha-targeted therapy (daclizumab) in multiple sclerosis. Proc Natl Acad Sci U S A 2006 Apr; 103(15): 5941–6.

122 Saraste M, Irjala H, Airas L. Expansion of CD56 Bright natural killer cells in the peripheral blood of multiple sclerosis patients treated with interferon-beta. Neurol Sci 2007 Jun; 28(3): 121–6.

123 Rinaldi L, Laroni, A., Ranzato, F., Calabrese, M., Perini, P., Sanzari, M., Plebani, M-, Battistin L., Gallo P. Regulatory CD56 bright natural killer cells expanded during cyclophosphamide therapy in multiple sclerosis. Mult Scler 2007 2007; Sept 2007-Supplement 2 (13): S35.

124 Malaviya R, Twesten NJ, Ross EA, Abraham SN, Pfeifer JD. Mast cells process bacterial Ags through a phagocytic route for class I MHC presentation to T cells. J Immunol 1996 Feb; 156(4): 1490–6.

125 Stelekati E, Orinska Z, Bulfone-Paus S. Mast cells in allergy: innate instructors of adaptive responses. Immunobiology 2007; 212(6): 505–19.

126 Christy AL, Brown MA. The multitasking mast cell: positive and negative roles in the progression of autoimmunity. J Immunol 2007 Sep; 179(5): 2673–9.

127 Olsson Y. Mast cells in plaques of multiple sclerosis. Acta Neurol Scand 1974; 50(5): 611–18.

128 Toms R, Weiner HL, Johnson D. Identification of IgE-positive cells and mast cells in frozen sections of multiple sclerosis brains. J Neuroimmunol 1990 Dec; 30(2–3): 169–77.

129 Rozniecki JJ, Hauser SL, Stein M, Lincoln R, Theoharides TC. Elevated mast cell tryptase in cerebrospinal fluid of multiple sclerosis patients. Ann Neurol 1995 Jan; 37(1): 63–6.

130 Trojano M, Pellegrini F, Fuiani A, et al. New natural history of interferon-beta-treated relapsing multiple sclerosis. Ann Neurol 2007 Apr; 61(4): 300–6.

131 Furtado GC, Pina B, Tacke F, et al. A novel model of demyelinating encephalomyelitis induced by monocytes and dendritic cells. J Immunol 2006 Nov; 177(10): 6871–9.

132 Bjartmar C, Wujek JR, Trapp BD. Axonal loss in the pathology of MS: consequences for understanding the progressive phase of the disease. J Neurol Sci 2003 Feb; 206(2): 165–71.

133 Trapp BD, Wujek JR, Criste GA, et al. Evidence for synaptic stripping by cortical microglia. Glia 2007 Mar; 55(4): 360–8.

134 Basso AS, Frenkel D, Quintana FJ, et al. Reversal of axonal loss and disability in a mouse model of progressive multiple sclerosis. J Clin Invest 2008 Apr; 118(4): 1532–43.

135 Pitt D, Werner P, Raine CS. Glutamate excitotoxicity in a model of multiple sclerosis. Nat Med 2000 Jan; 6(1): 67–70.

136 Smith T, Groom A, Zhu B, et al. Autoimmune encephalomyelitis ameliorated by AMPA antagonists. Nat Med 2000 Jan; 6(1): 62–6.

137 Waxman SG. Mechanisms of disease: sodium channels and neuroprotection in multiple sclerosis-current status. Nat Clin Pract Neurol 2008 Mar; 4(3): 159–69.

138 Bakshi R, Thompson AJ, Rocca MA, Pelletier D, Dousset V, Barkhof F, et al. MRI in multiple sclerosis: current status and future prospects. Lancet Neurol 2008 Jul; 7(7): 615–25.

139 Bakshi R, Neema M, Healy B, et al. Predicting clinical progression in multiple sclerosis with the Magnetic Resonance Disease Severity Scale. Arch Neurol 2008 November 2008; 65(11): 1449–53.

140 Comabella M, Balashov K, et al. Elevated interleukin-12 in progressive multiple sclerosis correlates with disease activity and is normalized by pulse cyclophosphamide therapy. J Clin Invest 1998 Aug; 102(4): 671–8.

141 Khoury SJ, Guttmann CR, Orav EJ, et al. Longitudinal MRI in multiple sclerosis: correlation between disability and lesion burden. Neurology 1994 Nov; 44(11): 2120–4.

142 Khoury SJ, Guttmann CR, Orav EJ, et al. Changes in activated T cells in the blood correlate with disease activity in multiple sclerosis. Arch Neurol 2000 Aug; 57(8): 1183–9.

143 Achiron A, Gurevich M, Friedman N, et al. Blood transcriptional signatures of multiple sclerosis: unique gene expression of disease activity. Ann Neurol 2004 Mar; 55(3): 410–17.

144 Corvol JC, Pelletier D, Henry RG, et al. Abrogation of T cell quiescence characterizes patients at high risk for multiple sclerosis after the initial neurological event. Proc Natl Acad Sci USA 2008 Aug; 105(33): 11839–44.

145 Birnbaum G, Cree B, Altafullah I, et al. Combining beta interferon and atorvastatin may increase disease activity in multiple sclerosis. Neurology 2008 Oct; 71(18): 1390–5.

146 Gauthier SA, Glanz BI, Mandel M, et al. A model for the comprehensive investigation of a chronic autoimmune disease: the multiple sclerosis CLIMB study. Autoimmun Rev 2006 Oct; 5(8): 532–6.

147 Weiner HL. The challenge of multiple sclerosis: how do we cure a chronic heterogeneous disease? Ann Neurol 2009 Mar; 0: 239–48.

148 Lassmann H, Brück W, Lucchinetti C. Heterogeneity of multiple sclerosis pathogenesis: implications for diagnosis and therapy. Trends Mol Med 2001; 7: 115–21.

CHAPTER 2

Biomarkers

Manuel Comabella[1] and Samia J. Khoury[2]

[1]Centre d'Esclerosi Múltiple de Catalunya, CEM-Cat, Unitat de Neuroimmunologia Clínica, Hospital Universitari Vall dHebron (HUVH), Barcelona, Spain
[2]Partners Multiple Sclerosis Center, Center for Neurologic Diseases, Brigham and Women's Hospital and Department of Neurology, Harvard Medical School, Boston, MA, USA

Introduction

In 2001, an expert working group proposed the following terms and definitions for biomarkers [1]:

- *Biological marker (biomarker)*: "A characteristic that is objectively measured and evaluated as an indicator of normal biological processes, pathogenic processes, or pharmacologic responses to a therapeutic intervention."
- *Clinical endpoint*: "A characteristic or variable that reflects how a patient feels, functions, or survives."
- *Surrogate endpoint*: "A biomarker that is intended to substitute for a clinical endpoint. A surrogate endpoint is expected to predict clinical benefit (or harm or lack of benefit or harm) based on epidemiologic, therapeutic, pathophysiologic, or other scientific evidence."

Surrogate endpoints are a subset of biomarkers, and though all surrogate endpoints are considered biomarkers, only a few biomarkers will achieve a surrogate endpoint status. This is due to the fact that biomarkers should not only strongly and significantly correlate with the clinical endpoint, but also must fully capture the net effect of the treatment on the true clinical endpoint [2]. In a complex disease like multiple sclerosis (MS), in which different pathophysiological mechanisms contribute to disease phenotype, an individual biomarker will most likely capture one of the many ongoing pathogenic processes rather than the full effect, for instance, of a therapeutic intervention. Both complex disease characteristics and conditions for surrogacy of a biomarker certainly explain that, to date, there is no single biomarker that fulfills the criteria of a surrogate endpoint in MS [3]. This may be attributed to stringent conditions to establish surrogacy in the setting of a complicated disease.

Multiple Sclerosis: Diagnosis and Therapy, First Edition. Edited by Howard L. Weiner and James M. Stankiewicz. © 2012 John Wiley & Sons, Ltd.
Published 2012 by John Wiley and Sons, Ltd.

MS is quite a heterogeneous disease with respect to clinical manifestations, disease course, brain magnetic resonance imaging (MRI) findings, composition of lesion pathology, and response to treatment. In this setting, and despite the above-mentioned difficulties in finding surrogate endpoints in MS, there is a strong need for biomarkers that reliably capture these different aspects of disease heterogeneity. In this regard, biomarkers in MS may help in (i) MS diagnosis and disease stratification; (ii) prediction of disease course; (iii) identification of new therapies beneficial for the disease; (iv) and personalized therapy based on the prediction of treatment response and identification of patients at high risk for side effects.

This chapter will focus on the main diagnostic, prognostic, process-specific, and treatment-related molecular biomarkers that have been proposed for the disease, and will also include candidate biomarkers arising from the application of new high-throughput technologies such as genomics and proteomics for biomarker discovery. Finally, a brief description of MRI and optical coherence tomography as imaging biomarkers will also be covered in this chapter.

Body fluid sources of biomarkers

Insomuch as cerebrospinal fluid (CSF) circulates in the subarachnoid space in close proximity to sites of inflammatory lesions, biomarkers detected in the CSF are likely to be more specific and sensitive to central nervous system (CNS) pathology compared with biomarkers identified in peripheral blood or urine. However, inflammatory lesions distal to the CSF outflow pathways of the fourth ventricle are less likely to induce changes in lumbar CSF compared to lesions located closer to the CSF pathways. In addition, CSF collection is a relatively invasive procedure which restricts its use beyond diagnostic purposes for biomarker discovery, and limits the number of CSF samples available to monitor biomarker changes in longitudinal studies.

Biomarkers identified in peripheral blood are of significant clinical value because blood collection is minimally invasive to the patient. However, the use of blood as a source to determine biomarkers has several disadvantages, including diurnal variation of many soluble markers, and influence of systemic events such as viral infections in the levels of measured biomarkers. Additionally, blood biomarkers may show a lack of sensitivity to detect local pathological changes taking place in the CNS of MS patients.

The major advantage of urine-tested biomarkers is the ease with which urine can be obtained. Nonetheless, levels of biomarkers can be negatively influenced by local processes such as symptomatic or asymptomatic urinary tract infections.

Molecular biomarkers

Table 2.1 shows a summary of the different categories of biomarkers and candidate molecules that have been proposed for MS.

TOP TIPS 2.1: Biomarker categories in multiple sclerosis

- *Diagnostic biomarkers* allow separation of MS patients from healthy individuals and patients with other neurological or autoimmune conditions.
- *Predictive biomarkers* allow determination of the risk of conversion to MS at the time of the CIS or during the early phases of the disease.
- *Process-specific biomarkers* are associated with the different pathophysiological processes described in MS: inflammation, demyelination, oxidative stress, glial activation/dysfunction, remyelination/repair, neuroaxonal damage.
- *Treatment-related biomarkers* capture the effect of treatment and allow discrimination of responders and nonresponders to a particular therapy.

Diagnostic biomarkers

Diagnostic biomarkers should allow discrimination between MS patients and healthy individuals or patients with other neurological or autoimmune diseases. This category also includes biomarkers that have the potential to distinguish between patients belonging to different clinical subtypes or stratify patients into subgroups characterized by distinct pathogenetic mechanisms.

TOP TIPS 2.2: Processes associated with biomarker development

- *Biomarker discovery:* exploratory biomarkers
- *Biomarker validation:* known biomarkers
- *Regulatory approval:* regulatory biomarkers
- *Translation into clinical practice*

Oligoclonal bands: The only biomarker that is currently used in the diagnostic procedure of MS is the determination of immunoglobulin G (IgG) in CSF. Qualitative assessment is carried out by isoelectric focusing and immunoblotting/immunofixation for detection of oligoclonal bands (OBs) [4]. OBs only indicate the presence of an abnormal humoral immune response in the CNS of MS patients and are not specific for the disease. Sometimes, OBs are negative when determined near disease onset and emerge during follow-up [5]. However, once OBs are present, they persist over time.

Neuromyelitis optica: (NMO) is an inflammatory autoimmune demyelinating disease of the CNS that selectively targets the optic nerves and spinal

Table 2.1 Summary of proposed molecular biomarkers in MS

Category	Biomarkers
Diagnostic biomarkers	– IgG oligoclonal bands; aquaporin-4 antibodies; heat-shock proteins
Predictive biomarkers	– IgG and IgM oligoclonal bands; anti-MBP and anti-MOG antibodies; CHI3L1; fetuin-A; TOB1; anti-EBNA1
Process-specific biomarkers	
1. Inflammation	– Cytokines; chemokines; adhesion molecules; MMPs; osteopontin; sHLA-I and sHLA-II
2. Demyelination	– MBP and degradation products; CNPase; 7-oxygenated steroids
3. Oxidative stress	– NO and metabolites
4. Glial activation/dys-function	– S100b; GFAP
5. Remyelination/repair	– NCAM; CNTF; BDNF; NGF; Nogo-A
6. Neuroaxonal damage	– NSE; Nf and anti-Nf antibodies; tau; 14-3-3; NAA
Treatment response	
1. IFN-b	– GPC5; NPAS3; GRIA3; IFN-γ; TRAIL; IL-8; sHLA-I; VLA-4; VCAM-1; IL-10; TIMP-1; IL-17F; apoptosis-related molecules; type I IFNs; MxA
2. GA	– HLA-DRB1*1501; TRBβ; CTSS

MOG: myelin oligodendrocyte glycoprotein; MBP: myelin basic protein; CHI3L1: chitinase 3-like 1; TOB1: transducer of ERBB2, 1; EBNA: nuclear antigen 1 of the Epstein–Barr virus; MMPs: matrix metalloproteinases; sHLA-I and sHLA-II: soluble HLA class I and II; CNPase: 2′:3′-cyclic nucleotide 3′-phosphodiesterase; NO: nitric oxide; GFAP: glial fibrillary acidic protein; NCAM: neural cell adhesion molecule; CNTF: ciliary neurotrophic factor; BDNF: brain-derived neurotrophic factor; NGF: nerve growth factor; NSE: neuron-specific enolase; Nf: neurofilaments; NAA: N-acetyl aspartic acid; GPC5: glypican 5; NPAS3: neuronal PAS domain protein 3; GRIA3: glutamate receptor ionotropic AMPA 3; TRAIL: TNF-related apoptosis inducing ligand; VLA-4: very late antigen-4; VCAM-1: vascular cell adhesion molecule 1; TIMP-1: tissue inhibitor of matrix metalloproteinase-1; MxA: Myxovirus resistance protein A; TRBβ: T-cell receptor β; CTSS: cathepsin S.

cord and often leads to significant disability [6]. Recently, a highly sensitive and specific autoantibody biomarker for NMO (NMO-IgG) was found in the serum of patients with definite NMO [7] and proposed to be included in the diagnostic criteria of the disease [8]. NMO-IgG targets aquaporin-4, a water channel that is in astrocyte foot processes and plays important roles in brain water homeostasis. NMO-IgG antibodies are the first clinically validated biomarkers that allow the classification of a subgroup of patients with inflammatory demyelinating disorders, and the distinction of patients with NMO from patients with classical MS.

Antigen microarrays: Antigen microarrays identify patterns of antibody reactivity that may help to discriminate between MS patients and controls or between different clinical subtypes of MS. By using this approach, Quintana, et al. [9] identified specific serum autoimmune signatures that distinguished MS patients from healthy donors and patients with other neurological or autoimmune conditions, and an upregulated response to heat-shock proteins in relapsing-remitting MS (RRMS) patients that was not observed in patients with progressive forms of MS.

Predictive biomarkers

Predictive biomarkers may be used to determine the risk of conversion to MS at the time of the first clinical manifestations of MS or clinically isolated syndromes (CIS) or during the early phases of the disease.

Within this group, we should first mention the prognostic value of IgG OB, whose presence in CSF from CIS patients is associated with an increased risk of conversion to clinically definite MS (CDMS) [10]. Isoelectric focusing also allows for the detection of IgM OB, whose presence in early phases of the disease has been associated with an increased likelihood of conversion to CDMS, more relapses, and higher EDSS scores compared with patients without IgM OB [11]. Furthermore, the presence of IgM reacting against myelin lipids strongly correlates with early appearance of a second relapse and greater disability [12].

Insomuch as MS is an autoimmune demyelinating disease, autoantibodies reactive against myelin proteins – such as myelin oligodendrocyte glycoprotein (MOG), myelin basic protein (MBP), or myelin-associated glycoprotein (MAG) – have been studied as predictive biomarkers. In a first study [13], increased serum levels of IgM anti-MOG and anti-MBP antibodies at the time of the CIS event were found to be highly predictive of conversion to CDMS. However, this finding could not be replicated in later studies [14–17].

Many epidemiological and experimental observations point to an important role of the Epstein–Barr virus (EBV) in the pathogenesis of MS. In a recent study, elevated immune responses toward the nuclear antigen 1 of the EBV (EBNA1) were observed in serum of patients with CIS and associated with an increased risk of conversion to MS based on McDonald criteria, although they did not constitute an independent risk factor of OB [18]. However, additional studies in larger cohorts of CIS patients are needed to evaluate whether the titer of EBNA1 antibodies may play a role as independent factors for MS conversion.

New methodologies such as genomics and mass spectrometry-based proteomics have also been applied to identify biomarkers associated with conversion to MS. In this regard, a microarray study in naïve CD4 + T cells from CIS patients identified a gene expression signature in patients at high risk for conversion to CDMS. In particular, consistent down-regulation of *TOB1* (transducer of ERBB2, 1) – a gene that codes for a transcription factor involved in cell growth regulation – was characteristic of patients who rapidly converted to CDMS [19].

Regarding proteomics, fetuin-A, a negative acute-phase reactant, was found to be increased in CSF samples from patients who remained as CIS compared with patients who converted to MS. This finding was validated by an alternate technique (ELISA) [20]. In a more recent proteomic study, CHI3L1 (chitinase 3-like 1), a member of the chitinase family that binds chitin but lacks chitinase activity, was found to be overexpressed in CSF from CIS patients who converted to CDMS compared with patients who continued as CIS. Furthermore, increased CSF CHI3L1 levels were associated with a shorter time to CDMS and higher EDSS scores during follow-up [21].

Process-specific biomarkers

This category includes biomarkers related with the different pathophysiological processes that have been described in the disease.

Inflammation

Cytokines: Cytokines are key regulators of inflammation that have been implicated in the immunopathogenesis of MS. CSF and blood levels of pro-inflammatory cytokines are usually found to be elevated in MS patients compared with healthy individuals and controls with other neurological disorders [22–28]. Furthermore, upregulation of pro-inflammatory cytokines like TNF-α, lymphotoxin, IL-2, IL-17, and IFN-γ, and downregulation of anti-inflammatory cytokines such as IL-4 and IL-10 in peripheral blood and CSF of MS patients has been observed during or preceding clinical exacerbations compared with patients in remission [22, 23, 27, 29–32]. Differences in cytokine levels have also been reported between MS patients with different clinical forms of the disease and, for instance, higher levels of IL-12 and IL-15 and lower levels of IL-10 were observed in patients with chronic progressive forms compared with patients with RRMS forms of the disease [32, 35]. In some studies, increased levels of pro-inflammatory cytokines correlated with clinical and radiological disease activity, whereas other studies failed to show such correlations. Despite the many reports of altered cytokine levels in MS, these findings lack specificity, as they are also observed in other inflammatory neurological disorders, and thus cytokine levels are not routinely tested in MS.

Chemokines: Chemokines regulate recruitment and migration of inflammatory cells from peripheral blood to the CNS. Levels of CXCL10 (formerly interferon γ-induced protein; IP-10), CXCL12, CXCL13 have been found to be increased, and levels of CCL2 (formerly monocyte chemoattractant protein 1; MCP-1) decreased, in CSF and blood samples of MS patients when compared with controls with other neurological diseases [36–38].

Upregulation of CCL3 (formerly macrophage inflammatory protein 1a; MIP-1a), CCL5 (formerly RANTES), CXCL8 (formerly IL-8), CXCL9 (formerly monokine induced by gamma interferon; MIG), CXCL10, and downregulation of CCL2 have been observed during relapses [39–41]. Similar to cytokines, these findings are not specific for MS.

Adhesion molecules: Adhesion molecules are cell surface proteins required for the migration of inflammatory cells through the blood–brain barrier. Adhesion molecules also exist in a soluble form, released from activated cells, which are not only markers indicative of cell activation but they also function to inhibit cell contact and migration. Higher levels of sL-Selectin, sVCAM-1 (vascular cell adhesion molecule-1), and sICAM-1 (intercellular cell adhesion molecule-1) have been reported in MS patients than in control subjects and patients with non-inflammatory neurological disorders [42–44]. Levels of sICAM-1, sPECAM-1 (platelet/endothelial cell adhesion molecule), sP-Selectin and sE-Selectin were found to be increased in blood and CSF during relapses [45–47]. In some studies, levels of sPECAM-1, sICAM-1, sL-Selectin, sVCAM-1 were elevated in patients with gadolinium (Gd)-enhancing lesions on MRI [42, 44, 46, 48, 49].

MMPs: Matrix metalloproteinases (MMPs) constitute a family of proteolytic enzymes which degrade the extracellular matrix both in physiological and pathological conditions. MMPs have also been involved in myelin breakdown, pro-inflammatory cytokine release, and axonal damage. MMP9 is one of the most studied MMPs in MS, and its levels have consistently been reported to be elevated in CSF or serum of RRMS patients compared with healthy controls when measured by means of several methods [50–52]. MMP9 appears to be related with clinical disease activity, and raised MMP9 levels are usually found in patients during relapses compared with patients in remission [53–59], although other investigators failed to show such differences [60]. Furthermore, MMP-9 levels also correlated with radiological disease activity, and serum levels were found to be increased in patients with Gd-enhancing lesions [61]. Differences between clinical forms of MS have also been reported for MMP9, and lower levels were found in patients with progressive forms of MS compared to RRMS forms [57, 62–64].

The main MMP-9 inhibitor, TIMP-1 (tissue inhibitor of matrix metalloproteinase-1), does not seem to be elevated in relation to MMP-9, a finding that suggests an imbalance toward an increased proteolytic activity [54, 55].

Increased CSF levels of MMP-9 are not specific for MS and are also found elevated in many other inflammatory neurological conditions. In addition, MMP-9 levels have been reported to be highly correlated with a CSF cell count [65].

Osteopontin: This is a pro-inflammatory cytokine produced by both immune and non-immune cells that was initially found to be highly expressed in demyelinating plaques from MS brain tissue [66]. In later studies in MS, increased plasma osteopontin levels were found in RRMS patients during clinical exacerbations compared with patients in clinical remission [67, 68], and in secondary progressive MS (SPMS) patients compared with other clinical forms of MS and healthy individuals [68]. In CSF studies, osteopontin was significantly elevated in patients with MS and other inflammatory diseases compared with patients with non-inflammatory neurological disorders [69]. Similar to plasma studies, osteopontin levels were higher in RRMS with active disease [70]. Despite these observations, osteopontin does not appear to be a specific marker for MS, as raised levels are also found in patients with other neurological and non-neurological disorders.

HLA: Human leukocyte antigen class I (HLA-I) molecules in soluble form are receiving increasing attention in MS. Soluble HLA-A, B and C (sHLA-I) antigens occur naturally in body fluid and can act as anti-inflammatory as well as pro-inflammatory molecules. Non-classical class I soluble HLA-G (sHLA-G) molecules are structurally related to HLA class I antigens and are considered to exert tolerogenic functions. CSF concentrations of sHLA-I and sHLA-G have been found to be elevated in MS patients compared with patients with other neurological disorders [71, 72]. Interestingly, whereas CSF and serum levels of sHLA-I were related to clinical and MRI disease activity, those of sHLA-G were more associated with clinical and MRI disease remission [73–75]. Soluble HLA class II (sHLA-II) molecules have been investigated to a lesser extent in MS, with discordant results. In one study, serum sHLA-II concentrations were reported to be elevated in MS patients during clinical exacerbations compared with patients in remission and healthy controls [76]. In another study, sHLA-II levels were lower in MS patients than in healthy controls and patients with other neurological disorders [77].

Demyelination

Myelin basic protein (MBP) and its degradation products have been systematically studied in MS. During acute demyelination, MBP and/or its fragments are released into the CSF, and levels are especially elevated during clinical attacks [78]. This increase can last for a period of 5–6 weeks after the onset of a clinical exacerbation, and raised CSF MBP levels have been found to correlate with Gd enhancement on brain MRI [79]. Although MBP can also be detected in urine, levels fluctuate widely and do not seem to parallel acute myelin damage or correlate with CSF MBP. However, urinary MBP has been proposed as a predictor of the transition from the RRMS form to the

SPMS form of the disease [80]. Despite these observations, it should be highlighted that increased CSF MBP concentrations are not specifically seen in demyelination associated with MS, and are also detectable in other CNS disorders such as ischemic processes and infectious diseases [81].

CSF and blood levels of other myelin proteins have also been investigated in MS. For instance, CNPase (2′:3′-cyclic nucleotide 3′-phosphodiesterase) activity in serum and CSF was found to be similar between MS patients and controls [82]. In addition, breakdown products of cholesterol such as 7-oxygenated steroids (7-ketocholesterol) were reported to be highly elevated in CSF samples from MS patients and capable of inducing neuronal damage via activation of microglial poly(ADP-ribose)-polymerase; PARP-1) [83]. However, differences in the technique used to measure 7-oxygenated steroids may lead to different results [84].

Oxidative stress

Nitric oxide (NO) is produced by the enzyme nitric oxide synthase (NOS), which is highly expressed by macrophages and upregulated in acute demyelinating MS lesions. Raised NO levels are known to have deleterious effects including blood–brain barrier disruption, oligodendrocyte injury, axonal degeneration, and impairment of nerve conduction.

NO and its metabolites (nitrate and nitrite) have been reported to be elevated in the CSF, serum/plasma, and urine of patients with MS and other inflammatory neurological diseases compared to patients with non-inflammatory neurological disorders [85–93]. NO and its metabolites were found to be increased during relapses [91–94]. Additionally, NO metabolites were increased in patients with mild disability compared with patients with advanced disease, correlated with the volume of Gd-enhanced lesions on MRI, and were higher at baseline in patients who later showed progression on the EDSS during a 3-year follow-up [95]. These findings suggest that raised levels of NO or its products may be used as prognostic markers in MS, although additional studies in larger cohorts of patients are needed.

Glial activation/dysfunction

CSF S100b levels: S100b is an acidic calcium binding protein found in astrocytes and Schwann cells. Increased levels of S100b in CSF are observed in conditions associated with astrocytosis or gliosis. CSF S100b levels have been found to be elevated in MS patients, especially during clinical exacerbations, and raised levels may persist for several weeks after the relapse onset [93, 96–99]. S100b levels in CSF were higher in patients with progressive forms of MS, especially in primary progressive (PPMS) patients, compared with RRMS patients and controls [100]. However, CSF S100B levels do not appear to correlate with either disability or MRI findings in patients with PPMS [101]. In additional, other studies failed to show differences in CSF S100b levels between patients with MS or CIS and controls [102, 103].

CSF GFAP levels: Glial fibrillary acidic protein (GFAP) is the major structural component of the glial intermediate filament of astrocytes, and its CSF levels are increased in conditions associated with astrogliosis. Several studies have shown increased CSF GFAP concentrations in MS patients compared with control subjects [102, 104, 105]. In a longitudinal study [105], CSF levels of GFAP were found to increase during a 24-month follow-up period and correlate with clinical deficit scores. However, CSF GFAP levels remained unchanged during clinical relapses [105]. CSF concentrations of GFAP appear to be higher in patients with SPMS, in whom GFAP levels have been found to correlate with disability as measured by the EDSS [100, 102].

Remyelination/Repair

NCAM: The neural cell adhesion molecule (NCAM) is a glycoprotein present in the plasma membrane of neural and glial cells with roles in myelination and remyelination. It has been shown that CSF NCAM levels are low in MS patients during remission and rise in the weeks following a clinical exacerbation, paralleling clinical improvement [106, 107].

CNTF: The ciliary neurotrophic factor (CNTF) is a growth factor expressed in astrocytes with roles in oligodendrocyte survival. Increased levels of CNTF were found in the CSF of MS patients after a clinical exacerbation [108].

BDNF: The brain-derived neurotrophic factor (BDNF) is mainly expressed in neurons but also in immune cells and has roles in CNS neurogenesis, neuroprotection, and neuroregeneration. CSF and blood BDNF levels have been found to be lower in MS patients compared with controls [109–113], although some studies failed to show such differences [114, 115]. Comparisons of BDNF levels between MS patients in relapse and remission evidenced higher levels of BDNF during relapses [109, 112, 116]. Furthermore, BDNF secretion by activated immune cells significantly correlated with higher inflammatory activity as measured by MRI [117].

NGF: The nerve growth factor (NGF) is involved in the regulation of growth and the differentiation of neurons. In some studies, CSF and serum NGF levels were increased in MS patients compared with controls [114, 118], whereas in other studies NGF was only detected in a small percentage of patients [115, 119].

Altogether, these findings may indicate a role for neurotrophic factors, particularly BDNF and NCAM in stimulating CNS recovery during the acute phases of the disease.

Nogo-A: Nogo-A is highly expressed in mature oligodendrocytes and has roles inhibiting neurite outgrowth. Soluble Nogo-A was specifically detected in the CSF of MS patients but not in controls with other inflammatory and non-inflammatory disorders [120]. However, the validity of these findings has been called into question mainly alluding to a lack of specificity of the antibodies used for western blot in the original study [121]. Anti-Nogo-A antibodies have also been determined in MS, and serum IgM anti-Nogo-A antibodies were found to be significantly increased in MS patients and controls with other inflammatory and non-inflammatory neurological disorders compared with healthy donors. Additionally, an increased intra-thecal production of IgG anti-Nogo-A antibodies was observed in RRMS patients compared with patients with chronic progressive MS and controls with other inflammatory disorders [122]. These findings are, therefore, non-specific, as anti-Nogo-A antibodies were observed in both MS patients and controls. Other investigators failed, however, to detect serum anti-Nogo-A antibodies in MS patients and controls [123].

Neuroaxonal damage

Axonal damage has been shown to be already present in the early phases of the disease and is a major cause of permanent disability in MS patients. Candidate biomarkers of neurodegeneration comprise neuron-specific proteins that are released into body fluids as a consequence of the axonal damage occurring in the CNS of MS patients. It is expected that biomarkers of neurodegeneration lack specificity for MS, as they are also found in other neurodegenerative disorders characterized by axonal loss. Neuroaxonal damage biomarkers may become attractive surrogate endpoints to evaluate the efficacy of neuroprotective agents.

CSF NSE: Neuron-specific enolase (NSE) is an enzyme expressed in mature neurons and cells of neuronal origin. CSF NSE levels are usually normal in subjects with MS [98, 102, 124]. However, in a recent study, CSF and serum NSE levels were reported to be lower in CIS patients when compared with controls, finding that suggests a reduced neuronal metabolic activity in early phases of the disease [103].

CSF Nf levels: Neurofilaments (Nf) are structural neuron-specific proteins composed of three subunits that differ in molecular size: light (Nf-l), medium (Nf-m), and heavy (Nf-h). The axonal diameter is influenced by the amount of phosphorylation of neurofilaments.

Several studies have shown that CSF Nf-l levels are elevated in MS patients compared to healthy individuals and patients with other inflammatory and non-inflammatory neurological disorders [102, 105, 125–129]. In some studies, raised CSF levels of Nf-L correlated with the EDSS score and progression index [105, 125, 126, 129], whereas other investigators failed to show such correlations [102]. When CSF Nf-l concentrations were analyzed in patients with different clinical forms of MS, levels were found to be higher in patients with SPMS and PPMS compared to patients with RRMS [126], or in patients with SPMS compared to patients with RRMS and PPMS [105]. Other studies, however, did not show differences between RRMS and SPMS patients [102, 129]. In a recent study [129], CSF Nf-l levels were also measured in a group of patients with CIS and found to be significantly lower when compared with RRMS patients, and increased in CIS patients who later converted to CDMS. CSF levels of Nf-l are higher during clinical exacerbations compared to remission, and levels have been shown to drop gradually with time [102, 105, 125, 129].

Fewer studies have measured CSF levels of Nf-h in MS patients [93, 129–131]. In a 3-year follow-up study [130], CSF Nf-h levels at baseline were increased in patients with progressive forms of MS compared to RRMS patients. During follow-up, a higher proportion of patients with SPMS and PPMS forms presented an increase in CSF Nf-h levels compared to patients with the RRMS form. CSF levels of Nf-h correlated with neurological disability [130]. This is in agreement with a recent study by Teunissen, et al. [129] who found raised CSF Nf-h levels in patients with SPMS when compared with RRMS. CSF Nf-h levels have been reported to increase during clinical exacerbations [129, 131].

Antibodies against Nf have also been determined in MS. An increased frequency of anti-Nf-l and anti-Nf-h antibodies was observed in the CSF and serum of MS patients when compared with healthy controls and patients with other neurological diseases [132–134], and levels correlated with MRI measures of inflammation and brain atrophy [132]. In contrast, a more recent study found that increased anti-Nf-l and anti-Nf-m antibodies in the CSF of MS patients did not correlate with any clinical variables [135, 136]. When comparing clinical forms, serum anti-Nf-l antibodies were reported to be increased in patients with PPMS compared with patients with SPMS ($p < 0.05$) and RRMS (trend) [134]. Although the CSF and serum anti-Nf-l antibody responses significantly correlated, the mean CSF anti-Nf-l antibody levels were similar between the different clinical forms of MS [134]. In contrast, in another study [133] intrathecal production of anti-Nf-l antibodies was significantly elevated in patients with progressive forms of MS (PPMS and SPMS).

Tau protein: Tau protein is found in neuronal axons where it promotes the assembly and stabilization of microtubules. An accumulation of tau proteins in neurons occurs in various neurological disorders including Alzheimer disease, Creutzfeldt–Jakob disease, and traumatic brain injury. In these conditions, increased total and/or phosphorylated tau is detected in CSF reflecting the degree of ongoing axonal damage.

Several studies have reported increased CSF levels of total or phosphorylated tau protein in MS and CIS patients compared to controls [131, 137–141]. In other studies, however, CSF tau levels were found to be similar between patients with CIS and MS and controls [129, 142–144]. When the CSF levels of tau protein were compared between patients in relapse and remission, one study showed raised CSF tau concentrations in patients during relapses [145], whereas in another study tau levels did not appear to be influenced by the proximity of the lumbar punctures to the relapse event [146]. In a 3-year follow-up study, patients with higher baseline CSF tau levels progressed faster on the neurological disability, and levels correlated with increased disability at the end of the follow-up [146]. CSF tau levels were found to be increased in patients with Gd-enhancing lesions on the MRI [139]. Altogether, these findings suggest that CSF tau levels appear to be influenced by the inflammatory activity and may be useful to predict the short-term progression of the disease.

CSF 14-3-3:   The 14-3-3 protein family comprises several phosphoserine-binding proteins that are expressed abundantly in neurons and glial cells and play roles in neuronal intracellular trafficking and signal transduction. 14-3-3 proteins have been associated with several neurodegenerative diseases, and raised CSF 14-3-3 levels are a marker for Creutzfeldt–Jakob disease.

In CIS patients, the detection of 14-3-3 in CSF by western blot was associated with a shorter time to conversion to CDMS and to reach an EDSS equal or higher than 2 compared to CIS patients with a negative assay [147]. In another study [143], the percentage of CIS and MS patients with immunoreactivity on western blot for the 14-3-3 protein was similar, and differences in the mean EDSS score during follow-up were higher in patients with positive immunoreactivity. In a similar study by Satoh, et al. [148], patients with immunoreactivity for the 14-3-3 protein showed more severe disability. In contrast, in another study, CSF 14-3-3 protein was detected in a very low percentage (2 out of 22) of MS patients and there was no relation with the progression index [149]. When CSF 14-3-3 was measured by a different technique (ELISA), protein levels were detected in a higher percentage of MS patients compared to patients with inflammatory neurological disorders, and in none of patients with non-inflammatory neurological disorders. The differences, however, were not statistically significant [138].

CSF NAA: N-acetyl aspartic acid (NAA) is an amino acid that is almost exclusively found in neurons and neuronal processes, with some expression in oligodendrocytes. NAA is usually identified in MR spectroscopy studies of the normal and MS brain. In MS patients, NAA as measured by MR spectroscopy is significantly decreased in lesions and in normal-appearing white matter and concentrations inversely correlate with EDSS scores [150].

In a few studies, NAA concentrations have been measured in CSF samples. In a first study [151], CSF NAA was measured by gas chromatography mass spectrometry and the concentration was found to be similar between MS patients and controls with other neurological disorders. However, CSF NAA levels were significantly lower in patients with SPMS compared to patients with RRMS. Additionally, NAA concentrations correlated with EDSS and MRI measures such as T2 lesion load and black hole lesion load [151]. In a more recent study by the same group [129], original findings were confirmed and patients with SPMS had significantly lower CSF NAA concentrations compared to CIS and RRMS patients. In the latter groups, NAA levels were comparable to those found in patients with inflammatory neurological disorders and controls without neurological diseases, the findings suggesting that CSF NAA levels are not useful in identifying axonal damage in the early phases of the disease. However, NAA levels appear to decrease in later and progressive phases of MS [129].

Treatment response biomarkers

The majority of response biomarkers that have been proposed for MS are related with interferon-beta treatment, and only a few are associated with the response to glatiramer acetate. These biomarkers can be detected at the gene, mRNA, and protein levels.

Interferon-beta (IFN-β)

Allelic variants: Genetic studies pursue the identification of allelic variants associated with the response to IFN-β treatment in MS patients. These studies genotyped polymorphisms located either in genes that belong to the type I IFN pathway, such as the IFN receptors 1 and 2 (*IFNAR1* and *IFNAR2*), or genes that are known to be induced by IFN-β [152–157]. In other studies, the influence in the response to IFN-β of HLA class I and class II alleles or the HLA-DR2 haplotype was analyzed [158–160]. Overall, results from these studies have shown either a lack of association or weak and unreplicated associations of candidate genes with IFN-β response.

To date, only two IFN-β pharmacogenomic whole-genome association studies have been published [161, 162]. Using a pooling-based strategy, Byun, et al. [161] genotyped responders and non-responders to IFN-β by means of the Affymetrix 100 K single nucleotide polymorphism (SNP) arrays. One of the main findings of the study was the high representation of genes encoding γ-aminobutyric or glutamate receptors among the SNPs that distinguished between responders and non-responders to IFN-β, data that suggests an interesting link between neuronal excitation and response to IFN-β. Furthermore, among the genes that best discriminated between responders and nonresponders, it was interesting to observe genes involved in neurogenesis and neuroprotection, such as *GPC5* (glypican 5) and *NPAS3* (neuronal PAS domain protein). Interestingly, *GPC5* was recently found to be associated with the response to IFN-β in an independent study [163].

In the study by Comabella, et al. [162], IFN-β responders and nonresponders were genotyped with the higher density Affymetrix 500 K SNP arrays. Unexpectedly, the strongest association signal corresponded to a polymorphism located in *GRIA3* (glutamate receptor ionotropic AMPA 3), a gene that codes for a glutamate receptor. This finding supports the potential connection between genes encoding neurotransmitter-gated channels and the response to IFN-β that was suggested in the study by Byun, et al. [161]. Interestingly, other genes that discriminated well between responders and nonresponders were the type I IFN-responsive genes *IFNAR2* or *ADAR* (adenosine deaminase, RNA-specific), suggesting an implication of the type I IFN pathway in the response to IFN-β treatment.

Similar genome-wide pharmacogenomic studies searching for genes associated with the response to other MS therapies have not yet been reported.

Proposed biomarkers: At the protein and mRNA levels, the following molecules have been proposed as biomarkers of response to IFN-β: (1) The presence of low baseline levels of IFN-γ was associated with a good response to IFN-β evaluated at 2 years of treatment [164]. (2) Increased proliferative responses against mitogens before treatment were associated with a good response to IFN-β [165]. (3) Good IFN-β responders were characterized by an early and sustained induction in TRAIL (TNF-related apoptosis-inducing ligand) expression that was not present in IFN-β nonresponders [166]. Furthermore, soluble TRAIL levels detected by ELISA in the serum of patients before starting treatment predicted response to treatment during the first year. (4) Patients with good response to treatment had a marked reduction in IL-8 expression, whereas nonresponders showed a lack of inhibition of IL-8 induced by IFN-β [167]. (5) During the first 3 months of treatment, sHLA-I levels were higher in patients who presented a good response to IFN-β [168]. (6) Good responders were characterized by lower expression of VLA-4 (very late antigen-4) and elevated serum levels of VCAM-1 during IFN-β treatment [169]. (7) Serum levels of IL-10 decreased in IFN-β nonresponders, which remained unchanged in patients who presented a good response to treatment [170]. (8) In responders, IFN-β resulted in an early and sustained increase in serum levels of TIMP-1 [171]. (9) Increased baseline serum levels of IL-17F were identified in a subgroup of nonresponders to IFN-β (defined by more steroid usage and more relapses compared to responders), findings that suggest that immune responses in nonresponders are mediated by Th17 cells [172]. (10) Finally, treatment of MS with IFN-β is associated with the development of neutralizing antibodies in a number of patients. It has been shown that persistent, high-titer neutralizing antibodies may reduce the clinical efficacy of IFN-β, especially with regards to relapses and MRI effects [173]. MxA (Myxovirus resistance protein A) has proven to be a sensitive measure of the biological response to IFN-β, and its activity is reduced during the development of neutralizing antibodies. However, its use as a response biomarker has been criticized for the lack of evidence of its role on disease pathogenesis and clinical response to IFN-β [174].

Identification of biomarkers: *Large*-scale transcriptomic studies have also been performed to identify biomarkers of response to IFN-β. By applying a complex statistical analysis to gene expression data obtained by RT-PCR in 70 genes involved in immune regulation, Baranzini, et al. [175] identified gene triplets that were highly predictive of the response to IFN-β at baseline. Interestingly, many of the triplets were composed of apoptosis-related genes. Using whole-genome gene expression microarrays, van Baarsen, et al. [176] reported that the baseline expression of a set of 15 type I IFN-responsive genes inversely correlated with the individual pharmacological response to IFN-β. Finally, in a more recent study,, et al.on a subgroup of patients who would not respond to IFN-β Comabella, et al. [177] identified a baseline gene expression signature characterized by over-expression of type I IFN-responsive genes.

Summary: Though results from these studies are promising and many different treatment-related biomarkers have been proposed, it is important to highlight the need for replication studies in large cohorts of treated patients with long clinical and/or radiological follow-ups, in order to validate response biomarkers. Furthermore, efforts should also be made to better define the clinical and radiological criteria of response and treatment failure to each MS therapy.

Glatiramer acetate

The influence of allelic variants in the response to glatiramer acetate (GA) has remained far less explored and limited to only two studies. In a first study [178], the HLA-DRB1*1501 allele was found to be associated with GA efficacy. In a more recent study [179], the selection of a panel of candidate genes was based on their implication in the MS pathogenesis and GA's mode-of-action. Although attractive genes such as *TRBβ* (T cell receptor β) and *CTSS* (cathepsin S) were proposed as candidates associated with the response to GA, the previous association with the HLA-DRB1*1501 could not be confirmed.

Imaging biomarkers

Table 2.2 shows a summary of the imaging biomarkers proposed for MS.

Magnetic resonance imaging

MRI is one of the most extensively used methods to monitor both disease activity and progression in MS patients, and a widely measured surrogate endpoint in clinical trials. Imaging markers, such as the presence of black holes, the number and volume of T1 and T2 lesions, and the number and volume of Gd-enhancing lesions, have been proposed as prognostic biomarkers in MS [180], and are used as surrogate endpoints in phase II clinical trials. Nevertheless, one limitation of MRI is that imaging measures are only partially informative of the underlying pathogenetic processes. Thus, changes in MRI measures are usually associated with the main pathological processes of inflammation and axonal degeneration, whereas remyelination and regeneration are inadequately captured by MRI [181]. T1 lesions are more associated with axonal loss and tissue damage. T2 lesions are, however, less specific and may reflect the presence of edema, demyelination, inflammation, astrogliosis, or axonal loss [180, 182]. Markers of brain

Table 2.2 Imaging biomarkers in MS

Technique	Markers
T1	Number and volume of T1 lesions; presence of black holes
T2	Number and volume of T2 lesions
Gd	Number and volume of Gd-enhancing lesions
Brain volume	Brain parenchymal fraction; grey matter volume; white matter volume; cervical spinal cord volume; regional volumes
Magnetization transfer	Magnetization transfer ratio
MR spectroscopy	NAA, glutamate, glutamine, GABA, choline, creatinine, myoinositol, ascorbic acid
Diffusion MRI	Mean diffusivity; diffusion tensor
Functional MRI	Regional activation
Fractal dimension	White matter FD; gray matter FD
Optical coherence tomography	Thickness of the RNFL; macular volume

MRI: Magnetic resonance imaging; Gd: gadolinium; NAA: N-acetyl aspartic acid; GABA: γ-Amino-butyric acid; RNFL: retinal nerve fiber layer atrophy include the brain parenchymal fraction, volume of gray and white matter, and cervical spinal cord and regional volumes [180]. Brain atrophy measures modestly correlate with brain inflammation markers, and are yet to be validated as prognostic markers for the disease.

Newer nonconventional MRI techniques, such magnetization transfer imaging, MR spectroscopy, diffusion-weighted imaging, functional MRI, and fractal dimension analysis may provide complementary information to conventional MRI [183–186]. However, nonconventional techniques are used in a research setting and their implementation in the daily clinical practice is not straightforward. This topic is covered more extensively by Neema and colleagues in Chapter 6.

Optical coherence tomography

OCT is a noninvasive, noncontact, accurate, and reproducible technique that provides high-resolution measurements of the thickness of the retinal nerve fiber layer (RNFL), which contains only nonmyelinated axons. A recent study showed correlations between RNFL thickness and MRI brain atrophy measures, such as brain parenchymal fraction [187], suggesting that RNFL measured by OCT may become a surrogate marker for the assessment of brain atrophy in MS. RNFL thickness has also been shown to: (a) correlate with cognitive impairment, mainly when evaluated by the symbol digit modality test [188]; (b) negatively correlate with disability as assessed by EDSS [189]; and (d) had the potential to predict disease activity in terms of presence of new relapses and changes in the EDSS over time [190].

Conclusion

As a summary of biomarkers, it is important to emphasize that although the field of biomarkers is very active in MS and the number of biomarkers proposed for the disease grows rapidly, more efforts are still needed to standardize collection techniques and measurement methods and, more importantly, to validate candidate biomarkers. The ultimate goal in this biomarker validation process is to translate discoveries into clinical practice in order to provide benefit to the MS patient.

References

1 Biomarkers Definitions Working Group. Biomarkers and surrogate endpoints: preferred definitions and conceptual framework. Clin Pharmacol Ther 2001; 69: 89–95.
2 Prentice RL. Surrogate endpoints in clinical trials: definition and operational criteria. Stat Med 1989; 8: 431–40.

3 Bielekova B, Martin R. Development of biomarkers in multiple sclerosis. Brain 2004; 127(Pt 7): 1463–78.

4 Andersson M, Alvarez-Cermeño J, Bernardi G, Cogato I, Fredman P, Frederiksen J, et al. Cerebrospinal fluid in the diagnosis of multiple sclerosis: a consensus report. J Neurol Neurosurg Psychiat 1994; 57: 897–902.

5 Davies G, Keir G, Thompson EJ, Giovannoni G. The clinical significance of an intrathecal monoclonal immunoglobulin band: a follow-up study. Neurology 2003; 60: 1163–6.

6 Wingerchuk DM, Hogancamp WF, O'Brien PC, Weinshenker BG. The clinical course of neuromyelitis optica (Devic's syndrome). Neurology 1999; 53: 1107–14.

7 Lennon VA, Wingerchuk DM, Kryzer TJ, Pittock SJ, Lucchinetti CF, Fujihara K, et al. A serum autoantibody marker of neuromyelitis optica: distinction from multiple sclerosis. Lancet 2004; 364: 2106–12.

8 Wingerchuk DM, Lennon VA, Pittock SJ, Lucchinetti CF, Weinshenker BG. Revised diagnostic criteria for neuromyelitis optica. Neurology 2006; 66: 1485–9.

9 Quintana FJ, Farez MF, Viglietta V, Iglesias AH, Merbl Y, Izquierdo G, et al. Antigen microarrays identify unique serum autoantibody signatures in clinical and pathologic subtypes of multiple sclerosis. Proc Natl Acad Sci USA 2008; 105: 18889–94.

10 Tintore M, Rovira A, Rio J, Tur C, Pelayo R, Nos C, et al. Do oligoclonal bands add information to MRI in first attacks of multiple sclerosis? Neurology 2008; 70: 1079–83.

11 Villar LM, Masjuan J, González-Porqué P, Plaza J, Sádaba MC, Roldán E, et al. Intrathecal IgM synthesis predicts the onset of new relapses and a worse disease course in MS. Neurology 2002; 59: 555–9.

12 Villar LM, Sádaba MC, Roldán E, Masjuan J, González-Porqué P, Villarrubia N, et al. Intrathecal synthesis of oligoclonal IgM against myelin lipids predicts an aggressive disease course in MS. J Clin Invest 2005; 115: 187–94.

13 Berger T, Rubner P, Schautzer F, Egg R, Ulmer H, Mayringer I, et al. Antimyelin antibodies as a predictor of clinically definite multiple sclerosis after a first demyelinating event. N Engl J Med 2003; 349: 139–45.

14 Kuhle J, Pohl C, Mehling M, Edan G, Freedman MS, Hartung HP, et al. Lack of association between antimyelin antibodies and progression to multiple sclerosis. N Engl J Med 2007; 356: 371–8.

15 Lim ET, Berger T, Reindl M, Dalton CM, Fernando K, Keir G, et al. Anti-myelin antibodies do not allow earlier diagnosis of multiple sclerosis. Mult Scler 2005; 11: 492–4.

16 Pelayo R, Tintoré M, Montalban X, Rovira A, Espejo C, Reindl M, et al. Antimyelin antibodies with no progression to multiple sclerosis. N Engl J Med 2007; 356: 426–8.

17 Pittock SJ, Reindl M, Achenbach S, Berger T, Bruck W, Konig F, et al. Myelin oligodendrocyte glycoprotein antibodies in pathologically proven multiple sclerosis: frequency, stability and clinicopathologic correlations. Mult Scler 2007; 13: 7–16.

18 Lünemann JD, Tintoré M, Messmer B, Strowig T, Rovira A, Perkal H, et al. Elevated Epstein-Barr virus-encoded nuclear antigen-1 immune responses predict conversion to multiple sclerosis. Ann Neurol 2010; 67: 159–69.

19 Corvol JC, Pelletier D, Henry RG, Caillier SJ, Wang J, Pappas D, et al. Abrogation of T cell quiescence characterizes patients at high risk for multiple sclerosis after the initial neurological event. Proc Natl Acad Sci USA 2008; 105: 11839–44.

20 Tumani H, Lehmensiek V, Rau D, Guttmann I, Tauscher G, Mogel H, et al. CSF proteome analysis in clinically isolated syndrome (CIS): candidate markers for conversion to definite multiple sclerosis. Neurosci Lett 2009; 452: 214–17.

21 Comabella M, Fernández M, Martin R, Rivera-Vallvé S, Borrás E, Chiva C, et al. Cerebrospinal fluid chitinase 3–like 1 levels are associated with conversion to multiple sclerosis. Brain 2010; 133: 1082–93.

22 Rieckmann P, Albrecht M, Kitze B, Weber T, Tumani H, Broocks A, et al. Cytokine mRNA levels in mononuclear blood cells from patients with multiple sclerosis. Neurology 1994; 44: 1523–6.

23 Navikas V, He B, Link J, Haglund M, Söderström M, Fredrikson S, et al. Augmented expression of tumor necrosis and lymphotoxin in mononuclear cells in multiple sclerosis and optic neuritis. Brain 1996; 119: 213–23.

24 Navikas V, Matusevicius D, Söderström M, Fredrikson S, Kivisäkk P, Ljungdahl A, et al. Increased interleukin-6 mRNA expression in blood and cerebrospinal fluid mononuclear cells in multiple sclerosis. J Neuroimmunol 1996; 64: 63–9.

25 Monteyne P, Van Laere V, Marichal R, Sindic CJ. Cytokine mRNA expression in CSF and peripheral blood mononuclear cells in multiple sclerosis: detection by RT-PCR without in vitro stimulation. J Neuroimmunol 1997; 80: 137–42.

26 Matusevicius D, Kivisäkk P, Navikas V, Söderström M, Fredrikson S, Link H. Interleukin-12 and perforin mRNA expression is augmented in blood mononuclear cells in multiple sclerosis. Scand J Immunol 1998; 47: 582–90.

27 Matusevicius D, Kivisäkk P, He B, Kostulas N, Ozenci V, Fredrikson S, et al. Interleukin-17 mRNA expression in blood and CSF mononuclear cells is augmented in multiple sclerosis. Mult Scler 1999; 5: 101–4.

28 Kivisäkk P, Matusevicius D, He B, Söderström M, Fredrikson S, Link H. IL-15 mRNA expression is up-regulated in blood and cerebrospinal fluid mononuclear cells in multiple sclerosis (MS). Clin Exp Immunol 1998; 111: 193–7.

29 Rieckmann P, Albrecht M, Kitze B, Weber T, Tumani H, Broocks A, et al. Tumor necrosis factor- messenger RNA expression in patients with multiple sclerosis is associated with disease activity. Ann Neurol 1995; 37: 82–7.

30 Philippé J, Debruyne J, Leroux-Roels G, Willems A, Dereuck J. In vitro TNF-alpha, IL-2 and IFN-gamma production as markers of relapses in multiple sclerosis. Clin Neurol Neurosurg 1996; 98: 286–90.

31 Ferrante P, Fusi ML, Saresella M, Caputo D, Biasin M, Trabattoni D, et al. Cytokine production and surface marker expression in acute and stable multiple sclerosis: altered IL-12 production and augmented signaling lymphocytic activation molecule (SLAM)–expressing lymphocytes in acute multiple sclerosis. J Immunol 1998; 160: 1514–21.

32 van Boxel-Dezaire AH, Hoff SC, van Oosten BW, Verweij CL, Dräger AM, Adèr HJ, et al. Decreased interleukin-10 and increased interleukin-12p40 mRNA are associated with disease activity and characterize different disease stages in multiple sclerosis. Ann Neurol 1999; 45: 695–703.

33 Nicoletti F, Patti F, Cocuzza C, Zaccone P, Nicoletti A, Di Marco R, et al. Eleveted serum levels of interleukin-12 in chronic progressive multiple sclerosis. J Neuroimmunol 1996; 70: 87–90.

34 Balashov KE, Smith DR, Khoury SJ, Hafler DA, Weiner HL. Increased interleukin 12 production in progressive multiple sclerosis: induction by activated CD4 + T cells via CD40 ligand. Proc Natl Acad Sci USA 1997; 94: 599–603.

35 van Boxel-Dezaire AH, Smits M, van Trigt-Hoff SC, Killestein J, van Houwelingen JC, Polman CH, et al. Cytokine and IL-12 receptor mRNA discriminate between different clinical subtypes in multiple sclerosis. J Neuroimmunol 2001; 120: 152–60.

36 Franciotta D, Martino G, Zardini E, Furlan R, Bergamaschi R, Andreoni L, et al. Serum and CSF levels of MCP-1 and IP-10 in multiple sclerosis patients with acute and stable

disease and undergoing immunomodulatory therapies. J Neuroimmunol 2001; 115: 192–8.

37 Mahad DJ, Howell SJ, Woodroofe MN. Expression of chemokines in the CSF and correlation with clinical disease activity in patients with multiple sclerosis. J Neurol Neurosurg Psychiat 2002; 72: 498–502.

38 Krumbholz M, Theil D, Cepok S, Hemmer B, Kivisäkk P, Ransohoff RM, et al. Chemokines in multiple sclerosis: CXCL12 and CXCL13 up-regulation is differentially linked to CNS immune cell recruitment. Brain 2006; 129: 200–11.

39 Miyagishi R, Kikuchi S, Fukazawa T, Tashiro K. Macrophage inflammatory protein-1 alpha in the cerebrospinal fluid of patients with multiple sclerosis and other inflammatory neurological diseases. J Neurol Sci 1995; 129: 223–7.

40 Sørensen TL, Tani M, Jensen J, Pierce V, Lucchinetti C, Folcik VA, et al. Expression of specific chemokines and chemokine receptors in the central nervous system of multiple sclerosis patients. J Clin Invest 1999; 103: 807–15.

41 Bartosik-Psujek H, Stelmasiak Z. The levels of chemokines CXCL8, CCL2 and CCL5 in multiple sclerosis patients are linked to the activity of the disease. Eur J Neurol 2005; 12: 49–4.

42 Hartung HP, Reiners K, Archelos JJ, Michels M, Seeldrayers P, Heidenreich F, et al. Circulating adhesion molecules and tumor necrosis factor receptor in multiple sclerosis: correlation with magnetic resonance imaging. Ann Neurol 1995; 38: 186–93.

43 Trojano M, Avolio C, Simone IL, Defazio G, Manzari C, De Robertis F, et al. Soluble intercellular adhesion molecule-1 in serum and cerebrospinal fluid of clinically active relapsing-remitting multiple sclerosis: correlation with Gd-DTPA magnetic resonance imaging-enhancement and cerebrospinal fluid findings. Neurology 1996; 47: 1535–41.

44 Giovannoni G, Lai M, Thorpe J, Kidd D, Chamoun V, Thompson AJ, et al. Longitudinal study of soluble adhesion molecules in multiple sclerosis: correlation with gadolinium enhanced magnetic resonance imaging. Neurology 1997; 48: 1557–65.

45 Sharief MK, Noori MA, Ciardi M, Cirelli A, Thompson EJ. Increased levels of circulating ICAM-1 in serum and cerebrospinal fluid of patients with active multiple sclerosis. Correlation with TNF-alpha and blood-brain barrier damage. J Neuroimmunol 1993; 43: 15–21.

46 Hartung HP, Michels M, Reiners K, Seeldrayers P, Archelos JJ, Toyka KV. Soluble ICAM-1 serum levels in multiple sclerosis and viral encephalitis. Neurology 1993; 43: 2331–5.

47 Kuenz B, Lutterotti A, Khalil M, Ehling R, Gneiss C, Deisenhammer F, et al. Plasma levels of soluble adhesion molecules sPECAM-1, sP-selectin and sE-selectin are associated with relapsing-remitting disease course of multiple sclerosis. J Neuroimmunol 2005; 167: 143–9.

48 Losy J, Niezgoda A, Wender M. Increased serum levels of soluble PECAM-1 in multiple sclerosis patients with brain gadolinium-enhancing lesions. J Neuroimmunol 1999; 99: 169–72.

49 Mössner R, Fassbender K, Kühnen J, Schwartz A, Hennerici M. Circulating L-selectin in multiple sclerosis patients with active, gadolinium-enhancing brain plaques. J Neuroimmunol 1996; 65: 61–5.

50 Cuzner ML, Davison AN, Rudge P. Proteolytic enzyme activity of blood leukocytes and cerebrospinal fluid in multiple sclerosis. Ann Neurol 1978; 4: 337–44.

51 Gijbels K, Masure S, Carton H, Opdenakker G. Gelatinase in the cerebrospinal fluid of patients with multiple sclerosis and other inflammatory neurological disorders. J Neuroimmunol 1992; 41: 29–34.

52 Kouwenhoven M, Ozenci V, Gomes A, Yarilin D, Giedraitis V, Press R, et al. Multiple sclerosis: elevated expression of matrix metalloproteinases in blood monocytes. J Autoimmun 2001; 16: 463–70.

53 Rosenberg GA, Dencoff JE, Correa N, Reiners M, Ford CC. Effect of steroids on CSF matrix metalloproteinases in multiple sclerosis. Relation to blood-brain barrier injury. Neurology 1996; 46: 1626–32.

54 Lee MA, Palace J, Stabler G, Ford J, Gearing A, Miller K. Serum gelatinase B, TIMP-1, TIMP-2 levels in multiple sclerosis. A longitudinal clinical and MRI study. Brain 1999; 122: 191–7.

55 Waubant E, Goodkin DE, Gee L, Bacchetti P, Sloan R, Stewart T, et al. Serum MMP-9 and TIMP-1 levels are related to MRI activity in relapsing multiple sclerosis. Neurology 1999; 7: 1397–401.

56 Lichtinghagen R, Seifert T, Kracke A, Marckmann S, Wurster U, Heidenreich F. Expression of matrix metalloproteinase-9 and its inhibitors in mononuclear blood cells of patients with multiple sclerosis. J Neuroimmunol 1999; 99: 19–26.

57 Galboiz Y, Shapiro S, Lahat N, Rawashdeh H, Miller A. Matrix metalloproteinases and their tissue inhibitors as markers of disease subtype and response to interferon-beta therapy in relapsing and secondary progressive multiple sclerosis patients. Ann Neurol 2001; 50: 443–51.

58 Mandler RN, Dencoff JD, Midani F, Ford CC, Ahmed W, Rosenberg GA. Matrix metalloproteinases and tissue inhibitors of metalloproteinases in cerebrospinal fluid differ in multiple sclerosis and Devic's neuromyelitis optica. Brain 2001; 124: 493–8.

59 Liuzzi GM, Trojano M, Fanelli M, Avolio C, Fasano A, Livrea P, et al. Intrathecal synthesis of matrix metalloproteinase-9 in patients with multiple sclerosis: implication for pathogenesis. Mult Scler 2002; 8: 222–8.

60 Leppert D, Ford J, Stabler G, Grygar C, Lienert C, Huber S, et al. Matrix metalloproteinase-9 (gelatinase B) is selectively elevated in CSF during relapses and stable phases of multiple sclerosis. Brain 1998; 121: 2327–34.

61 Waubant E, Goodkin D, Bostrom A, Bacchetti P, Hietpas J, Lindberg R, et al. IFN-beta lowers MMP-9/TIMP-1 ratio, which predicts new enhancing lesions in patients with SPMS. Neurology 2003; 60: 52–7.

62 Lindberg RL, De Groot CJ, Montagne L, Freitag P, van der Valk P, Kappos L, et al. The expression profile of matrix metalloproteinases (MMPs) and their inhibitors (TIMPs) in lesions and normal appearing white matter of multiple sclerosis. Brain 2001; 124: 1743–53.

63 Avolio C, Ruggieri M, Giuliani F, Liuzzi GM, Leante R, Riccio P, et al. Serum MMP-2 and MMP-9 are elevated in different multiple sclerosis subtypes. J Neuroimmunol 2003; 136: 46–53.

64 Sastre-Garriga J, Comabella M, Brieva L, Rovira A, Tintoré M, Montalban X. Decreased MMP-9 production in primary progressive multiple sclerosis patients. Mult Scler 2004; 10: 376–80.

65 Yushchenko M, Weber F, Mäder M, Schöll U, Maliszewska M, Tumani H, et al. Matrix metalloproteinase-9 (MMP-9) in human cerebrospinal fluid (CSF): elevated levels are primarily related to CSF cell count. J Neuroimmunol 2000; 110: 244–51.

66 Chabas D, Baranzini SE, Mitchell D, Bernard CC, Rittling SR, Denhardt DT, et al. The influence of the proinflammatory cytokine, osteopontin, on autoimmune demyelinating disease. Science 2001; 294: 1731–5.

67 Vogt MH, Lopatinskaya L, Smits M, Polman CH, Nagelkerken L. Elevated osteopontin levels in active relapsing-remitting multiple sclerosis. Ann Neurol 2003; 53: 819–22.

68 Comabella M, Pericot I, Goertsches R, Nos C, Castillo M, Blas Navarro J, et al. Plasma osteopontin levels in multiple sclerosis. J Neuroimmunol 2005; 158: 231–9.

69 Braitch M, Nunan R, Niepel G, Edwards LJ, Constantinescu CS. Increased osteopontin levels in the cerebrospinal fluid of patients with multiple sclerosis. Arch Neurol 2008; 65: 633–5.

70 Chowdhury SA, Lin J, Sadiq SA. Specificity and correlation with disease activity of cerebrospinal fluid osteopontin levels in patients with multiple sclerosis. Arch Neurol 2008; 65: 232–5.

71 Wiendl H, Feger U, Mittelbronn M, Jack C, Schreiner B, Stadelmann C, et al. Expression of the immune-tolerogenic major histocompatibility molecule HLA-G in multiple sclerosis: implications for CNS immunity. Brain 2005; 128: 2689–2704.

72 Fainardi E, Rizzo R, Melchiorri L, Stignani M, Castellazzi M, Tamborino C, et al. CSF levels of soluble HLA-G and Fas molecules are inversely associated to MRI evidence of disease activity in patients with relapsing-remitting multiple sclerosis. Mult Scler 2008; 14: 446–54.

73 Fainardi E, Granieri E, Tola MR, Melchiorri L, Vaghi L, Rizzo R, et al. Clinical and MRI disease activity in multiple sclerosis are associated with reciprocal fluctuations in serum and cerebrospinal fluid levels of soluble HLA class I molecules. J Neuroimmunol 2002; 133: 151–9.

74 Fainardi E, Rizzo R, Melchiorri L, Vaghi L, Castellazzi M, Marzola A, et al. Presence of detectable levels of soluble HLA-G molecules in CSF of relapsing-remitting multiple sclerosis: relationship with CSF soluble HLA-I and IL-10 concentrations and MRI findings. J Neuroimmunol 2003; 142: 149–58.

75 Fainardi E, Rizzo R, Melchiorri L, Castellazzi M, Paolino E, Tola MR, et al. Intrathecal synthesis of soluble HLA-G and HLA-I molecules are reciprocally associated to clinical and MRI activity in patients with multiple sclerosis. Mult Scler 2006; 12: 2–12.

76 Ott M, Seidl C, Westhoff U, Stecker K, Seifried E, Fischer PA, et al. Soluble HLA class I and class II antigens in patients with multiple sclerosis. Tissue Antigens 1998; 51: 301–4.

77 Filaci G, Contini P, Brenci S, Gazzola P, Lanza L, Scudeletti M, et al. Soluble HLA class I and class II molecule levels in serum and cerebrospinal fluid of multiple sclerosis patients. Hum Immunol 1997; 54: 54–62.

78 Lamers KJ, de Reus HP, Jongen PJ. Myelin basic protein in CSF as indicator of disease activity in multiple sclerosis. Mult Scler 1998; 4: 124–6.

79 Barkhof F, Frequin ST, Hommes OR, Lamers K, Scheltens P, van Geel WJ, et al. A correlative triad of gadolinium-DTPA MRI, EDSS, and CSF-MBP in relapsing multiple sclerosis patients treated with high-dose intravenous methylprednisolone. Neurology 1992; 42: 63–7.

80 Whitaker JN. Myelin basic protein in cerebrospinal fluid and other body fluids. Mult Scler 1998; 4: 16–21.

81 Whitaker JN, Williams PH, Layton BA, McFarland HF, Stone LA, Smith ME, et al. Correlation of clinical features and findings on cranial magnetic resonance imaging with urinary myelin basic protein-like material in patients with multiple sclerosis. Ann Neurol 1994; 35: 577–85.

82 Clapshaw PA, Müller HW, Wiethölter H, Seifert W. Simultaneous measurement of 2': 3' cyclic-nucleotide 3' phosphodiesterase and RNase activities in sera and spinal fluids of multiple sclerosis patients. J Neurochem 1984; 42: 12–15.

83 Diestel A, Aktas O, Hackel D, Hake I, Meier S, Raine CS, et al. Activation of microglial poly(ADP-ribose)–polymerase-1 by cholesterol breakdown products

during neuroinflammation: a link between demyelination and neuronal damage. J Exp Med 2003; 198: 1729–40.

84 Leoni V, Lütjohann D, Masterman T. Levels of 7–oxocholesterol in cerebrospinal fluid are more than one thousand times lower than reported in multiple sclerosis. J Lipid Res 2005; 46: 191–5.

85 Johnson AW, Land JM, Thompson EJ, Bolaños JP, Clark JB, Heales SJ. Evidence for increased nitric oxide production in multiple sclerosis. J Neurol Neurosurg Psychiat 1995; 58: 107.

86 Giovannoni G, Heales SJ, Silver NC, O'Riordan J, Miller RF, Land JM, et al. Raised serum nitrate and nitrite levels in patients with multiple sclerosis. J Neurol Sci 1997; 145: 77–81.

87 Giovannoni G, Silver NC, O'Riordan J, Miller RF, Heales SJ, Land JM, et al. Increased urinary nitric oxide metabolites in patients with multiple sclerosis correlates with early and relapsing disease. Mult Scler 1999; 5: 335–41.

88 Brundin L, Morcos E, Olsson T, Wiklund NP, Andersson M. Increased intrathecal nitric oxide formation in multiple sclerosis; cerebrospinal fluid nitrite as activity marker. Eur J Neurol 1999; 6: 585–90.

89 Peltola J, Ukkonen M, Moilanen E, Elovaara I. Increased nitric oxide products in CSF in primary progressive MS may reflect brain atrophy. Neurology 2001; 57: 895–6.

90 Yuceyar N, Taş kiran D, Sağduyu A. Serum and cerebrospinal fluid nitrite and nitrate levels in relapsing-remitting and secondary progressive multiple sclerosis patients. Clin Neurol Neurosurg 2001; 103: 206–11.

91 Danilov AI, Andersson M, Bavand N, Wiklund NP, Olsson T, Brundin L. Nitric oxide metabolite determinations reveal continuous inflammation in multiple sclerosis. J Neuroimmunol 2003; 136: 112–18.

92 Acar G, Idiman F, Idiman E, Kirkali G, Cakmakçi H, Ozakbaş S. Nitric oxide as an activity marker in multiple sclerosis. J Neurol 2003; 250: 588–92.

93 Rejdak K, Petzold A, Stelmasiak Z, Giovannoni G. Cerebrospinal fluid brain specific proteins in relation to nitric oxide metabolites during relapse of multiple sclerosis. Mult Scler 2008; 14: 59–66.

94 Sellebjerg F, Giovannoni G, Hand A, Madsen HO, Jensen CV, Garred P. Cerebrospinal fluid levels of nitric oxide metabolites predict response to methylprednisolone treatment in multiple sclerosis and optic neuritis. J Neuroimmunol 2002; 125: 198–203.

95 Rejdak K, Eikelenboom MJ, Petzold A, Thompson EJ, Stelmasiak Z, Lazeron RH, et al. CSF nitric oxide metabolites are associated with activity and progression of multiple sclerosis. Neurology 2004; 63: 1439–45.

96 Michetti F, Massaro A, Murazio M. The nervous system-specific S-100 antigen in cerebrospinal fluid of multiple sclerosis patients. Neurosci Lett 1979; 11: 171–5.

97 Massaro AR, Michetti F, Laudisio A, Bergonzi P. Myelin basic protein and S-100 antigen in cerebrospinal fluid of patients with multiple sclerosis in the acute phase. Ital J Neurol Sci 1985; 6: 53–6.

98 Lamers KJ, van Engelen BG, Gabreëls FJ, Hommes OR, Borm GF, Wevers RA. Cerebrospinal neuron-specific enolase, S-100 and myelin basic protein in neurological disorders. Acta Neurol Scand 1995; 92: 247–51.

99 Rejdak K, Petzold A, Kocki T, Kurzepa J, Grieb P, Turski WA, et al. Astrocytic activation in relation to inflammatory markers during clinical exacerbation of relapsing-remitting multiple sclerosis. J Neural Transm 2007; 114: 1011–15.

100 Petzold A, Eikelenboom MJ, Gveric D, Keir G, Chapman M, Lazeron RH, et al. Markers for different glial cell responses in multiple sclerosis: clinical and pathological correlations. Brain 2002; 125: 1462–73.

101 Lim ET, Petzold A, Leary SM, Altmann DR, Keir G, Thompson EJ, et al. Serum S100B in primary progressive multiple sclerosis patients treated with interferon-beta-1a. J Negat Results Biomed 2004; 3: 4.

102 Malmeström C, Haghighi S, Rosengren L, Andersen O, Lycke J. Neurofilament light protein and glial fibrillary acidic protein as biological markers in MS. Neurology 2003; 61: 1720–5.

103 Hein Née Maier K, Köhler A, Diem R, Sättler MB, Demmer I, Lange P, et al. Biological markers for axonal degeneration in CSF and blood of patients with the first event indicative for multiple sclerosis. Neurosci Lett 2008; 436: 72–6.

104 Rosengren LE, Lycke J, Andersen O. Glial fibrillary acidic protein in CSF of multiple sclerosis patients: relation to neurological deficit. J Neurol Sci 1995; 133: 61–5.

105 Norgren N, Sundström P, Svenningsson A, Rosengren L, Stigbrand T, Gunnarsson M. Neurofilament and glial fibrillary acidic protein in multiple sclerosis. Neurology 2004; 63: 1586–90.

106 Massaro AR, Albrechtsen M, Bock E. N-CAM in cerebrospinal fluid: a marker of synaptic remodelling after acute phases of multiple sclerosis? Ital J Neurol Sci 1987; Suppl 6: 85–8.

107 Massaro AR, Tonali P. Cerebrospinal fluid markers in multiple sclerosis: an overview. Mult Scler 1998; 4: 1–4.

108 Massaro AR, Soranzo C, Carnevale A. Cerebrospinal-fluid ciliary neurotrophic factor in neurological patients. Eur Neurol 1997; 37: 243–6.

109 Sarchielli P, Greco L, Stipa A, Floridi A, Gallai V. Brain-derived neurotrophic factor in patients with multiple sclerosis. J Neuroimmunol 2002; 132: 180–8.

110 Azoulay D, Vachapova V, Shihman B, Miler A, Karni A. Lower brain-derived neurotrophic factor in serum of relapsing remitting MS: reversal by glatiramer acetate. J Neuroimmunol 2005; 167(1–2): 215–18.

111 Castellano V, White LJ. Serum brain-derived neurotrophic factor response to aerobic exercise in multiple sclerosis. J Neurol Sci 2008; 269: 85–91.

112 Frota ER, Rodrigues DH, Donadi EA, Brum DG, Maciel DR, Teixeira AL. Increased plasma levels of brain derived neurotrophic factor (BDNF) after multiple sclerosis relapse. Neurosci Lett 2009; 460: 130–2.

113 Azoulay D, Urshansky N, Karni A. Low and dysregulated BDNF secretion from immune cells of MS patients is related to reduced neuroprotection. J Neuroimmunol 2008; 195: 186–93.

114 Gold SM, Schulz KH, Hartmann S, Mladek M, Lang UE, Hellweg R, et al. Basal serum levels and reactivity of nerve growth factor and brain-derived neurotrophic factor to standardized acute exercise in multiple sclerosis and controls. J Neuroimmunol 2003; 138: 99–105.

115 Gielen A, Khademi M, Muhallab S, Olsson T, Piehl F. Increased brain-derived neurotrophic factor expression in white blood cells of relapsing-remitting multiple sclerosis patients. Scand J Immunol 2003; 57: 493–7.

116 Caggiula M, Batocchi AP, Frisullo G, Angelucci F, Patanella AK, Sancricca C, et al. Neurotrophic factors and clinical recovery in relapsing-remitting multiple sclerosis. Scand J Immunol 2005; 62: 176–82.

117 Weinstock-Guttman B, Zivadinov R, Tamaño-Blanco M, Abdelrahman N, Badgett D, Durfee J, et al. Immune cell BDNF secretion is associated with white matter volume in multiple sclerosis. J Neuroimmunol 2007a; 188: 167–74.

118 Jiang Y, Yang Y, Zhang B, Peng F, Bao J, Hu X. Cerebrospinal fluid levels of iodothyronines and nerve growth factor in patients with multiple sclerosis and neuromyelitis optica. Neuro Endocrinol Lett 2009; 30: 85–90.

119 Massaro AR, Soranzo C, Bigon E, Battiston S, Morandi A, Carnevale A, et al. Nerve growth factor (NGF) in cerebrospinal fluid (CSF) from patients with various neurological disorders. Ital J Neurol Sci 1994; 15: 105–8.

120 Jurewicz A, Matysiak M, Raine CS, Selmaj K. Soluble Nogo-A, an inhibitor of axonal regeneration, as a biomarker for multiple sclerosis. Neurology 2007; 68: 283–7.

121 Lindsey JW, Crawford MP, Hatfield LM. Soluble Nogo-A in CSF is not a useful biomarker for multiple sclerosis. Neurology 2008; 71: 35–7.

122 Reindl M, Khantane S, Ehling R, Schanda K, Lutterotti A, Brinkhoff C, et al. Serum and cerebrospinal fluid antibodies to Nogo-A in patients with multiple sclerosis and acute neurological disorders. J Neuroimmunol 2003; 145: 139–47.

123 Onoue H, Satoh JI, Ogawa M, Tabunoki H, Yamamura T. Detection of anti-Nogo receptor autoantibody in the serum of multiple sclerosis and controls. Acta Neurol Scand 2007; 115: 153–60.

124 Cunningham RT, Morrow JI, Johnston CF, Buchanan KD. Serum neurone-specific enolase concentrations in patients with neurological disorders. Clin Chim Acta 1994; 230: 117–24.

125 Lycke JN, Karlsson JE, Andersen O, Rosengren LE. Neurofilament protein in cerebrospinal fluid: a potential marker of activity in multiple sclerosis. J NeurolNeurosurg Psychiat 1998; 64: 402–24.

126 Semra YK, Seidi OA, Sharief MK. Heightened intrathecal release of axonal cytoskeletal proteins in multiple sclerosis is associated with progressive disease and clinical disability. J Neuroimmunol 2002; 122: 132–9.

127 Norgren N, Rosengren L, Stigbrand T. Elevated neurofilament levels in neurological diseases. Brain Res 2003; 987: 25–31.

128 Haghighi S, Andersen O, Odén A, Rosengren L. Cerebrospinal fluid markers in MS patients and their healthy siblings. Acta Neurol Scand 2004; 109: 97–9.

129 Teunissen CE, Iacobaeus E, Khademi M, Brundin L, Norgren N, Koel-Simmelink MJ, et al. Combination of CSF N-acetylaspartate and neurofilaments in multiple sclerosis. Neurology 2009; 72: 1322–9.

130 Petzold A, Eikelenboom MJ, Keir G, Grant D, Lazeron RH, Polman CH, et al. Axonal damage accumulates in the progressive phase of multiple sclerosis: three year follow up study. J Neurol Neurosurg Psychiat 2005; 76: 206–11.

131 Brettschneider J, Petzold A, Junker A, Tumani H. Axonal damage markers in the cerebrospinal fluid of patients with clinically isolated syndrome improve predicting conversion to definite multiple sclerosis. Mult Scler 2006; 12: 143–8.

132 Eikelenboom MJ, Petzold A, Lazeron RH, Silber E, Sharief M, Thompson EJ, et al. Multiple sclerosis: Neurofilament light chain antibodies are correlated to cerebral atrophy. Neurology 2003; 60: 219–23.

133 Silber E, Semra YK, Gregson NA, Sharief MK. Patients with progressive multiple sclerosis have elevated antibodies to neurofilament subunit. Neurology 2002; 58: 1372–81.

134 Ehling R, Lutterotti A, Wanschitz J, Khalil M, Gneiss C, Deisenhammer F, et al. Increased frequencies of serum antibodies to neurofilament light in patients with primary chronic progressive multiple sclerosis. Mult Scler 2004; 10: 601–6.

135 Bartos A, Fialová L, Soukupová J, Kukal J, Malbohan I, Pitha J. Antibodies against light neurofilaments in multiple sclerosis patients. Acta Neurol Scand 2007; 116: 100–7.

136 Bartos A, Fialová L, Soukupová J, Kukal J, Malbohan I, Pit'ha J. Elevated intrathecal antibodies against the medium neurofilament subunit in multiple sclerosis. J Neurol 2007; 254: 20–5.

137 Kapaki E, Paraskevas GP, Michalopoulou M, Kilidireas K. Increased cerebrospinal fluid tau protein in multiple sclerosis. Eur Neurol 2000; 43: 228–32.

138 Bartosik-Psujek H, Archelos JJ. Tau protein and 14-3-3 are elevated in the cerebrospinal fluid of patients with multiple sclerosis and correlate with intrathecal synthesis of IgG. J Neurol 2004; 251: 414–20.

139 Brettschneider J, Maier M, Arda S, Claus A, Süssmuth SD, Kassubek J, et al. Tau protein level in cerebrospinal fluid is increased in patients with early multiple sclerosis. Mult Scler 2005; 11: 261–5.

140 Bartosik-Psujek H, Stelmasiak Z. The CSF levels of total-tau and phosphotau in patients with relapsing-remitting multiple sclerosis. J Neural Transm 2006; 113: 339–45.

141 Terzi M, Birinci A, Cetinkaya E, Onar MK. Cerebrospinal fluid total tau protein levels in patients with multiple sclerosis. Acta Neurol Scand 2007; 115: 325–30.

142 Jiménez-Jiménez FJ, Zurdo JM, Hernanz A, Medina-Acebrón S, de Bustos F, Barcenilla B, et al. Tau protein concentrations in cerebrospinal fluid of patients with multiple sclerosis. Acta Neurol Scand 2002; 106: 351–4.

143 Colucci M, Roccatagliata L, Capello E, Narciso E, Latronico N, Tabaton M, et al. The 14-3-3 protein in multiple sclerosis: a marker of disease severity. Mult Scler 2004; 10: 477–81.

144 Guimarães I, Cardoso MI, Sá MJ. Tau protein seems not to be a useful routine clinical marker of axonal damage in multiple sclerosis. Mult Scler 2006; 12: 354–6.

145 Süssmuth SD, Reiber H, Tumani H. Tau protein in cerebrospinal fluid (CSF): a blood-CSF barrier related evaluation in patients with various neurological diseases. Neurosci Lett 2001; 300: 95–8.

146 Martínez-Yélamos A, Saiz A, Bas J, Hernandez JJ, Graus F, Arbizu T. Tau protein in cerebrospinal fluid: a possible marker of poor outcome in patients with early relapsing-remitting multiple sclerosis. Neurosci Lett 2004; 363: 14–17.

147 Martínez-Yélamos A, Saiz A, Sanchez-Valle R, Casado V, Ramón JM, Graus F, et al. 14-3-3 protein in the CSF as prognostic marker in early multiple sclerosis. Neurology 2001; 57: 722–4.

148 Satoh J, Yukitake M, Kurohara K, Takashima H, Kuroda Y. Detection of the 14-3-3 protein in the cerebrospinal fluid of Japanese multiple sclerosis patients presenting with severe myelitis. J Neurol Sci 2003; 212: 11–20.

149 de Seze J, Peoc'h K, Ferriby D, Stojkovic T, Laplanche JL, Vermersch P. 14-3-3 Protein in the cerebrospinal fluid of patients with acute transverse myelitis and multiple sclerosis. J Neurol 2002; 249: 626–7.

150 De Stefano N, Guidi L, Stromillo ML, Bartolozzi ML, Federico A. Imaging neuronal and axonal degeneration in multiple sclerosis. Neurol Sci 2003; Suppl 5: S283–6.

151 Jasperse B, Jakobs C, Eikelenboom MJ, Dijkstra CD, Uitdehaag BM, Barkhof F, et al. N-acetylaspartic acid in cerebrospinal fluid of multiple sclerosis patients determined by gas-chromatography-mass spectrometry. J Neurol 2007; 254: 631–7.

152 Sriram U, Barcellos LF, Villoslada P, Rio J, Baranzini SE, Caillier S, et al. Pharmacogenomic analysis of interferon receptor polymorphisms in multiple sclerosis. Genes Immun 2003; 4: 147–52.

153 Cunningham S, Graham C, Hutchinson M, Droogan A, O'Rourke K, Patterson C, et al. Pharmacogenomics of responsiveness to interferon IFN-beta treatment in multiple sclerosis: a genetic screen of 100 type I interferon-inducible genes. Clin Pharmacol Ther 2005; 78: 635–46.

154 Leyva L, Fernández O, Fedetz M, Blanco E, Fernandez VE, Oliver B, et al. IFNAR1 and IFNAR2 polymorphisms confer susceptibility to multiple sclerosis but not to interferon-beta treatment response. J Neuroimmunol 2005; 163: 165–71.

155 Martínez A, de las Heras V, Mas Fontao A, Bartolomé M, de la Concha EG, Urcelay E, et al. An IFNG polymorphism is associated with interferon-beta response in Spanish MS patients. J Neuroimmunol 2006; 173: 196–9.

156 Weinstock-Guttman B, Tamano-Blanco M, Bhasi K, Zivadinov R, Ramanathan M. Pharmacogenetics of MXA SNPs in interferon-β treated multiple sclerosis patients. J Neuroimmunol 2007b; 182: 236–9.

157 O'Doherty C, Favorov A, Heggarty S, Graham C, Favorova O, Ochs M, et al. Genetic polymorphisms, their allele combinations and IFN-beta treatment response in Irish multiple sclerosis patients. Pharmacogenomics 2009; 10: 1177–86.

158 Villoslada P, Barcellos LF, Rio J, Begovich AB, Tintore M, Sastre-Garriga J, et al. The HLA locus and multiple sclerosis in Spain. Role in disease susceptibility, clinical course and response to interferon-beta. J Neuroimmunol 2002; 130: 194–201.

159 Fernández O, Fernández V, Mayorga C, Guerrero M, León A, Tamayo JA, et al. HLA class II and response to interferon-beta in multiple sclerosis. Acta Neurol Scand 2005; 112: 391–4.

160 Comabella M, Fernández-Arquero M, Río J, Guinea A, Fernández M, Cenit MC, et al. HLA class I and II alleles and response to treatment with interferon-beta in relapsing-remitting multiple sclerosis. J Neuroimmunol 2009; 210: 116–19.

161 Byun E, Caillier SJ, Montalban X, Villoslada P, Fernández O, Brassat D, et al. Genome-wide pharmacogenomic analysis of the response to interferon beta therapy in multiple sclerosis. Arch Neurol 2008; 65: 337–44.

162 Comabella M, Craig DW, Morcillo-Suárez C, Río J, Navarro A, Fernández M, et al. Genome-wide scan of 500, 000 single nucleotide polymorphisms in responders and non-responders to interferon-beta in multiple sclerosis. Arch Neurol 2009; 66: 972–8.

163 Cénit MD, Blanco-Kelly F, de las Heras V, Bartolomé M, de la Concha EG, Urcelay E, et al. Glypican 5 is an interferon-beta response gene: a replication study. Mult Scler 2009; 15: 913–17.

164 Petereit HF, Nolden S, Schoppe S, Bamborschke S, Pukrop R, Heiss WD. Low interferon gamma producers are better treatment responders: a two-year follow-up of interferon beta-treated multiple sclerosis patients. Mult Scler 2002; 8: 492–4.

165 Killestein J, Hintzen RQ, Uitdehaag BM, Baars PA, Roos MT, van Lier RA, et al. Baseline T cell reactivity in multiple sclerosis is correlated to efficacy of interferon-beta. J Neuroimmunol 2002; 133: 217–24.

166 Wandinger KP, Lunemann JD, Wengert O, Bellmann-Strobl J, Aktas O, Weber A, et al. TNF-related apoptosis inducing ligand (TRAIL) as a potential response marker for interferon-beta treatment in multiple sclerosis. Lancet 2003; 361: 2036–43.

167 Sturzebecher S, Wandinger KP, Rosenwald A, Sathyamoorthy M, Tzou A, Mattar P, et al. Expression profiling identifies responder and non-responder phenotypes to interferon-beta in multiple sclerosis. Brain 2003; 126: 1419–29.

168 Fainardi E, Rizzo R, Melchiorri L, Castellazzi M, Govoni V, Caniatti L, et al. Beneficial effect of interferon-beta 1b treatment in patients with relapsing-remitting multiple sclerosis is associated with an increase in serum levels of soluble HLA-I molecules during the first 3 months of therapy. J Neuroimmunol 2004; 148: 206–11.

169 Soilu-Hanninen M, Laaksonen M, Hanninen A, Eralinna JP, Panelius M. Down-regulation of VLA-4 on T cells as a marker of long term treatment response to interferon beta-1a in MS. J Neuroimmunol 2005; 167: 175–82.

170 Graber JJ, Ford D, Zhan M, Francis G, Panitch H, Dhib-Jalbut S. Cytokine changes during interferon-beta therapy in multiple sclerosis: correlations with interferon dose and MRI response. J Neuroimmunol 2007; 185: 168–74.

171 Comabella M, Río J, Espejo C, Ruiz de Villa M, Al-Zayat H, Nos C, et al. Changes in matrix metalloproteinases and their inhibitors during interferon-beta treatment in multiple sclerosis. Clin Immunol 2009; 130: 145–50.

172 Axtell RC, de Jong BA, Boniface K, van der Voort LF, Bhat R, De Sarno P, et al. T helper type 1 and 17 cells determine efficacy of interferon-beta in multiple sclerosis and experimental encephalomyelitis. Nat Med 2010; 16: 406–12.

173 Sorensen PS, Koch-Henriksen N, Ross C, Clemmesen KM, Bendtzen K. Danish Multiple Sclerosis Study Group. Appearance and disappearance of neutralizing antibodies during interferon-beta therapy. Neurology 2005; 65: 33–9.

174 Gilli F, Marnetto F, Caldano M, Sala A, Malucchi S, Capobianco M, et al. Biological markers of interferon-beta therapy: comparison among interferon-stimulated genes MxA, TRAIL and XAF-1. Mult Scler 2006; 12: 47–57.

175 Baranzini SE, Mousavi P, Rio J, Caillier SJ, Stillman A, Villoslada P, et al. Transcription-based prediction of response to IFN-beta using supervised computational methods. PLoS Biol 2005; 3: e2.

176 van Baarsen LG, Vosslamber S, Tijssen M, Baggen JM, van der Voort LF, Killestein J, et al. Pharmacogenomics of interferon-beta therapy in multiple sclerosis: baseline IFN signature determines pharmacological differences between patients. PLoS One 2008; 3: e1927.

177 Comabella M, Lünemann JD, Río J, Sánchez A, López C, Julià E, et al. A type I interferon signature in monocytes is associated with poor response to interferon-beta in multiple sclerosis. Brain 2009; 132: 3353–65.

178 Fusco C, Andreone V, Coppola G, Luongo V, Guerini F, Pace E, et al. HLADRB1*1501 and response to copolymer-1 therapy in relapsing-remitting multiple sclerosis. Neurology 2001; 57: 1976–79.

179 Grossman I, Avidan N, Singer C, Goldstaub D, Hayardeny L, Eyal E, et al. Pharmacogenetics of glatiramer acetate therapy for multiple sclerosis reveals drug-response markers. Pharmacogenet Genom 2007; 17: 657–66.

180 Miller DH. Biomarkers and surrogate outcomes in neurodegenerative disease: lessons from multiple sclerosis. NeuroRx 2004; 1: 284–94.

181 Charil A, Yousry TA, Rovaris M, Barkhof F, De Stefano N, Fazekas F, et al. MRI and the diagnosis of multiple sclerosis: expanding the concept of "no better explanation". Lancet Neurol 2006; 5: 841–52.

182 Barkhof F, Calabresi PA, Miller DH, Reingold SC. Imaging outcomes for neuroprotection and repair in multiple sclerosis trials. Nat Rev Neurol 2009; 5: 256–66.

183 Filippi M. Non-conventional MR techniques to monitor the evolution of multiple sclerosis. Neurol Sci 2001; 22: 195–200.

184 Pantano P, Mainero C, Caramia F. Functional brain reorganization in multiple sclerosis: evidence from fMRI studies. J Neuroimaging 2006; 16: 104–14.

185 Filippi M, Agosta F. Magnetization transfer MRI in multiple sclerosis. J Neuroimaging 2007; Suppl 1: 22S–26S.

186 Esteban FJ, Sepulcre J, de Miras JR, Navas J, de Mendizábal NV, Goñi J, et al. Fractal dimension analysis of grey matter in multiple sclerosis. J Neurol Sci 2009; 282: 67–71.

187 Gordon-Lipkin E, Chodkowski B, Reich DS, Smith SA, Pulicken M, Balcer LJ, et al. Retinal nerve fiber layer is associated with brain atrophy in multiple sclerosis. Neurology 2007; 69: 1603–9.

188 Toledo J, Sepulcre J, Salinas-Alaman A, García-Layana A, Murie-Fernandez M, Bejarano B, et al. Retinal nerve fiber layer atrophy is associated with physical and cognitive disability in multiple sclerosis. Mult Scler 2008; 14: 906–12.

189 Grazioli E, Zivadinov R, Weinstock-Guttman B, Lincoff N, Baier M, Wong JR, et al. Retinal nerve fiber layer thickness is associated with brain MRI outcomes in multiple sclerosis. J Neurol Sci 2008; 268: 12–17.

190 Sepulcre J, Murie-Fernandez M, Salinas-Alaman A, Garcia-Layana A, Bejarano B, Villoslada P. Diagnostic accuracy of retinal abnormalities in predicting disease activity in MS. Neurology 2007; 68: 1488–94.

CHAPTER 3

Epidemiology and Genetics

Philip L. De Jager

Program in Translational Neuro Psychiatric Genomics, Institute for the Neurosciences, Department of Neurology, Brigham & Women's Hospital, and Harvard Medical School, Boston, and Broad Institute of Harvard University and MIT, Cambridge, MA, USA

Introduction: risk factors

Our understanding of multiple sclerosis (MS) has advanced rapidly over the past decade; however, the inciting events of this chronic, disabling disease of the central nervous system remain elusive. Our working model is that environmental factors and stochastic events trigger MS in genetically susceptible individuals. Evidence for certain environmental risk factors is mounting, but the most rapid progress in the study of MS susceptibility has come from genetics in the past 3 years. Recent advances in genotyping technology and analytic methods have created a robust platform for gene discovery in MS, and continued developments in human genetic analysis promise insights into new classes of genetic variation in the near future. How these genetic risk factors interact with putative environmental risk factors is one of the fascinating questions that we can now begin to explore in the hope of shedding light on the earliest events involved in the onset of MS.

Distribution of MS in human populations

MS affects about 350,000 people in the United States and about 1.1 million people throughout the world [1]. Most MS patients develop the disease between 20 and 40 years of age, with a preponderance of women being affected [1]. While the overall prevalence rate is generally cited as approximately 1 in 1000 for populations of European ancestry, the lifetime risk in certain populations is as high as ~1 in 200 for women and slightly less for men [2–3]. Indeed, MS is between two to three times more prevalent in women, and this skewed gender distribution may be rising over time [4–5]. Much less is known about the prevalence of MS in non-European

---

Multiple Sclerosis: Diagnosis and Therapy, First Edition. Edited by Howard L. Weiner and James M. Stankiewicz.   © 2012 John Wiley & Sons, Ltd.
Published 2012 by John Wiley and Sons, Ltd.

populations and admixed populations such as African-Americans. Nonetheless, the available evidence suggests that prevalence is reduced, particularly in populations of African and East Asian ancestry [4, 6].

This difference in geographical distribution was noted early in the study of MS and is generally correct. It is unlikely to be solely explained by issues such as access to medical care and lack of familiarity with a diagnosis of MS in areas of low prevalence. Overall, MS prevalence demonstrates a latitude gradient, with an increased prevalence in northern latitudes of Europe and North America and in southern regions of Australia and New Zealand. However, there are notable exceptions to this general statement: for example, Sardinians have substantially higher rates of MS than other Italians, and Parsis are more commonly affected than other ethnic groups in South Asia [7]. These observations and others reporting reduced prevalence rates among African-Americans regardless of geography [8–9] suggest that the variable frequency of genetic susceptibility factors across human populations is likely to explain at least some of the geographical distribution of the disease.

There are a few observations that cannot be attributed to genetic factors. People who migrate to areas of greater MS prevalence tend to adopt the risk of their new homeland if they migrate in childhood, whereas those who migrate in later years retain the risk of their place of origin. Nor can genetics explain the differences in risk among those of common ancestry who migrate to areas of different MS prevalence [10]. It has also been argued that the recent decline in the latitude gradient and the relative increase in MS prevalence for white women in the United States and Canada must indicate exogenous factors, since genetic change does not occur over such a short period of time [2, 9, 11].

The much-quoted observation of change in risk depending on age at migration has been called into question. The cut-off for many years was assumed to be 15 years of age, but a study with a homogeneous Australian population demonstrated that when 15 years was used as the point of stratification, age of migration had no effect on MS susceptibility, suggesting that risk from migration must span a wider age range [12]. Overall, it is clear that neither genetic nor environmental risk factors are sufficient to independently explain the distribution of MS in different human populations; there is an active interplay between these two sets of risk factors.

Sunlight, vitamin D, and MS

The search for environmental agents tied to latitude that might directly affect risk of MS has been difficult. Norman and colleagues studied a US veteran population and reported that air pollution index, concentrations of minerals in ground water, temperature measures, measures of annual rainfall and average humidity, and amount of annual solar radiation, when analyzed by multiple regression, did not influence MS risk independently from latitude [13]. That study notwithstanding, much of the research for a latitude correlate has centered on the amount and duration of sunlight [14–15]. Studies measuring MS mortality as a function of occupation [16]; skin cancer rates in MS patients vs. sex-, age-, and location-matched controls [17]; and self-reported exposure to sunlight and risk of MS [18] all showed a protective role for sunlight. However, it should be noted that this evidence, while intriguing, might be misleading. The occupation and skin cancer-linkage studies that appear to show a relationship between less sunlight and MS risk may in fact reflect reverse causation—an epiphenomenon in which MS patients may preferentially avoid the sun as heat can exacerbate their symptoms, rather than sun exposure protecting against MS. Furthermore, case-control surveys can be confounded by recall bias if subjects with MS, aware of the posited relationship between sunlight and MS, misreport their exposure, relative to individuals without MS [19]. Nonetheless, increased sunlight exposure remains an attractive hypothesis that could contribute to the latitude gradient.

Exceptions to the latitude rule provide an important insight as to how sunlight might be acting to promote MS susceptibility. The first anomaly is the high prevalence of MS at low altitudes and the low MS rates at high altitudes in Switzerland [20]. The second is the high prevalence of MS inland and the lower MS prevalence along the coast in Norway [21–22]. Both of these phenomena can be convincingly explained by examining the role of vitamin D in this pathway [23]. UV light is stronger at higher altitudes, encouraging endogenous production of vitamin D3, and coastal residents eat more vitamin D-rich fish oils than do inland residents. The strongest support for the notion that the low levels of vitamin D are a risk factor for MS, however, comes from the results of two longitudinal investigations. In the first, a prospective study of dietary vitamin D intake and MS, women with supplemental intake ≥ 400 IU/day had a 60% reduced risk of MS [24]. In the second, a study among US military personnel, 25(OH)D levels were measured in healthy individuals who were followed for a diagnosis of MS. High levels of 25(OH)D were associated with a reduced risk of MS among whites (top vs bottom quintile of 25(OH)D RR $= 0.38$, 95% CI: 0.19–0.75) [25]. Epidemiological observations such as these are supported by experimental data showing that 1,25-dihydroxyvitamin D given exogenously prevents the onset of experimental autoimmune encephalomyelitis (EAE), the mouse model of MS [26–27]; while in vitamin D-deficient mice, the onset of EAE is accelerated [28]. Clinical data also support a role for vitamin D: MS patients have been found to have low serum concentrations of 25-hydroxyvitamin

D3 25(OH)D [29–30] and seasonal fluctuation of MS births and disease activity correlate with 25(OH)D seasonality [31–34].

Infectious agents and MS

Given the geographical distribution of MS, the change in risk among migrants of different age, and the possible occurrence of MS epidemics [10, 35], the hypothesis that MS results from exposure to an infectious agent was proposed early and has been repeatedly explored. Certainly, the idea that a virus could infect many people but only cause pathological manifestations in a few was already evident from poliomyelitis and provided a possible model for MS. This model of a viral cause was conceptually supported by observations that several viruses were associated with demyelinating encephalomyelitis both in human patients and in experimental animals and that high concentrations of IgG (oligoclonal bands) are found in many patients with MS [36].

Two competing hypotheses have aimed to explain the relationship of microbes to MS. The prevalence hypothesis argues that MS comes about as a result of a pathogen that is more common in areas of high MS prevalence. Alternatively, the hygiene hypothesis states that a heavy burden of microbial or parasitic infections creates a persistent effect on the immune system early in childhood, conferring protection against MS (and other autoimmune diseases). The effect on the immune system may include a shift from pro-inflammatory helper T cell (Th17) profile to a Th2 profile, such as that which is seen following helminthic infections and is associated with diminished inflammation in MS [4]. The hygiene hypothesis has generally been favored over the prevalence hypothesis in MS because it is better able to account for the latitude gradient, given recent increases in prevalence (improved hygiene), and changing risk among migrants [37].

Over the years various pathogens – such as human herpesvirus 6 (HHV6), *Chlamydia pneumoniae* and endogenous retroviruses – have been investigated for a possible connection to MS but none has been definitively linked with the disease [38]. The pathogen with the most robust evidence of association support it is the Epstein–Barr virus (EBV), the virus associated with infectious mononucleosis (IM), lymphoma, and nasopharyngeal carcinoma. The vast majority of adults have been infected with EBV. Interestingly, both IM and MS occur in adolescents and young adults and specifically target populations where EBV infection is known to occur at a later age (i.e. those with higher socioeconomic status and more education). IM also follows a similar latitude gradient to MS [39–40]. Thus, late infection with EBV, marked by the appearance of IM, is associated with MS risk; conversely, early infection with of EBV is seen in various parts of the world, such as Asia, where MS prevalence is low. MS risk was found to be associated with elevated levels of antibodies to the EBV nuclear antigen-1 (EBNA-1) many years prior to clinical manifestations of MS [41–45], and with a secondary boost in anti-EBNA-1 titers (i.e. not from primary EBV infection) occurring at some point between ages 17 and 29 [45]. One longitudinal study among US military personnel followed EBV seronegative individuals to determine whether risk of MS increases after primary EBV infection [46]; all of the EBV negative individuals who later developed MS became EBV positive prior to clinical onset compared with only 35.7% of controls, providing the strongest evidence to date that EBV infection increases the risk of MS.

At this point, epidemiological and serological studies suggest a role for EBV in MS susceptibility, but how can the hygiene hypothesis and a putative role for EBV be reconciled? The hygiene hypothesis argues that a large burden of microbes in early childhood shifts the immunological profile toward protection from MS. EBV alone is unlikely to be sufficient to explain such a shift. However, it is known that individuals who are seronegative for EBV (presumably members of the high hygiene group) have a very low risk of MS as long as they are EBV-negative [46]. On the other hand, individuals who are infected and develop IM, have a relative risk of MS of 2.3 compared with those who never developed IM (95% CI, 1.7–3.0) [47]. The EBV variant of the hygiene hypothesis [37] argues that good hygiene is detrimental from the MS perspective only insofar as it causes one to be infected with EBV later in life and hence have a higher chance of developing IM and MS.

Molecular evidence for the role of EBV in MS has extended these epidemiologic observations: Aloisi and colleagues have recently reported the presence of lymphoid follicles within the meninges of MS patients [48] These structures were noted to contain many B cells and plasma cells with evidence of EBV infection. A recent effort to validate this observation suggests, however, that EBV infection of such follicles may not be a general feature of MS [49], so further work on these technically challenging assays is needed to better characterize the extent of EBV infection in MS brains. The importance of B cell dysregulation in MS has been suggested by the recent successful phase II trial of rituximab (an anti-CD20 monoclonal antibody) in patients with relapsing-remitting disease [50]. So, evaluating EBV further in this context is critical. *In vitro* studies have suggested that, because of amino acid sequence homologies between EBV proteins and myelin basic protein, immune responses directed against EBV antigen could cross-react with self-antigen. In a genetically susceptible host in the right circumstances, the threshold of such autoreactive reactions may be lower. For example, immune response to EBV may be modulated by vitamin D, and suboptimal levels could lead to the activation of autoreactive T cells [51]. Thus, while definitive evidence for a role of EBV or another microbial trigger remains elusive, it is likely that one or, more likely, several different infectious agents may play a role in the initiation of the inflammatory process in MS.

Smoking and MS

There is substantial evidence that smoking is a risk factor for multiple sclerosis [52]. Four longitudinal studies were undertaken in the 1990s and early 2000s which, though varying in their definitions of smoking, all showed a relative risk of MS somewhere between 1.3 and 1.8 for smokers compared to subjects who had never smoked. [53]. The combined results from these four studies demonstrate a statistically significant association between a history of smoking and MS susceptibility ($p < 0.001$) [19]. Smoking is also linked to transition to secondary progressive disease in MS [54–55], and it has been noted that smoking may promote acute exacerbations of MS [56]. Furthermore, it was shown by Di Pauli and colleagues that smoking is also a risk factor for early conversion to MS after an initial demyelinating event [57]. These results suggest that toxins in the environment may contribute to various steps in the MS disease process and that behavioral modifications may yield important dividends to patients, particularly if it is accomplished early in their course.

TOP TIPS 3.1: Known environmental risk factors

1 Smoking
2 Infectious mononucleosis
3 Low vitamin D levels

Diet, neuro-endocrine and other factors

There is some evidence for the role of diet and hormones in MS risk; although, admittedly, it is not as robust as that for the aforementioned susceptibility factors. Given (1) the increasing ratio of females to males affected with MS, (2) symptom onset in young adulthood, and (3) the fact that women with MS appear to suffer somewhat fewer relapses in the second and third trimesters of pregnancy, sex hormones have been investigated for a possible role as modulators of MS risk. Progesterone appears to cause a switch from a Th1 to a Th2 immune response, while testosterone exerts anti-inflammatory and immunosuppressive effects in mouse models of autoimmunity [58]. The protection during pregnancy and the increased risk post-partum could be mediated by hormonal fluctuations of progesterone, estrogen, or other factors affected by pregnancy: for example, progesterone levels increase during gestation, reaching their peak during the third trimester, at which point evidence of protection from MS is the strongest, then plummet in the puerperium [59]. Further, it has been proposed that estradiol, the form of estrogen common in nonpregnant women, is deleterious with regard to MS, but that estriol, the predominant estrogen in pregnant women, is protective [60]. However, investigations of oral contraception use, parity, and age at first birth suggest that these beneficial effects from sex hormones are short-lived [19].

Researchers have also examined diet for a possible link to MS. Early epidemiological studies have suggested that diets high in saturated fats and low in polyunsaturated fats may increase risk; however, these studies are subject to recall bias [19]. As we have seen above, vitamin D deficiency has been implicated in MS pathogenesis, initially based in part on the observation that some populations whose geography would predispose them to the disease, instead have a relatively low prevalence. However, not all studies of nutrients have been limited to this particular fat-soluble vitamin. Certain polyunsaturated fats like omega-3 fatty acids may in fact play a small role in reducing the severity of disease, according to results from several randomized control trials [61–63], but results remain inconclusive.

Integrating environmental and genetic risk

With certain genetic factors now well established (such as the *HLA DRB1*1501* haplotype) [54], specific hypotheses can be tested to see whether subjects with different levels of genetic susceptibility to MS respond differently to environmental exposures or whether certain environmental factors are dependent on a particular genetic architecture. Given that HLA DRB1 is a co-receptor for EBV entry and that the *HLA DRB1*1501* allele may be able to present EBV antigen that mimic self-antigen, assessing the interaction of these two strong risk factors is of great interest. A recent study suggests that these two risk factors are largely independent and may be multiplicative. Specifically, individuals who have both risk factors (the *HLA DRB1*1501* allele and high levels of antibodies directed against the EBV protein EBNA-1) have a nine-fold increase in risk over individuals that have neither risk factor [65]. This observation has been validated in another cohort [66] which also supports the idea that there may be an interaction between these two risk factors. Interestingly, smoking appears to enhance the risk of MS associated with high anti-

EBNA-1 titers, and this effect appears to account for the increased risk of MS due to smoking in some cohorts. The same cohorts were also analyzed using *HLA DRB1*1501*, but this genetic risk factor did not influence the association between smoking, anti-EBNA-1 titers and MS risk [67]. These and other observations have led to approaches that integrate genetic and environmental risk factors to predict a diagnosis of MS. The one study published to date on this topic suggests that environmental and genetic risk factors offer nonredundant information for a diagnostic algorithm [68]. While our predictive model produces consistent results over several different subject cohorts, this algorithm that uses only 16 genetic variants is not yet performing well enough to be deployed clinically. Nonetheless, it demonstrates the way forward as we begin to integrate different risk factors; future versions of the algorithm will include the 50–100 common genetic variants and probably many rare variants that are thought to have a role in MS susceptibility. Furthermore, it will integrate interactions between risk factors that are thought to exist but have not yet been demonstrated, as it is likely that environmental factors may have differential effects in different subsets of subjects with MS and that taking the genetic architecture of subjects into account will clarify the role of environmental susceptibility factors.

Can we can consider exposure to sunlight and vitamin D levels in such models? Is their role similarly independent from genetic causes or can genetic predisposition account for their effect on MS risk? Researchers recently investigated the role of sun exposure using disease-discordant MZ twins. The avoidance of sunlight early in life seems to put people at risk for the future development of MS, independent of genetic susceptibility to MS [69]. Yet more evidence points in the direction of a complex interplay of genetic factors and vitamin D regulation: a recent study identified a novel MS susceptibility locus that includes the 1-alpha-hydroxylase (*CYP27B1*) gene involved in vitamin D metabolism. Diet, sun exposure, and genetics are all involved in vitamin D regulation. Since we know that serum levels of 25 (OH)D affect one's risk of MS, the exact degree to which diet and sunlight influence MS risk, apart from genetics, becomes more difficult to tease out without large sample sizes. Future epidemiological studies will benefit from knowledge of the genetic architecture of MS and will be better able to explore the independence, or interdependence, of genes and the environment.

Genetic susceptibility in MS

MS susceptibility is a genetically complex trait, with no simple Mendelian form described to date. While there are occasional families with large numbers of MS cases, unlike other neurodegenerative diseases such as

Alzheimer disease and Parkinson disease, no single gene has been discovered to explain the clustering of MS in such families. It is possible that rare genetic variants in different genes may explain some of this familial clustering; however, early evidence suggests that these multiplex families may simply harbor a larger proportion of common MS risk alleles than the families of sporadic MS cases [70]. To date, one thing is clear: many different genetic loci with incomplete penetrance contribute to an individual's risk of developing MS. The evidence indicates that each of these genes probably only exerts a modest influence [4]. This is consistent with the fact that heritability of MS is modest: the lifetime risk of developing MS for a sibling of an MS patient is 3%, which is similar to the rate for children whose parents have MS and is about 30 times greater than the risk to the general population. The identical twin of an MS patient has, on average, a 30% risk of developing MS, highlighting the important but not overwhelming role that genes play in the onset of MS. While susceptibility and age at which a patient develops symptoms show modest evidence of heritability, there is little evidence that a disease course is strongly heritable, so a patient's course is not very informative when considering what may happen to a family member who is newly diagnosed.

The search for susceptibility loci outside of the Major Histocompatibility Complex (MHC) initially relied on linkage studies of families with multiple cases of MS, without success. Around the turn of the century, it became clear that this lack of success was consistent with theoretical discussions that highlighted the lack of statistical power of the linkage approach in discovering genetic variants of modest effect for a common disease such as MS. Instead, an association-based approach, such as a simple case-control design, was put forward as the preferred method for gene discovery [71]. This realization led to the formation of the International MS Genetics Consortium (IMSGC), since, to be successful, an association study design requires very large sample sizes and very dense genotyping. In 2007, the collaboration came to fruition, and the first MS genome-wide association scan (GWAS) was performed by the IMSGC, resulting in the identification of two non-MHC susceptibility loci [72–73]. This ground-breaking discovery was possible because of a combination of newly developed resources such as the HapMap (a catalog of several million common human genetic variation), technological advances (including novel high-throughput genotyping platforms), and more powerful statistical methodologies. However, the critical strategic breakthrough with this study was the validation of the gene discovery strategy: a simple association study comparing allele frequencies in cases and controls proved successful when sufficient numbers of genetic markers and subjects were analyzed. The way forward was now clear: larger studies with more markers would enhance statistical power and lead to more discoveries.

The major histocompatibility complex (MHC)

Increasing sample sizes and high density genotyping panels have also led to new insights into the well-known MHC association with MS susceptibility. Human leukocyte antigen (HLA) genes, located within the MHC on chromosome 6p21, were first found to be associated with MS in 1972 [74]. Numerous linkage and association studies have since made this the most replicated finding in MS genetics [75]. In particular, the *HLA DRB1*1501* haplotype (also known by the *HLA DR2* and *HLA DR15* tissue types) has consistently demonstrated linkage and association with MS in different human populations [75]. However, other alleles within the MHC may separately confer MS risk. For example, Sardinians have a high concentration of *HLA DR3* and *HLA DR4* [76–77], which may account for their high rates of MS, and *HLA DR3* was found to be associated with susceptibility for MS in United Kingdom subjects [78].

Because of strong linkage disequilibrium (LD, the co-occurrence of alleles at two or more loci within individuals more frequently than would be expected by chance) within the MHC, as well as the strong effect size (odds ratio (OR) = 2.7 for one copy of the allele) [79–80] it remains unclear where the true susceptibility factor resides within the *HLA DRB1*1501* haplotype. In a study of African-Americans with MS, Oksenberg and colleagues show not only that *HLA DRB1*0301* (*HLA DR3*) and *HLA DRB1*1503* are associated with MS, but also that the *HLA DRB1*1501* allele confers MS risk independent of the tightly linked *HLA DQB1*0602* allele [81]. This pre-eminent role for *HLA DRB1*1501* is also seen in rare individuals of European descent where *HLA DRB1*1501* has been separated from *HLA DQB1*0602* [De Jager, unpublished result]. While the linkage disequilibrium in the MHC and allelic heterogeneity at *HLA DRB1* make it difficult to tease out a causal variant, it is clear that the *HLA DRB1*1501* allele is the strongest known MS susceptibility factor in the human genome and that the magnitude of its effect on MS susceptibility is unique for such a common allele.

More recently, larger sample sizes have enabled the resolution of susceptibility haplotypes that have effects independent of *HLA DRB1*1501* within the four megabases of the MHC. Specifically, it is now clear that the MHC class I region contributes to disease susceptibility. Multiple studies have validated the protective effect of the haplotype tagged by the *HLA A*02* allele [79], and the *HLA B*44* allele appears to tag another protective haplotype that has an effect independent of *HLA A*02* [82]. The previously reported association of *HLA C*05* appears to be secondary to these other two protective haplotypes [78]. Furthermore, other studies suggest that additional susceptibility alleles exist within the MHC, so further investigation with larger sample sizes will provide more insights into the role of this critical region of the genome. Nonetheless, we have already gained the critical insights that MHC class I molecules, and not just class II molecules, are involved in the onset of MS implicating, for example, CD8 + T cells and natural killer cells in the earliest events in MS.

Non-MHC MS susceptibility alleles

Several different GWAS have been conducted for MS susceptibility since the original study in 2007, and many of their results have been subsequently validated. Overall, outside of the MHC, the GWAS discovered the type of risk-associated variants that are targeted by this study design: genetic variants that are relatively common (frequency > 0.05) in the general population of European ancestry and have modest effects on disease susceptibility (odds ratio 1.1–1.25). The 19 susceptibility loci identified to date fit this pattern (Figure 3.1). It is now clear that there are no common variants of strong effect on susceptibility outside of the MHC. The *caveat* to this statement is that current genotyping arrays do not interrogate the entire human genome. Estimates vary, but roughly 80% of the common variation in the human genome has been explored to date for association with MS.

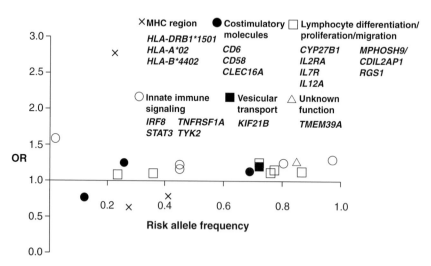

Figure 3.1 MS susceptibility allele spectrum. The validated MS susceptibility loci are divided in different categories based on their functional roles. Most of them are involved in immunological functions, even if it is not possible to exclude a potential role in the central nervous system function. Each dot represents one MS risk allele plotted by their frequency in European populations and their associated odds ratio (OR, odds ratio, the magnitude of the allele's affect).

Thus, we may still be surprised by what is lurking in the 20% of the genome that is more difficult to interrogate using current technologies. Nonetheless, the current GWAS strategy is an extremely powerful approach that has yet to deliver its full complement of susceptibility loci; 50–100 susceptibility loci may exist and will gradually be identified as study sample sizes increase. Ongoing efforts include a new meta-analysis of all existing MS GWASs that will incorporate data on over 15,000 subjects with MS and 30,000 controls, and will replicate results in an additional 10,000 subjects with MS and 10,000 controls. While this effort will have 99% power to discover common alleles with an odds ratio of 1.2, two or three times that number will be needed to identify the alleles with more modest effects (odds ratio >1.1). Thus, much remains to be done in investigating common variants with MS and a frank debate regarding the ultimate goal of gene discovery efforts in this arena is needed as loci with even more modest effects (odds ratio < 1.1) exist and can be robustly discovered, given large enough studies. The issue becomes one of prioritization of experimental strategies given limited resources.

A complementary area of investigation that will begin to bear fruit in the next few years involves the study of less common and rare variants (population frequency < 0.05) in MS. Next generation-sequencing technologies are rapidly maturing and are making the identification and study of such variants practical for the first time. Interest in these approaches is bolstered by the recent validation of two variants in this class that share the expected profile of being present in relatively few individuals in the general population but of having strong effects. Both sets of variants were discovered as part of targeted investigations of a given gene: the 92Q allele of *TNFRSF1A* is present in ~2% (odds ratio 1.6) and the MS associated *SIAE* alleles are present in <1% of individuals of European ancestry (odds ratio 8.6) [83]. Thus, rare variants with large effect sizes on MS susceptibility exist and are discoverable using genome-sequencing approaches. One final class of variant may exist but will not be discovered using current strategies: rare variants of modest effect will be extremely difficult to discover and validate as these variants would require extremely large sample sizes to be discovered.

The future of gene discovery in MS looks bright, but we already have important insights from the current complement of 19 susceptibility loci: *CBLB, CYP27B1, CD6, CD40, CD58, CD226, CLEC16A, CD80/TMEM39A, IL2RA, IL7R, IL12A, IRF8, KIF21B, MPHOSPH9/CDK2AP1, RGS1, SIAE, STAT3, TNFRSF1A*, and *TYK2*. Almost all of these loci contain genes with well-known immunologic functions, which suggests that the onset of MS is most likely to involve an immune dysregulation that secondarily triggers a degenerative process within the central nervous system. However, a definitive resolution of this question awaits the discovery of the full complement of susceptibility genes and a better grasp of the functional consequences of each locus on the human body. Given the known functions of the genes found in the MS susceptibility loci identified to date, we can make a few broad statements regarding which aspects of the immune system appear to be preferentially affected by MS risk alleles. For example, it appears that T cell activation is an important nexus for the effect of many of the variants, including those found in or near co-stimulatory genes (*CD6, CD40, CD58, CD80, CD226*) and those affecting signaling pathways involved in transmitting activation and proliferation signals (*CBLB, IL2RA, RGS1*). These and other molecules involved in the B cell arm of adaptive immunity (such as *SIAE*) are found along with several aspects of the innate immune system (*IRF8, STAT3, TNFRSF1A,* and *TYK2*), suggesting that the onset of MS is probably not due to the dysfunction of a single cell type but is instead due to systemic immune dysfunction. This observation is underscored by the fact that many of the susceptibility genes enumerated above have different functions at different levels of the immune system, and so tying the function of a risk allele to a single cell type is a useful but limited approximation as we begin to consider the sequence of events leading to the onset of MS.

So far, a few variants associated with MS susceptibility have been investigated in detail, and we are beginning to gain an appreciation of the possible mechanisms by which the risk-associated alleles are altering immune function. In several cases, such as the *CD58* and *CDK2AP1* loci, the level of RNA expression of a nearby gene is altered in the presence of the risk allele [84]; in the case of the *IL7R* locus, a more subtle alteration in the ratio of certain isoforms has been described [85]. Further, a broader effect on RNA expression of many genes in the type I interferon response pathway has been demonstrated in the case of the *IRF8* risk allele [86] This observation is not surprising given that *IRF8* is a transcription factor and is a known mediator of type I interferon responses. Finally, several *IL2RA* alleles appear to have independent effects on MS susceptibility and influence the level of soluble *IL2RA*. Thus, we are beginning to catalog the first few events that connect risk alleles to the onset of MS by a causal chain of events that will doubtlessly involve the interaction of many different risk alleles among themselves and with environmental factors such as smoking, EBV infection, and vitamin D nutrition.

Shared susceptibility loci among inflammatory diseases and evidence for allelic heterogeneity

The R92Q allele of *TNFRSF1A* that was discussed above illustrates another important aspect of the genetic architecture of MS: many of the loci are shared with other inflammatory diseases. This observation is consistent with the reported excess in inflammatory diseases among subjects with MS [87] and among family members who do not have MS themselves [88]. In the case of *TNFRSF1A*, the same allele influences risk for both MS and

TRAPS [86]. In contrast, the *IL12A* MS susceptibility allele is actually protective for celiac disease [89]. In the *IL2RA* locus, perhaps the best characterized locus to date [90] we find evidence for three variants with independent effects in MS and type 1 diabetes mellitus (DM-1) suscepti-bility: (1) an allele shared between DM-1 and MS (rs2104286); (2) an allele conferring susceptibility to DM-1 but protection from MS (rs11594656); and (3) a DM-1 allele not associated with MS susceptibility (rs41295061) [90]. This unsuspected complexity in the role of the *IL2RA* variants in autoimmunity suggests that identifying susceptibility loci is just the beginning of an arduous process of understanding multiple and conflicting effects of genetic variation found in a given gene. The task is further complicated by the extensive overlap among disease susceptibility loci that is seen today: 13 of 19 MS susceptibility loci discussed above are associated with more than one disease. Further evidence of sharing will probably emerge at many more loci as studies in other diseases reach a sufficient size to exclude the possibility that an allele of modest effect has a role in another disease. Thus, the emerging genetic architecture of inflam-matory disease is quite complex and will require the coordinated efforts of disease-specific consortia to elucidate the role of many loci in inflammatory diseases. A detailed genetic map of these diseases should prove valuable in understanding the shared pathophysiology of inflammatory disease and perhaps also in guiding therapeutic selection in MS. The latter could come in two forms: (1) diseases whose genetic architecture is most similar to MS may have a greater likelihood to respond to similar therapeutic interven-tion, thereby guiding the selection of therapies approved in another disease for testing in MS; or (2) this genetic information may help to identify those individuals who are most likely to develop certain inflammatory adverse events after an immunomodulatory intervention, such as thyroiditis and immune thrombocytopenic purpura, which are consequences of alemtu-zumab treatment [91].

Use of genetic risk factors in predictive models for multiple sclerosis

Since the genetic architecture of MS susceptibility is constituted primarily of loci of modest effect, analyzing the behavior of groups of susceptibility alleles could be informative. Recently, an aggregate measure of MS risk that combines weighted odds ratios from 16 genetic susceptibility loci (the weighted genetic risk score (wGRS) was created and used to predict a diagnosis of MS in three independent cohorts [68]. The results revealed that the wGRS can modestly but robustly predict MS risk. Figure 3.2 illustrates this by showing that the subjects with MS clearly have a greater load of susceptibility factors, on average, than do healthy people, although the 16 loci assessed so far are not sufficient to differentiate MS cases from

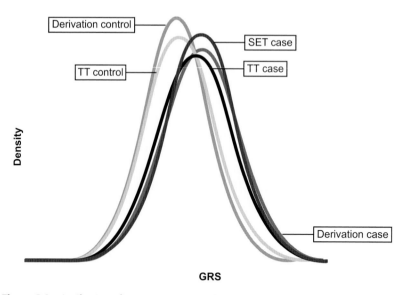

Figure 3.2 Distribution of wGRSs in cases and controls. A wGRS is calculated for each subject within each of the three different cohorts in this figure. Here, we illustrate the distribution of wGRSs in the derivation samples, with cases (curve labeled Derivation case) and controls (Derivation control). The TT sample collection is overlaid with cases (TT case) and controls (TT control). Finally, the Czech SET collection of CIS cases labeled SET case.

healthy controls. A noteworthy but unsurprising observation is that a group of subjects with a clinically isolated demyelinating syndrome appear to have an architecture of genetic risk that is indistinguishable from that of subjects with MS (Figure 3.2).

With only 16 loci assayed in this version of the wGRS (out of the likely 50 to 100 loci that should emerge from current studies), it is too early to say whether a purely genetic algorithm will have clinical utility [92], particularly since we do not yet understand the role that less common variants of large effect (such as *TNFRSF1A* R92Q and the *SIAE* alleles) may play. It is likely that a predictive algorithm incorporating these risk alleles as well as other dimensions of information will eventually emerge. In fact, prediction of a case of MS is enhanced by the inclusion of nongenetic risk factors, such as sex, smoking, and anti-Epstein–Barr virus titers [68] This suggests that an algorithm using MS susceptibility loci might provide useful information if used in the context of a diagnostic algorithm that incorporates other data, such as environmental risk factors or, ultimately, blood biomarker or imaging data. However, genetic data in the context of the diagnostic evaluation of a sporadic MS case may be of marginal utility unless imaging is not available to support the clinical evaluation. A more useful application of this predictive score may ultimately be for individuals who are at higher risk to develop the disease, such as the first-degree relatives of patients with MS [70]. The identification of individuals during the clinically silent phase of the disease could be extremely helpful in guiding the selection of those subjects who would benefit most from early imaging screening and eventually early treatment.

The next decade of multiple sclerosis risk factors

During the past 10 years, a dramatic change has occurred in our understanding of MS genetic and environmental risks, with 18 of the risk alleles discussed in this review having been discovered in just the past 3 years. A robust method to discover common variants of modest effect, the association study, is now available, and many collaborations are maximizing the yield of this method by increasing the number of genotyped individuals. Many more loci will doubtlessly emerge as systems analyses and integrated analyses of genetic and other data are deployed to uncover pathways that have a predilection for being targeted by MS susceptibility alleles [93]. Overall, the study of the human genome has yielded strong dividends in the field of MS, and a new generation of studies to assess other classes of genetic variation is already starting. The next decade promises to deliver a robust assessment of rare variants, using whole genome sequencing, and to finally validate loci affecting treatment and disease course as investigators begin to perform joint analyses across datasets. In parallel, the arduous studies to identify environmental risk factors have returned robust evidence that elaborated many observations first made in the past century, and we now have good evidence for several different processes such as vitamin D metabolism and EBV infection that are being targeted for molecular investigations in the context of our understanding of MS pathophysiology. The convergence of the success of these two disciplines outlines an exciting field of investigation where immunology, epidemiology, and genetics will now converge to allow insights into the sequence of molecular events that lead to the onset of MS. Given the technologies and methods available today, it looks likely that this new generation of studies will quickly inform existing efforts to develop algorithms that support clinical decisions. While it is too early to say whether personalized medicine will appear in MS, it is likely that genetic and environmental information will be incorporated into some aspects of the management of the disease in the coming decade.

References

1 Hauser SL, Goodin DS. Multiple sclerosis and other demyelinating diseases. In: Kasper DL, Braunwald E, Hauser S, Longo D, Jameson LJ, Fauci AS (eds.), Harrison's Principles of Internal Medicine, 16th edn. McGraw-Hill Professional; 2004, pp. 2461–71.

2 Hernán MA, Olek MJ, Ascherio A. Geographic variation of MS incidence in two prospective studies of US women. Neurology 1999 Nov; 53(8): 1711–18.

3 Koch-Henriksen N, Hyllested K. Epidemiology of multiple sclerosis: incidence and prevalence rates in Denmark 1948–64 based on the Danish Multiple Sclerosis Registry. Acta Neurol Scand 1988 Nov; 78(5): 369–80.

4 Compston A, Coles A. Multiple sclerosis. Lancet 2008 Oct; 372(9648): 1502–17.

5 Ascherio A, Munger K. Epidemiology of multiple sclerosis: from risk factors to prevention. Semin Neurol 2008 Feb; 28(1): 17–28. Review.

6 Smestad C, Sandvik L, Holmoy T, Harbo HF, Celius EG. Marked differences in prevalence of multiple sclerosis between ethnic groups in Oslo, Norway. J Neurol 2008; 249–55.

7 Rosati G. The prevalence of multiple sclerosis in the world: an update. Neurol Sci 2001; 22: 117–39.

8 Kurtzke JF, Beebe GW, Norman JE Jr., Epidemiology of multiple sclerosis in US veterans. 1. Race, sex, and geographic distribution. Neurology 1979; 29: 1228–35.

9 Wallin MT, Page WF, Kurtzke JF. Multiple sclerosis in US veterans of the Vietnam era and later military service: race, sex, geography. Ann Neurol 2004 Jan; 55(1): 65–71.

10 Gale CR, Martyn CN. Migrant studies in multiple sclerosis. Prog Neurobiol 1995; 47: 425–48.

11 Orton SM, Herrera BM, Yee IM, et al for the Canadian Collaborative Study Group. Sex ratio of multiple sclerosis in Canada: a longitudinal study. Lancet Neurol 2006 Nov; 5(11): 932–6.

12 Hammond SR, English DR, McLeod JG. The age-range of risk of developing multiple sclerosis: evidence from a migrant population in Australia. Brain 2000; 123(5): 968–74.

13 Norman JE Jr, Kurtzke JF, Beebe GW. Epidemiology of multiple sclerosis in US veterans: 2. Latitude, climate, and the risk of multiple sclerosis. J Chronic Dis 1983; 36(8): 551–9.

14 Ascherio A, Munger KL, Simon KC. Vitamin D and multiple sclerosis. Lancet Neurol 2010; 9(6): 599–612. Review.

15 Hayes CE, Cantorna MT, DeLuca HF. Vitamin D and multiple sclerosis. Proc Soc Exp Biol Med 1997; 216: 21–7.

16 Freedman DM, Dosemeci M, Alavanja MC. Mortality from multiple sclerosis and exposure to residential and occupational solar radiation: a case-control study based on death certificates. Occup Environ Med 2000; 57: 418–21.

17 Goldacre MJ, Seagroatt V, Yeates D, Acheson ED. Skin cancer in people with multiple sclerosis: a record linkage study. J Epidemiol Community Health 2004; 58: 142–4.

18 Van der Mei IA, Ponsonby AL, Dwyer T, et al. Past exposure to sun, skin phenotype and risk of multiple sclerosis: a case-control study. BMJ 2003; 327: 316–21.

19 Ascherio A, Munger K. Environmental risk factors for multiple sclerosis. Part II. Noninfectious factors. Ann Neurol 2007 Jun; 61(6): 504–13.

20 Kurtzke JF. On the fine structure of the distribution of multiple sclerosis. Acta Neurol Scand 1967; 43: 257–82.

21 Swank RL, Lerstad O, Strom A, Backer J. Multiple sclerosis in rural Norway: its geographic and occupational incidence in relation to nutrition. N Engl J Med 1952; 246: 722–8.

22 Westlund K. Distribution and mortality time trend of multiple sclerosis and some other diseases in Norway. Acta Neurol Scand 1970; 46: 455–83.

23 Goldberg P. Multiple sclerosis: vitamin D and calcium as environmental determinants of prevalence (A viewpoint) part 1: sunlight, dietary factors and epidemiology. Int J Environ Stud 1974; 6: 19–27.

24 Munger: Neurol 2004 –

25 Cantorna MT, Hayes CE, DeLuca HF. 1, 25-Dihydroxyvitamin D3 reversibly blocks the progression of relapsing encephalomyelitis, a model of multiple sclerosis. Proc Natl Acad Sci USA 1996; 93: 7861–4.

26 Munger KL, Levin LI, Hollis BW, Howard NS, Ascherio A. Serum 25-hydroxyvitamin D levels and risk of multiple sclerosis. JAMA 2006; 296: 2832–8.

27 Lemire JM, Archer DC. 1, 25 dihydroxyvitamin D3 prevents the in vivo induction of murine experimental autoimmune encephalomyelitis. J Clin Invest 1991; 87: 1103–7.

28 Pedersen LB, Nashold FE, Spach KM, Hayes CE. 1, 25-dihydroxyvitamin D3 reverses experimental autoimmune encephalomyelitis by inhibiting chemokine synthesis and monocyte trafficking. J Neurosci Res 2007 Aug 15; 85(11): 2480–90.

29 Nieves J, Cosman F, Herbert J, Shen V, Lindsay R. High prevalence of vitamin D deficiency and reduced bone mass in multiple sclerosis. Neurology 1994; 44: 1687–92.

30 Ozgocmen S, Bulut S, Ilhan N, Gulkesen A, Ardicoglu O, Ozkan Y. Vitamin D deficiency and reduced bone mineral density in multiple sclerosis: effect of ambulatory status and functional capacity. J Bone Miner Metab 2005; 23: 309–13.

31 Willer CJ, Dyment DA, Sadovnick AD, Rothwell PM, Murray TJ, Ebers GC. Timing of birth and risk of multiple sclerosis: population based study. BMJ 2005; 330: 120.

32 Sotgiu S, Pugliatti M, Sotgiu MA, et al. Seasonal fluctuations of multiple sclerosis births in Sardinia. J Neurol 2006; 253: 38–44.

33 Embry AF, Snowdon LR, Vieth R. Vitamin D and seasonal fluctuations of gadolinium-enhancing magnetic resonance imaging lesions in multiple sclerosis. Ann Neurol 2000; 48: 271–2.

34 Auer DP, Schumann EM, Kumpfel T, Gossl C, Trenkwalder C. Seasonal fluctuations of gadolinium-enhancing magnetic resonance imaging lesions in multiple sclerosis. Ann Neurol 2000; 47; 276–7.

35 Kurtzke JF, Hyllested K. Multiple sclerosis in the Faroe Islands. I. Clinical and epidemiological features. Ann Neurol 1979 Jan; 5(1): 6–21.

36 Gilden DH. Infectious causes of multiple sclerosis. Lancet Neurol 2005 Mar; 4(3): 195–202.

37 Ascherio A, Munger K. Environmental risk factors for multiple sclerosis. Part I: The role of infection. Ann Neurol 2007 Apr; 61(4): 288–99.

38 Giovannoni G, Cutter GR, Lunemann J, et al. Infectious causes of multiple sclerosis. Lancet Neurol 2006; 5: 887–94.

39 Warner HB, Carb RI. Multiple sclerosis and Epstein-Barr virus. Lancet 1981; 2: 1290.

40 Niederman JC, Evans AS. Epstein–Barr virus. In: Evans Epidemiology and Control, 4th edn. New York: Plenum Medical Book Company; 1997, pp. 253–283.

41 Ascherio A, Munger KL, Lennette ET, Spiegelman D, Hernán MA, Olek MJ, et al. Epstein–Barr virus antibodies and risk of multiple sclerosis: a prospective study. JAMA 2001; 286(24): 3083–8.

42 DeLorenze GN, Munger KL, Lennette ET, Orentreich N, Vogelman JH, Ascherio A. Epstein–Barr virus and multiple sclerosis: evidence of association from a prospective study with long-term follow up. Arch Neurol 2006; 63(6): 839–44.

43 Sundström P, Juto P, Wadell G, Hallmans G, Svenningsson A, Nyström L, Dillner J, Forsgren L. An altered immune response to Epstein–Barr virus in multiple sclerosis: a prospective study. Neurology 2004; 62(12): 2277–82.

44 Levin LI, Munger KL, Rubertone MV et al. Multiple sclerosis and Epstein-Barr virus. JAMA 2003; 289: 1533–6.

45 Levin LI, Munger KL, Rubertone MV, et al. Temporal relationship between elevation of Epstein Barr virus antibody titers and initial onset of neurological symptoms in multiple sclerosis. JAMA 2005; 293: 2496–2500.

46 Levin 2010 –

47 Thacker EL, Mirzaei F, Ascherio A. Infectious mononucleosis and risk for multiple sclerosis: a meta-analysis. Ann Neurol 2006 Mar; 59(3): 499–503.

48 Serafini B, Rosicarelli B, Franciotta D, et al. Dysregulated Epstein-Barr virus infection in the multiple sclerosis brain. J Exp Med 2007 Nov; 204(12): 2899–912.

49 Willis SN, Stadelmann C, et al. Epstein–Barr virus infection is not a characteristic feature of multiple sclerosis brain. Brain 2009; 132(Pt 12): 3318–28.

50 Hauser SL, Waubant E, Arnold DL, et al. B-cell depletion with rituximab in relapsing-remitting multiple sclerosis. N Engl J Med 2008 Feb; 358(7): 676–88.

51 Holmoy T. Vitamin D modulates the immune response to Epstein-Barr virus: Synergistic effect of risk factors in multiple sclerosis. Med Hypotheses 2008; 70(1): 66–9.

52 Riise T, Nortvedt MW, Ascherio A. Smoking is a risk factor for multiple sclerosis. Neurology 2003; 61: 1122–24.

53 Marrie RA, Cutter G, Tyry T, Campagnolo D, Vollmer T. Smoking status over two years in patients with multiple sclerosis. Neuroepidemiology 2008 Nov; 32(1): 72–9.

54 Hernán MA, Jick SS, Logroscino G, Olek MJ, Ascherio A, Jick H. Cigarette smoking and the progression of multiple sclerosis. Brain 2005; 128: 1461–1465.

55 Healy Arch Neurol 2009.

56 Courville CB, Maschmeyer JE, DeLay CP. Effects of smoking on the acute exacerbations of multiple sclerosis. Bull Los Angeles Neurol Soc 1964; 29: 1–6.

57 Di Pauli F, Reindl M, Ehling R, et al. Smoking is an early risk factor for conversion to clinically definite multiple sclerosis. Mult Scler 2008; 14: 1026–30.

58 Whitacre CC, Reingold SC, O'Loony PA. A gender gap in autoimmunity. Science 1999; 283: 1277–8.

59 Whitacre CC. Sex differences in autoimmune disease. Nat Immunol 2001; 2: 777–80.

60 Tanzer J. Estrogen effect in multiple sclerosis more nuanced than described 2008; 63(2): 263. Letter.

61 Dworkin RH, Bates D, Millar JHD, Paty DW. Linoleic acid and multiple sclerosis: a reanalysis of three double-blind trials. Neurology 1984; 34: 1441–5.

62 Bates D, Cartlidge NE, French JM, et al. A double-blind controlled trial of long chain n-3 polyunsaturated fatty acids in the treatment of multiple sclerosis. J Neurol Neurosurg Psychiatry 1989; 52: 18–22.

63 Weinstock-Guttman B, Baier M, Park Y, et al. Low fat dietary intervention with omega–3 fatty acid supplementation in multiple sclerosis patients. Prostaglandins Leukot Essent Fatty Acids 2005; 73: 397–404.

64 Oksenberg JR, Baranzini SE, Sawcer S, Hauser SL. The genetics of multiple sclerosis: SNPs to pathways to pathogenesis. Nat Rev Genet 2008 Jul; 9(7): 516–26.

65 De Jager PL, Simon KC, Munger KL, Rioux JD, Hafler DA, Ascherio A. Integrating risk factors: HLA-DRB1*1501 and Epstein-Barr virus in multiple sclerosis. Neurology 2008 Mar; 70(13 Pt 2): 1113–18.

66 Sundström P, Nystrom M, et al. Antibodies to specific EBNA-1 domains and HLA DRB1*1501 interact as risk factors for multiple sclerosis. J Neuroimmunol 2009; 215(1–2): 102–7.

67 Simon KC, van der Mei IA, et al. Combined effects of smoking, anti-EBNA antibodies, and HLA-DRB1*1501 on multiple sclerosis risk. Neurology 2010; 74(17): 1365–71.

68 De Jager PL, Chibnik LB, et al. Integration of genetic risk factors into a clinical algorithm for multiple sclerosis susceptibility: a weighted genetic risk score. Lancet Neurol 2009; 8(12): 1111–19.

69 Islam T, Gauderman WJ, Cozen W, Mack TM. Childhood sun exposure influences risk of multiple sclerosis in monozygotic twins. Neurology 2007 Jul; 69(4): 381–8.

70 Gourraud PA, McElroy JP, et al. Aggregation of multiple sclerosis genetic risk variants in multiple and single case families. Ann Neurol 2011; 69(1): 65–74.

71 Orton SM, Morris AP, Herrera BM, et al. Evidence for genetic regulation of vitamin D status in twins with multiple sclerosis. Am J Clin Nutr 2008 Aug. 88(2): 441–7.

72 Hafler DA, Compston A, Sawcer S, et al. for the International Multiple Sclerosis Genetics Consortium. Risk alleles for multiple sclerosis identified by a genome-wide study. N Engl J Med 2007; 357: 851–62.

73 Baranzini SE, Wang J, Gibson RA, et al. Genome-wide association analysis of susceptibility and clinical phenotype in multiple sclerosis. Hum Mol Genet 2008 Nov 14 (Epub).

74 Jersild C, Svejgaard A, Fog T. HL-A antigens and multiple sclerosis. Lancet; 1972; 1: 1240–1.

75 Fernando MM, Stevens CR, Walsh EC, et al. Defining the role of the MHC in autoimmunity: a review and pooled analysis. PloS Genet 2008 Apr 25; 4(4): e1000024. Review.

76 Marrosu MG, Murru MR, Costa G, et al. Multiple sclerosis in Sardinia is associated and in linkage disequilibrium with HLA-DR3 and HLA-DR4 alleles. Am J Hum Genet 1997; 61: 454–7.

77 Marrosu MG, Murru MR, Costa G, Murru R, Muntoni F, Cucca F. DRB1-DQA1-DQB1 loci and multiple sclerosis predisposition in the Sardinian population. Hum Mol Genet 1998; 7: 1235–7.

78 Yeo TW, De Jager PL, Gregory SG, et al. A second major histocompatibility complex susceptibility locus for multiple sclerosis. Ann Neurol 2007 Mar; 61(3): 228–36.

79 Fogdell-Hahn A, Ligers A, Gronning M, Hillert J, Olerup O. Multiple sclerosis: a modifying influence of HLA class I genes in an HLA class II associated autoimmune disease. Tissue Antigens 2000 Feb; 55(2): 140–8.

80 Barcellos LF, Oksenberg JR, Begovich AB, et al. HLA-DR2 dose effect on susceptibility to multiple sclerosis and influence on disease course. Am J Hum Genet 2003; 72: 710–716.

81 Okenberg JR, Barcellos LF, Cree BA, et al. Mapping multiple sclerosis susceptibility to the HLA-DR locus in African-Americans. Am J Hum Genet 2004 Jan; 74(1): 160–167.

82 Healy BC, Liguori M, et al. HLA B*44: protective effects in MS susceptibility and MRI outcome measures. Neurology 2010; 75(7): 634–40.

83 Surolia I, Pirnie SP, et al. Functionally defective germline variants of sialic acid acetylesterase in autoimmunity. Nature 2010; 466(7303): 243–7.

84 De Jager, PL, Baecher-Allan C, et al. The role of the CD58 locus in multiple sclerosis. Proc Natl Acad Sci USA 2009; 106(13): 5264–9.

85 Gregory, SG, Schmidt S, et al. Interleukin 7 receptor alpha chain (IL7R) shows allelic and functional association with multiple sclerosis. Nat Genet 2007; 39(9): 1083–91.

86 De Jager, PL, Jia X, et al. Meta-analysis of genome scans and replication identify CD6, IRF8 and TNFRSF1A as new multiple sclerosis susceptibility loci. Nat Genet 2009; 41(7): 776–82.

87 Henderson, RD, Bain CJ, et al. The occurrence of autoimmune diseases in patients with multiple sclerosis and their families. J Clin Neurosci 2000; 7(5): 434–7.

88 Barcellos LF, Kamdar BB, et al. Clustering of autoimmune diseases in families with a high-risk for multiple sclerosis: a descriptive study. Lancet Neurol 2006; 5(11): 924–31.

89 Hunt KA, Zhernakova A, et al. Newly identified genetic risk variants for celiac disease related to the immune response. Nat Genet 2008; 40(4): 395–402.

90 Maier LM, Lowe CE, et al. IL2RA genetic heterogeneity in multiple sclerosis and type 1 diabetes susceptibility and soluble interleukin-2 receptor production. PLoS Genet 2009; 5(1): e1000322.

91 Coles AJ, Compston DA, et al. Alemtuzumab vs. interferon beta-1a in early multiple sclerosis. N Engl J Med 2008; 359(17): 1786–801.

92 Sawcer S, Ban M, et al. What role for genetics in the prediction of multiple sclerosis? Ann Neurol 2010; 67(1): 3–10.

93 Baranzini SE, Galwey NW, et al. Pathway and network-based analysis of genome-wide association studies in multiple sclerosis. Hum Mol Genet 2009; 18(11): 2078–90.

CHAPTER 4

Diagnosis

James M. Stankiewicz, Varun Chaubal, and Guy J. Buckle

Partners Multiple Sclerosis Center, Brigham and Women's Hospital and Department of Neurology, Harvard Medical School, Boston, MA, USA

Introduction

At present significant delays to the diagnosis of multiple sclerosis (MS) remain [1]. This may be related to the wide range of symptoms that can occur from inflammation in any number of possible places in the brain or spinal cord. Even disease progression can vary between relapsing-remitting or insidiously progressive. This variety can confuse clinicians trying to differentiate between MS or other neurologic disease. In this chapter we discuss diagnostic considerations and include a discussion of diseases that can have an overlapping appearance with the hope of helping clinicians to become more secure in approach.

Initial presentation (clinically isolated syndrome)

The majority of patients with MS will at some point present with a stereotyped constellation of symptoms and signs constituting a first clinical "attack" of demyelination, often referred to as a clinically isolated syndrome (CIS). A CIS typically comprises unilateral optic neuritis, partial transverse myelitis, or a brainstem-cerebellar syndrome (see below). The majority of patients presenting with a CIS will also have characteristic lesions on brain MRI not accounting for their clinical presentation and indicative of prior asymptomatic episodes of inflammatory demyelination. The management of these patients should be based on their risk of having a second attack and thus converting to relapsing-remitting MS (RRMS), also termed clinically definite MS (CDMS).

Multiple Sclerosis: Diagnosis and Therapy, First Edition. Edited by Howard L. Weiner and James M. Stankiewicz. © 2012 John Wiley & Sons, Ltd.
Published 2012 by John Wiley and Sons, Ltd.

Using modern imaging criteria, it is now also possible to make a diagnosis of MS prior to a second clinical attack by demonstrating new asymptomatic lesions on MRI (i.e. dissemination in time), and most disease modifying therapies (DMTs) are utilized in both RRMS and a CIS with characteristic abnormal MRI findings [Figure 4.1].

Optic neuritis

In the Optic Neuritis Treatment Trial (ONTT) [2], the cumulative probability of developing MS by 15 years after onset of optic neuritis was 50% (95% confidence interval, 44–56%) and strongly related to presence of lesions on the baseline non-contrast-enhanced brain (MRI). Twenty-five percent of patients with no lesions on baseline brain MRI developed MS during follow-up compared to 72% of patients with one or more lesions. Within a 5-year time window the risk of conversion was 51% in patients with three or more MRI lesions, with patients generally experiencing only mild disability [3].

Brainstem–cerebellar

Morrissey et al. [4] demonstrated that at 5 years follow-up 67% of patients with initial brainstem symptoms and lesions elsewhere experienced another event that qualified them for a diagnosis of MS. All Five patients with a normal brain MRI at presentation did not convert. A recent study by Tintore et al. [5] followed 246 patients with a clinically isolated syndrome affecting either the optic nerve, brainstem, or spinal cord with and without brainstem or cerebellar lesions present on MRI. At a median follow-up almost 8 years 71% of patients with infratentorial lesions were likely to have a second attack, with a third reaching an EDSS of at least 3. Without infratentorial lesions only 30% had a second attack with 12% reaching an EDSS of at least 3.

Transverse myelitis

An important distinction to make in the setting of transverse myelitis is to determine whether it is partial or compete. Lipton and Teasdall [6] showed that the rate of conversion in the setting of complete transverse myelitis is low while Ford et al. [7] carried out a prospective follow-up study on 15 patients hospitalized with a diagnosis of acute partial transverse myelopathy of unknown etiology. Twelve of the 15 [80%] developed clinically definite or lab-supported definite MS by the end of a mean follow-up period of 38.5 months. The presence of CNS periventricular white matter lesions by cranial MRI at onset increased the likelihood of development of MS to 93%. Morrissey et al. [4] found that 59% of patients experiencing a myelitis with abnormal brain MRI were likely, after 5 years, to be diagnosed with MS after a second event, while only 9% of patients with normal brain MRI were.

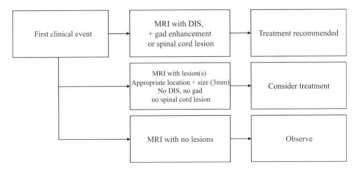

Figure 4.1 A suggested approach to clinically isolated syndrome with regards to treatment.

In a patient population with 86% abnormal brain MRIs, Gajafatto et al. [8] found that at median follow-up of 6.2 years 79% were likely to convert to MS, with patients with pyramidal presentations more likely to be disabled at follow-up. With almost 50% of patients having abnormal brain MRIs at the time of acute partial transverse myelitis, Sellner et al. [9] found a 44% conversion rate with a mean follow-up of nearly 4 years. Increased risk of MS was seen in patients achieving a high disability associated with the myelitis, a family history of disease, abnormalities on brain MRI, oligoclonal banding or elevated IgG index in the CSF.

Rate of conversion of all CISs and likelihood of disability

At 5 years Morrissey et al. [4] found that 72% of patients presenting with a clinically isolated syndrome involving the optic nerve, brainstem, or spinal cord experienced a second attack. They also found that 13% of patients with 1–3 MRI lesions achieved an EDSS of at least 3, while 45% of patients with ≤4 lesions reached this endpoint. A follow-up study after a mean of 20.2 years demonstrated that 82% of patients with abnormal MRI eventually converted to MS, but only 21% of patients with baseline normal MRIs. At 20 years 58% were classified as relapsing-remitting, 39% benign (EDSS ≤ 3) and 42% secondary progressive. Patients with secondary progression had a threefold faster growth rate of T2 MRI lesions [10].

Making the diagnosis

The majority of MS cases can be diagnosed by clinical, or a combination of clinical and imaging parameters, provided these are properly applied and that other causes of CNS inflammatory white matter disease (so-called "MS mimickers") are ruled out, usually by history, appropriate blood tests, and occasionally by CSF analysis. A CSF analysis which is positive for markers of abnormal intrathecal immunoglobulin synthesis (increased IgG index, synthesis rate, and/or oligoclonal bands) can be useful for predicting conversion to MS. A recent study of 415 patients with clinically isolated syndrome undergoing CSF analysis showed that 61% of patients had oligoclonal bands and that this banding doubled the risk of developing MS, independent of MRI. The presence of these bands did not, however, help to predict disability at a mean follow-up of 50 months [11]. Recent IgG oligoclonal banding techniques have shown an increase in sensitivity to 91% and specificity to 94% for conversion of clinically isolated syndrome patients to MS [12], though it may not be widely available. Because lumbar puncture can be uncomfortable for patients and cases are often straight-forward, we reserve it for unusual presentations of MS with atypical features on MRI, as well as in primary progressive MS, where imaging may be unrevealing, especially early in the disease course. It is also worth noting, as discussed below, that oligoclonal banding can be seen in other neurologic diseases that can mimic MS, so vigilance remains important. Visual-evoked potential (VEP) recordings are usually unnecessary in the setting of acute optic neuritis but can be useful in documenting a prior episode of retrobulbar neuritis when they show a unilaterally prolonged P100 latency with preserved wave form; beyond this, further evoked potential (EP) studies are not often helpful or reliable.

Diagnostic criteria

Initial criteria used to diagnose MS were based on clinical features alone and required demonstration of CNS lesions disseminated in space and time by objective abnormalities on the neurological examination, as well as the elimination of alternative diagnoses which might present with a similar clinical picture, ultimately rendering MS a diagnosis of exclusion, as is still the case today. In 1983 the "Poser Criteria" [13] were proposed, which used paraclinical findings (neuroimaging, evoked potentials, and spinal fluid analysis) to supplement clinical evidence for the diagnosis in situations where strict clinical criteria were not met. An international panel chaired by W. Ian McDonald met in July 2000 to review pre-existing criteria for the diagnosis of MS and to incorporate modern imaging techniques into a diagnostic scheme that would allow the physician to satisfy a requirement for dissemination of lesions in time and/or space without having to wait for a second clinical manifestation of disease, as had previously been the norm [14]. The resulting "McDonald Criteria" were cumbersome, but, if properly applied, had a sensitivity of 83%, specificity of 83%, negative predictive value of 89%, and an accuracy of 83% for clinically definite MS at

> **BOX 4.1   2010 McDonald Revisions (current criteria); criteria for dissemination in space**
>
> DIS can be demonstrated by $\geq$1 T2 lesion[a] in at least 2 of 4 areas of the CNS:
> - Periventricular
> - Juxtacortical
> - Infratentorial
> - Spinal cord[b]
>   [a] Gadolinium enhancement of lesions is not required for DIS.
>   [b] If a subject has a brainstem or spinal cord syndrome, the symptomatic lesions are excluded from the criteria and do not contribute to lesion count.
>   DIS = dissemination in space; CNS = central nervous system.
>
> *Source*: Polman et al. [17]

3 years in patients initially presenting with a clinically isolated syndrome (CIS), suggestive of demyelinating disease [15]. A revision in 2005 further simplified the possibility of making a definitive diagnosis of MS after either a monosymptomatic presentation or a progressive course from the outset (primary progressive MS) [16]. Recently, an additional revision has been accepted. The 2010 "Dublin" revisions greatly simplify diagnosis, but preserve sensitivity and specificity [17]. Now dissemination in space requires only one or more T2 lesion(s) in at least two of four locations (juxtacortical, periventricular, infratentorial, and spinal cord) (Box 4.1). Dissemination in time requires either a new T2 lesion on a follow-up scan or a nonsymptomatic enhancing lesion in the brain or spinal cord on the initial scan (Box 4.2). A caveat to this is that a lesion does not contribute to dissemination in space if it is symptomatic and in the brainstem or spinal cord.

> **BOX 4.2   2010 McDonald Revisions (current criteria); criteria for dissemination in time**
>
> DIT can be demonstrated by:
> 1 A new T2 and/or gradolinium-enhancing lesion(s) on follow-up MRI with reference to a baseline scan, irrespective of the timing of the baseline MRI.
> 2 Simultaneous presence of asymptomatic gadolinium-enhancing and nonenhancing lesions at any time.
>   MRI = magnetic resonance imagining; DIT = dissemination in time.
>
> *Source*: Polman et al. [17].

Nearly all subsequent clinical trials in RRMS have relied on the 2005 McDonald criteria for inclusion, and most of the FDA-approved therapies for RRMS have also received FDA approval for initiation at the time of a CIS if the initial MRI findings are suggestive of prior asymptomatic inflammation. Since initiation of treatment at the time of a CIS in patients with abnormal MRI findings has been shown to delay the onset of a second clinical attack, i.e. clinically definite MS (CDMS), most MS specialists now advocate early treatment, at the time of a CIS, if the baseline MRI shows at least two characteristic lesions indicative of prior asymptomatic demyelination. Earlier recognition allows for treatment to be at least considered after a first clinical episode and to tailor the follow-up approach with the patient. It should also be re-emphasized that the McDonald criteria do not absolutely require an MRI in order to diagnose MS. Two or more attacks with objective clinical evidence of two or more CNS lesions will suffice. In contradistinction, the criteria also do not provide for a diagnosis of MS based on imaging alone. At least one attack with objective clinical evidence of a CNS lesion on examination (CIS) is required before paraclinical data (chiefly MRI) come into play. Furthermore, it cannot be overemphasized that there must be no better explanation for any clinical or paraclinical abnormalities in order for the diagnosis to be secure, i.e. "MS mimickers" must be ruled out.

A common obfuscation in the application of the McDonald criteria seems to arise from the dual meaning of the word "lesion." In the context of the initial clinical presentation, "lesion" refers to a demonstrable clinical abnormality of the CNS on neurological examination and not to an area of signal abnormality on MRI. Unfortunately (but perhaps unavoidably), "lesion" is also commonly used to define an area of signal abnormality seen on MRI. In our experience the most common difficulty, however, arises from the failure to differentiate MRI lesions that are typical for MS from those that are "nonspecific" and are frequently noted as incidental findings on routine imaging of patients with headache, vertigo, and a variety of other common conditions. While the McDonald criteria address, to some extent, the issues of lesion size (>3 mm) and location (infratentorial, juxtacortical, periventricular, spinal cord) in satisfying a requirement for dissemination in space, the issue of lesion morphology (rounded, ovoid, etc.) is not well-addressed in any of the criteria. Also, while the criteria fairly carefully spell out what is needed to satisfy a requirement for dissemination in time, they do not specifically address the issue of a follow-up to a CIS with a normal initial brain MRI. It is our clinical practice generally to repeat an MRI 6 months after initial presentation. In patients with more suspicious and fulminant initial presentations we will repeat an MRI as early as 3 months from the initial event.

TOP TIPS 4.1: Diagnosis of MS

- MS may still be diagnosed without ancillary data if two separate attacks have occurred in time and clinical findings are evident.
- Patients with primary progressive MS may have normal appearing brain and spinal cord MRI initially.
- CSF should be obtained in atypical cases.

Radiologically isolated syndrome

Recently a group of patients scanned for unrelated reasons, but found to have MRIs that look radiologically like MS, have been identified and followed. Lebrun et al. [18] reported that when a repeat brain MRI was obtained (mean time 6 months, range 3–30 months), 77% of this group developed new lesions. A clinical event occurred in 37% of patients with a time from the initial MRI to the event of 2.3 years (range 0.8–5 years). Further analysis [19] determined that patients with abnormal visual-evoked potentials, gadolinium enhancement, or of a younger age, were more likely to convert clinically, while the oligoclonal bands, elevated CSF IgG index, and number of T2 lesions were not predictive. Okuda et al. [20] reported radiologic progression in 59% of patients with a median follow-up of 2.7 years (range 0.1–26 years), and clinical progression in 30% with a median follow-up of 5.4 years (range 1.1–9.8 years). Gadolinium enhancement was also predictive of a follow-up event. Siva et al. [21] found that 37% of patients developed clinically definite MS with a median time to development of 28.4 months (range 2.6–11.9 years.) By way of comparison, patients developing an optic neuritis with MRI possessing ≥ 3 lesions converted to clinically definite MS 51% of the time within 5 years [3]. It remains a difficult question whether to offer treatment to asymptomatic patients with suspicious MRIs. Generally we prefer to follow these patients off medication, an approach that is supported by a recent finding that 72% of patients already had criteria

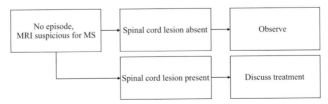

Figure 4.2 A suggested approach to radiologically isolated syndrome with regards to treatment. Spinal cord lesions greatly increase the risk of another event, even in patients with "radiologically isolated syndrome."

of dissemination to space and time before a clinical event [18]. One could consider treatment in limited circumstances (Figure 4.2). For example, a rationale might exist for the treatment of an asymptomatic patient with both brain and cervical spine lesions. Recent work found that 84% of patients with this profile were categorized as either clinically isolated syndrome or primary progressive MS after a mean of 1.6 years with an odds of conversion 75-fold higher than those with no spinal cord lesions – an impressive result [22].

MRI negative multiple sclerosis

Boster et al. [23] followed 109 patients referred to an MS center with symptoms suggestive of MS, normal examinations, and otherwise negative testing. Work-ups included brain MRI, screening bloods, and CSF. After following patients for a mean of 4.4 years the group found that none of these patients converted to MS. In fact patients remained clinically well preserved with continued normal examinations, MRIs, and CSF. Because this presentation to an MS clinic is not uncommon we find this work reassuring. Some caveats are probably worth keeping in mind. We have seen clearly abnormal spinal cord imaging return to normal in some patients with time. It is also possible for primary progressive patients to have normal imaging initially. In primary progressives, if signal intensity changes are not evident in the spinal cord, often atrophy will be present. It is reasonable to continue to follow patients with symptoms suggestive of MS, but an attempt should be made to limit unnecessary diagnostic evaluations.

Differential diagnosis

Though MS is common in the second and third decades of life and typically presents with readily recognizable symptoms, signs, and test findings, it remains possible to mistake other diseases for MS. Variable neurologic presentations and lack of definitive serologic or radiologic findings contribute to occasional misdiagnosis. A proper differential diagnosis rests on categorizing the presentation as either relapsing or progressive. For example, amyotrophic lateral sclerosis might mimic primary progressive MS, but would hardly be confused with relapsing disease.

Relapsing disease

Various autoimmune, infectious, and vasculitic diseases can look similar to MS and have a waxing, waning course. In general, the distinction from MS is clear, but challenging cases do occur from time to time. Certain "red flags" can help appropriately to raise suspicion for an alternate relapsing diagnosis. An expert panel was recently convened and released guidelines [24]. Though a systematized approach can be helpful, it is no substitute for clinical experience. For this reason, we discuss potential MS mimics and potential areas of confusion below. Due to space considerations we do not attempt to offer a complete description of individual diseases, but rather treat each with an eye toward helping to distinguish them from multiple sclerosis.

Autoimmune

Neuromyelitis optica (NMO):   The natural history of NMO is a stepwise decline of motor, sensory, visual, and sphincter function. An optic neuritis with complete visual loss, or recurrent optic neuritis, should raise suspicions for NMO. A complete myelitis with tetra- or paraparesis with bowel and bladder involvement should also elevate suspicion. The average age of onset is older than that for MS (in the late 30s); cases have been reported in pediatric and geriatric populations. Involvement is 10 times more frequent in women, and more common in non-Caucasian populations. About a fifth

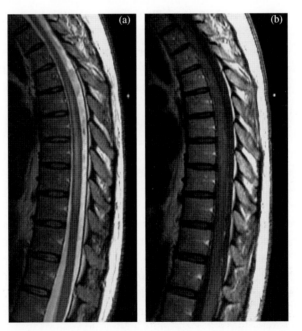

Figure 4.3 *Neuromyelitis optica.* Sagittal T2 (A) and T1 post-gadolinium (B) sections taken from a 53-year-old female with neuromyelitis optica. An example of a T2 longitudinally extensive lesion typical of neuromyelitis optica. The lesion exhibits subtle enhancement after the administration of gadolinium.

of cases are monophasic and rarely a more gradual progression can occur. Brainstem involvement can arise, including potentially fatal inflammation of medullary respiratory centers. Intractable hiccups or nausea develops in about 20% of patients. Encephalopathy, hypothalamic dysfunction, and cognitive impairment can also be infrequently associated. MRI of the brain initially often is normal, but with time will tend to show nonspecific lesions. MRI of the spinal cord typically reveals cord lesions involving three or more vertebral segments (Figure 4.3). Rarely a posterior-reversible encephalopathy syndrome (PRES)-like presentation can be seen. Serum can be sent for NMO IgG antibody. Different assays are available, with the most common indirect immunofluorescence method having an estimated sensitivity of 86%, and a specificity of 91% [25]. In patients that are seronegative it is not clear that CSF testing for NMO IgG adds value. CSF pleocytosis and elevated protein are common, but oligoclonal banding is absent in the majority of cases.

Neurosarcoidosis: Sarcoid involves the nervous system in approximately 5% of cases. Conversely, Systemic sarcoidosis is seen in 90% of patients presenting with neurosarcoidosis [26]. A useful recent retrospective study by Joseph et al. [27] of 30 patients with definite or probable neurosarcoid, showed that though women more commonly develop sarcoid, men with sarcoid are more likely to have nervous system involvement. Headaches (27%), visual failure (27%), ataxia (20%), and vomiting (23%) were frequently observed. Cough and dyspnea occurred in about 15% of patients. Seizures were observed in patients 17% of the time. Importantly, cranial neuropathy occurred in 80% of patients. On a cautionary note, only 29% of patients assayed for serum angiotensin-converting enzyme (ACE) had elevations. Though underwhelming, this was actually a more robust finding than in another recent study [28]. Another report considering 11 patients with probable neurosarcoidosis found a sensitivity and specificity of CSF-ACE activity of 55% and 94%, respectively [29]. Joseph et al. further reported that CSF oligoclonal banding was observed in 27% of cases and was always accompanied by elevations of CSF protein. Either parenchymal or meningeal enhancement was demonstrated in 13/14 cases undergoing MRI. Unfortunately the authors did not present the number of patients with meningeal enhancement, as this feature may help to separate this entity from MS. Others have reported leptomeningeal enhancement (36% of patients) and periventricular T2-hyperintensities (46%) [30]. Joseph et al. also reported that about half of patients had abnormal chest x-rays. It is unclear whether chest CT adds additional value [27–28]. Gallium scanning was revealing in about two-thirds of patients. Ten of 13 patients (77%) had a positive Kveim test, of whom 6 also had CNS tissue confirmation. Optic nerve involvement was observed in 37% of patients. Spinal cord involvement occurred in 5 of 30 patients. Cognitive impairment was observed in 20% of patients. A definitive diagnosis is ultimately made by biopsy, which reveals characteristic noncaseating granulomatous pathology. Corticosteroids represent the mainstay of treatment.

Behçet disease: Neuro-Behçet disease is rare, but can present with recurrent brainstem involvement that can be difficult to distinguish clinically from MS. In the largest published series of patients with neuro-Behçet disease [31], 51% of patients had brainstem involvement, and 14% had spinal cord involvement (Figure 4.4). The most frequent presenting symptoms were hemiparesis (60%), behavioral changes (54%), sphincter disturbance (48%), and headache (49%). All patients had oral ulcerations, 94% of patients had genital ulcerations, 66% had eye involvement, 56% had arthritis, and 33% had thrombophlebitis. Over half of patients with primary nervous system involvement have either basal ganglia or brainstem lesions. Elevated opening pressures were occasionally observed, as was pleocytosis. Oligoclonal banding was not seen. The largest collected group of Caucasians presenting with Behçet disease noted that systemic features (oral ulceration, intraocular inflammation, and skin lesions) were almost always present during attacks. Headache was observed in 86% of patients, cranial nerve findings in 55%, ataxia in 41%, and sensory changes in 27%. This population presented more frequently with seizure (27% vs

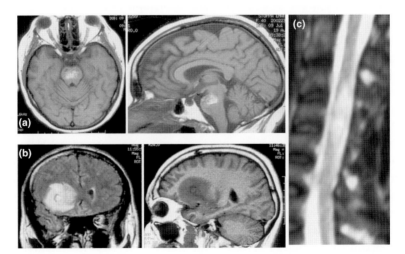

Figure 4.4 *Neuro-Behçet syndrome*. Patients with neuro-Behçet's: (A) Axial and sagittal T1-weighted SE MR images showing a large pontomesencephalic lesion in a 41-year-old. (B) Coronal FLAIR MR and sagittal T1-weighted SE MR images showing an extensive subcortical lesion in the right frontotemporal region in a 26-year-old man. (C) Sagittal T2-weighted FSE MR image demonstrating spinal cord involvement at C3–C5 level. (Reproduced from La Monaco et al. [57] with permission from Springer.)

0–5%) and optic neuritis (9% vs 1%) than previously studied non-western cohorts [32]. Only 5 of 22 patients showed elevation in ESR or CRP. MRI showed abnormalities in 10 out of 16 patients. Two of 16 had transverse sinus occlusions. Neuroimaging findings in others would probably not have been distinguishable from MS. Of 3 patients undergoing spinal MRI, 2 showed T2 intramedullary signal change. CSF pleocytosis occurred in half the cases in which it was obtained, while CSF oligoclonal banding was uniformly absent in this cohort. Though rare, it is possible for neuro-Behçet disease to occur without evidence of mucosal ulceration [33]. Diagnosis is ultimately made on clinical grounds, though pathergy testing can be supportive.

Systemic lupus erthematosis: Neuropsychiatric manifestations occur in about 60% of patient with systemic lupus erthematosis (SLE). SLE can be confused with MS (or more precisely, Devic syndrome) when it presents with optic neuritis or myelopathy but most typically presents with symptoms less often seen with MS – encephalopathy, headache, peripheral neuropathy, or seizures. Systemic involvement including malar rash, photosensitivity, arthritis, fever, or chills indicate the appropriate diagnosis in combination with abnormal serologies. Monocular visual loss due to optic neuropathy is typically severe and painless. Transverse myelopathy can occur, most frequently in an antiphospholipid antibody setting. CSF also does not reliably distinguish lupus from MS. Oligoclonal banding can be seen roughly half the time. Protein and cell counts can be elevated above what is seen in MS, but this is inconsistent. MRI often does not effectively distinguish MS and SLE, though MS-atypical stroke-like vascular distribution abnormalities can occur. Affected spinal cord can show extensive involvement, potentially imitating Devic syndrome. Abnormally high antinuclear antibodies (ANA) and ESR are found in lupus. Though different studies have shown different prevalences of ANA positivity, it is clear that ANA can return elevated in MS. A prospective study of MS patients found ANA positivity in 59% of patients, while antidouble-stranded DNA was present in 28% of patients, and antiphospholipid antibody in one-third [34]. Our experience fits better with a study showing that 22% of MS patients had antinuclear antibodies, with titers typically falling in the 1:80 to 1:160 range [35]. A good general rule of thumb is that when titers are persistent and high, serious consideration should be given to a diagnosis of lupus. It is important to distinguish between MS and SLE because treatment with interferon beta can worsen SLE.

Antiphospholipid syndrome: APLS typically affects young women and occurs frequently in patients with SLE [36]. A history of thrombosis, miscarriages, pregnancy morbidity, livedo reticularis, or thrombocytopenia should suggest the diagnosis. Stroke, seizures, TIA, neuropsychiatric involvement, or headache occur commonly in SLE and APLS and should also raise suspicions. Ischemic optic neuropathy is more prevalent than optic neuritis in this population. It is usually unilateral, abrupt, and recovers poorly. Fundoscopic examination demonstrates atypical optic disc swelling. Symptoms that mimic MS can occur, however. SLE patients developing a transverse myelitis are more likely to have APLS than patients without it [37]. Myelitis, if it occurs, is most often >2 vertebral levels and affects the thoracic area. This stands in contrast with the cervical predilection in MS-related myelitis. Brain MRI findings can mimic those of MS, though periventricular involvement is less often seen. Because there is a coincidence of SLE and antiphospholipid syndrome, ANA and ANCA testing can be positive. CSF oligoclonal bands are most often absent. Anticardiolipin antibodies are typically elevated in active disease. Repeatedly negative antiphospholipid testing makes a diagnosis of antiphospholipid syndrome unlikely.

Sjögren syndrome: Nervous system involvement occurs in approximately 20% of patients with Sjögren syndrome (SS) [38]. A retrospective study by Delalande et al. [39] of 82 patients meeting diagnostic criteria for SS who had neurologic involvement found that SS could either mimic relapsing or progressive disease. Average age of onset was 53 years old. Neurologic symptoms preceded diagnosis in the vast majority (81%) of patients. Peripheral nervous system involvement was common (62%), predominantly of a sensory type, though multiple mononeuropathies (9%), myositis ($n = 2$), and polyradiculopathies ($n = 1$) were also observed. Central nervous system involvement was seen in 68% of patients, brain was affected in 40%, and spinal cord in 35%. Seizures occurred in 9%; cognitive dysfunction in 11%. Cranial nerve involvement occurred in 20% of patients and affected the trigeminal, facial, or cochlear nerves. Thirty percent of patients had oligoclonal bands. Optic nerve symptoms occurred in 16% of patients, though visual-evoked potentials were abnormal in 61% of the patients tested. Of patients undergoing brain MRI, 70% presented white matter lesions and 40% met the radiologic criteria for MS. Another caution is that anti-Ro/SS-A or anti-La/SS-B antibodies were detected in 21% of patients at the diagnosis of SS and in only 43% of patients after repeated testing. ANA was actually present more often than SS-A and SS-B (54%). Also of note, 53% of patients had sicca symptoms at neurologic presentation, though xerostomia and xerophthalmia occurred in over 90% of patients in follow-up. Raynaud disease (43%) and cutaneous involvement (41%) was also reasonably common. DeSeze et al. [40] performed rigorous diagnostic testing including salivary gland biopsy, Schirmer testing, salivary gland scintigraphy, and anti-Ro/SS-A and anti-La/SS-B serologies in patients diagnosed with primary progressive multiple sclerosis complaining of either xerostomia or xerophthalmia and found that 16% of patients actually met diagnostic criteria for Sjögren syndrome. A portion of this cohort was then later assayed for anti-alpha fodrin antibody, a new test with potentially better sensitivity and specificity for SS, and found that 90% of SS patient with nervous system involvement had either SS-A, SS-B, or anti-alpha fodrin antibody positivity [41]. Immunosuppression has been used with success in Sjogren populations with neurologic involvement.

Infectious

Lyme disease: Lyme infection may be divided into acute and chronic phases. Neurologic manifestations occurring acutely with *B. burgdorferi* infection include aseptic meningitis, prominent thoracic or abdominal belt-like radicular pain, or meningitic symptoms. When cranial neuropathy occurs it most often involves the seventh cranial nerve. Polyneuropathy is also seen. Because of the systemic features, frequent recollection of tic bite, and the presence of erythema migrans, acute lyme infection is not often confused with MS, though the clinician should be aware that serologic testing early in the infection can be unrevealing and should be repeated 6 weeks after exposure. The distinction between chronic lyme infection and MS can be more challenging. Lyme-induced recurrent cranial nerve palsies can mimic relapsing MS, while spastic paraparesis and cerebellar ataxia (though exceedingly rare in lyme disease) can be confused with progressive MS. Tic bites, while more readily recalled in acute infection, may be more difficult to recall in retrospect. CSF findings can overlap with MS, with oligoclonal banding and pleocytosis being frequently present. MRI findings can also be similar to MS, with white matter lesions evident. Some comfort might be taken from a recent prospective study of serologic testing in lyme disease that showed a sensitivity of 100% and specificity of 99% in patients with chronic lyme disease [42]. Criteria for diagnosis have been established by the American Academy of Neurology. Some patients suffering from persistent fatigue, myalgias, arthralgias, paresthesias, and neurocognitive disturbances with negative lyme testing undergo treatment despite a lack of scientific evidence that chronic lyme disease exists without standard serologic confirmation [43], or that lyme-related treatment could aid these symptoms [44–45].

Vasculitic

Vasculitis: Vasculitis may present systemically or may be limited to the central nervous system. Systemic vasculitis tends to cause peripheral neuropathies or mononeuritis multiplex, though oculomotor palsies can occur. When the central nervous system is involved, manifestations include fatigue, fever, night sweats, and headaches. Seizures or encephalopathy can occur. MRI can show MS-indistinguishable white matter lesions, but might also show evidence of infarct, hemorrhage, or meningeal enhancement. Multiple punctate-enhancing lesions are infrequently seen, but are relatively characteristic. CSF analysis frequently reveals leukocytosis. Primary CNS vasculitis may have no systemic manifestations, normal serologies, and normal or relatively bland CSF [46]. For this reason a high index of suspicion is necessary. It is important to establish a diagnosis as vasculitis can often be rapidly progressive and does not respond to standard MS treatments. Cerebral MRA or a conventional angiogram can result in false positives. Despite its low sensitivity, leptomeningeal and brain biopsy has the highest specificity (87%) and the highest positive predictive value (80%) [47].

Metabolic

Mitochondrial: Cerebral autosomal dominant arteriopathy with subcortical infarcts and leukoencephalopathy (CADASIL) can mimic MS by presenting episodically. CADASIL presents with prominent headache, stroke-like episodes, and diffuse and extensive white matter changes on MRI. Anterior temporal and external capsule involvement (infrequent in MS) helps radiologically to distinguish CADASIL from MS. Microhemorrhage may also occur [48]. CSF bands are also rarely, if ever, present. A family history of stroke at a relatively young age is common, though sporadic occurrence of CADASIL does occur. Diagnosis is made if genetic testing reveals the presence of Notch3 mutation in the appropriate clinical setting.

Leber disease: Leber's must be considered in the setting of recurrent optic neuritis. The mutation is passed only by the mother and affects only men. It generally presents painlessly, is binocular and chronically progressive. Other symptoms such as parkinsonism, dystonia, seizures, myoclonus, polyneuropathy, ataxia, or encephalopathy can occur. It is reported that some patients presenting with predominantly optic nerve disease with MRI findings typical for MS and oligoclonal CSF banding, have the genetic mutation seen in Leber disease [49–50]. Diagnosis is made by detection of a point mutation in mitochondrial DNA.

Progressive MS

Progressive MS tends to occur in an older age group, with more motor disability. Diseases that have an insidious course are discussed below.

Infectious

HTLV-1: Human T cell leukemia virus (HTLV-1] presents as a chronic progressive myelopathy in an age group similar to progressive MS. It can be contracted sexually, via blood transfusion, or by intravenous drug abuse. Though it is prevalent in the West Indies and Japan, only a small proportion of those carrying antibodies to HTLV-1 will develop symptoms. Back and leg pain are common with bladder symptoms presenting early. Hyperreflexia and spasticity are present and impressive in advanced disease, though ankle jerks can be dropped. Lower extremity sensation is almost always affected. Both serum and CSF bands are typically present. Visual potentials can be slowed. MRI can show white matter involvement though typically the posterior fossa is relatively spared. Thoracic cord atrophy is frequently observed, and occasional intramedullary T2 hyperintensity may be found. Antibodies to HTLV-1 can be found both in serum and CSF. Because HTLV-1 is common in some populations, distinguishing HTLV-1 morbidity from that of an HTLV-1 infected patient with MS can be difficult. Recent work suggests that HTLV-1 proviral DNA loads in CSF and peripheral blood differentiate MS from HTLV-1 related myelopathy [51].

Whipple disease: Caused by infection with the bacteria *Tropheryma whippelii*, the classic finding in Whipple disease is oculomasticatory myorhythmia. This presents as intermittent synchronous movements of the eyes, face, and lower jaw and occurs in 20% of patients. Neurologic symptoms rarely precede systemic symptoms. A review of 84 cases [52] identified cognitive change with or without encephalopathy as the most common finding, though a majority of patients also had supranuclear vertical gaze palsies. Cranial nerve abnormalities, or myoclonus occurred in 25% of patients, seizures in 23%, and ataxia in 20%. Systemic features included migratory polyarthralgia (48%), weight loss (46%), chronic diarrhea (45%), fever of unknown origin (40%), and malaise (29%). Over half of patients have focal MRI abnormalities. PCR reactive to the infectious entity reveals the diagnosis in the appropriate setting, but brain biopsy may be required to confirm cerebral involvement. Brain MRI can appear normal, or can be MS-like with white matter or enhancing lesions. Gray matter involvement can occur, but is atypical for MS. CSF oligoclonal bands are at times present. Identification allows treatment with appropriate antibiotics, but response to treatment is variable.

Metabolic

B12 deficiency: Subacute combined degeneration due to B12 deficiency can be confused with MS, though cervical lesions seen with B12 deficiency tend to be longer than seen with MS and are predominantly posterior. A prospective study by Shorvon et al. [53] of 50 patients with B12 deficiency and megaloblastic anemia found that two-thirds had nervous system involvement, the most common finding being peripheral neuropathy with a quarter of patients having cognitive impairment or psychiatric involvement. Spinal cord involvement was rare. Classically, reflexes are increased with bilaterally present Babinski sign though ankle jerks are lost. In reality, it is not often this clear-cut. If the serum vitamin-B12 concentration is equivocal, a raised plasma homocysteine or methylmalonic acid concentration can confirm the presence of deficiency. Studies looking for a more direct relationship between B12 deficiency and MS have been unsuccessful [54].

Copper deficiency: Copper deficiency presents like B12 deficiency. The largest series of patients with neurologic involvement attributed to copper deficiency found that patients most frequently complained of gait difficulty and lower extremity parasthesias [55]. Gait was somewhat spastic in appearance, typically with brisk reflexes, upgoing toes, and diminished ankle jerks. Anemia was frequent. CSF was normal, except for mild protein elevation. MRI revealed elongated spinal cord abnormalities in 2 of 13 patients, brain MRI showed non-specific T2 hyperintensities in 3 of 13 patients. Either zinc overload or malabsorption could be responsible for copper deficiency. Both serum ceruloplasmic or copper levels might be reduced. It is important to identify this because copper therapy can prevent further clinical progression

Paraneoplastic

Two common paraneoplastic presentations can look demyelinating in nature on initial presentation: paraneoplastic cerebellar degeneration or paraneoplastic limbic encephalitis. Cerebellar degeneration typically begins with gait unsteadiness but rapidly progresses to include dysarthria, diplopia, and dysphagia. Cancers most often responsible for this include small cell lung cancer, gynecologic cancers, breast tumors, or Hodgkin lymphoma. MRI is often unrevealing early, can show cerebellar atrophy late. Anti-Yo, anti-Hu, and anti-Tr are most frequently associated. Though the presentation of limbic encephalitis is not particularly like MS (mood and sleep disturbances, seizures, hallucinations, cognitive impairment), the presence of MRI T2/FLAIR hyperintensities in the temporal lobe can lead to confusion. With this presentation small-cell lung cancer, testicular germ-cell neoplasms, thymoma, Hodgkin lymphoma, or teratoma are most often found. Hu and ma2 are most frequently involved with the limbic variant. Presence of unintended weight loss, pruritis, and fevers should raise suspicion for a paraneoplastic process. CSF analysis typically shows a lymphocytic pleocytosis, elevated protein, and oligoclonal bands. Seventy percent of patients with paraneoplastic syndrome present with neurologic abnormalities. Evidence of cancer by whole body CT or 19 fluorodeoxyglucose-labeled position emission tomography was seen at initial evaluation 70–80% of the time. Survival is generally poor. For further detail the excellent review by Dalmau and Rosenfeld [56] is recommended.

Genetic

Spinocerebellar ataxias: Many genetically distinct variants have been reported. The classic spinocerebellar ataxia presentation involves dysequilibrium, progressive incoordination of gait and limbs, speech and eye movement abnormalities, though spasticity, extrapyramidal signs, ophthalmoplegia, dementia, deafness, or optic atrophy can occur. Heredity spastic paraplegic variants can present at a similar age to MS and a clear-cut family history is not always easily obtainable. Pes cavus, though not always present, should increase suspicion of this diagnosis, as should spasticity out of proportion to weakness, spasticity with preserved vibratory sensation, or hyper-reflexia with diminished ankle jerks. Visual-evoked potentials are frequently abnormal, and evidence of optic atrophy and cerebellar involvement can be seen, adding to potential confusion. CSF most often lacks oligoclonal bands. Nerve conduction/electromyogram testing can reveal peripheral sensory nerve involvement. MRI can show atrophy, particularly of the cerebellum and brainstem. Genetic testing is currently available for over 20 distinct types.

Friedriech ataxia: Patients typically present in childhood, though diagnosis has been made in the seventh decade. Friedriech ataxia (FA) presents most often with a mix of progressive sensory and cerebellar ataxia. Weakness occurs later, so that generally 10–15 years after presentation patients are unable to stand and have difficulty sitting without support. Hypertrophic cardiomyopathy, skeletal deformities such as kyphoscoliosis, talipes cavus, and diabetes are common. In a large study by Harding et al. [57] reflexes were diminished in 70% of patients, but toes were upgoing in nearly 90% of patients. Muscle atrophy was observed in about half the patients examined. MRI reveals medullary and spinal cord involvement. A little less than half of FA patients can also have MRI white matter hyperintensities. The disease is associated with a GAA-trinucleotide repeat expansion in the first intron of the FRDA gene on chromosome 9.

Amyotrophic lateral sclerosis, primary lateral sclerosis: Though a mix of upper and lower motor neuron findings is not likely to suggest MS, early presentation can be predominantly upper motor, leading to potential confusion. A high signal may be found in the motor tracts on a brain MRI, but otherwise the MRI tends to be unremarkable. A symmetric presentation with only motor signs should suggest this as a possibility. Nerve conduction studies and electromyogram testing in sufficiently advanced disease is definitive. A presentation lacking lower motor neuron findings, and salient family history in the setting of a progressive spastic tetraparesis, should prompt consideration of progressive lateral sclerosis. Delayed motor conduction can help to make this diagnosis.

Celiac sprue: Progressive spinal and cerebellar deterioration might be confused with MS, but atypical features such as myoclonus, encephalopathy, seizure, or peripheral neuropathy should suggest an alternate cause. Systemic features include weight loss, abdominal distention, chronic diarrhea, and steatorrhea. Patients may have brainstem involvement and MRI can show both enhancing and T2 hyperintensities [58]. Antigliadin antibodies have been associated but as they can also be seen in normals, duodenal biopsy is recommended.

Leukodystrophies: These typically present in children, but when adrenoleukodystrophy (ALD) and metachromatic leukodystrophy (MLD) occur in adults they present similarly to progressive multiple sclerosis with a slowly worsening myelopathy. The presence of Addisonian features, including abdominal pain and bronzing of the skin, along with a family history and absence of CSF oligoclonal bands, should elevate suspicion for ALD. Cranial MRI in adult-onset ALD most often shows corticospinal tract involvement, though white matter lesions can also be seen [59]. Neurologic features other than myelopathy include cognitive decline and behavioral disturbances. MRI in adult-onset MLD patients show classic signs of leukodystrophy with symmetric periventricular white matter abnormalities and relative sparing of U-fibers, accompanied by cortical and subcortical atrophy [60]. Both MLD and ALD show clinical and electrophysiologic evidence of peripheral neuropathy. Very long-chain fatty acids can be sent to confirm the diagnosis in ALD. Diagnosis of MLD is made by demonstration of aryl-sulfatase A deficiency.

TOP TIPS 4.2: Differential diagnosis

- It is important to maintain clinical suspicions for other diseases, even at follow-up.
- Serological testing for MS mimics is rarely revealing and often gives a false sense of security.
- The absence of ankle jerks should prompt further investigation.
- Lyme disease with neurologic involvement should not be diagnosed without, at a minimum, a positive serum titer, and ideally with a positive CSF titer.

Conclusion

MS can present with a wide variety of symptoms and signs, and there remains no substitute for clinical judgment. One must remain alert to alternate possible diagnoses, both at the initial visit and at follow-up. MRI is a remarkably sensitive paraclinical test used to demonstrate both the acute and chronic changes in CNS signal characteristics that are typically seen in MS. As such, it is used increasingly as both a diagnostic tool to establish dissemination in time and space, a prognostic tool at the time of a CIS, and as a tool to monitor disease activity and the effectiveness of treatments. Ultimately, conventional (proton) MRI is not specific to any disease process and can be misleading if not interpreted in the proper clinical context. The typical "laundry list" differential generated by the radiologist in response to common nonspecific T2 signal changes in the white matter is daily proof of this and is almost never helpful. For this reason it is the obligation of the diagnosing and treating neurologist to consider all clinical data and personally review the MRI scans. Conventional measures of disease burden or activity – such as T2 lesion number or volume, or gadolinium enhancement – do not correlate particularly well with symptoms or disability on cross-sectional studies, much less at the office visit. One should not be drawn into the type of simple structure/function explanation that characterizes other CNS lesions. Surprising numbers of MS lesions may be found in supposedly "eloquent" areas of the CNS, including the brainstem and spinal cord, without any corresponding symptoms or signs on examination. One must incorporate the MRI into an overall picture of the patient that also includes clinical measures of disease activity, such as relapse rate, disability progression, and cognitive and psychosocial parameters when deciding when to initiate or change treatment. Longitudinal studies and improving MRI techniques are beyond the scope of this chapter and are addressed in Chapter 6. These will undoubtedly shed new light on the disease process, but will also raise new questions, as increased sensitivity shows us pathologic processes in what we even now tentatively deem the "normal appearing" brain tissue.

References

1 Fernandez O, Fernandez V, Arbizu T, Izquierdo G, Bosca I, Arroyo R, et al. Characteristics of multiple sclerosis at onset and delay of diagnosis and treatment in Spain (The Novo Study). J Neurol 2010 Sep; 257(9): 1500–7.

2 Visual function 15 years after optic neuritis: a final follow-up report from the Optic Neuritis Treatment Trial. Ophthalmology 2008 Jun; 115(6): 1079–82 e5.

3 The 5-year risk of MS after optic neuritis. Experience of the optic neuritis treatment trial. Optic Neuritis Study Group. Neurology 1997 Nov; 49(5): 1404–13.

4 Morrissey SP, Miller DH, Kendall BE, Kingsley DP, Kelly MA, Francis DA, et al. The significance of brain magnetic resonance imaging abnormalities at presentation with clinically isolated syndromes suggestive of multiple sclerosis. A 5-year follow-up study. Brain 1993 Feb; 116(Pt 1): 135–46.

5 Tintore M, Rovira A, Arrambide G, Mitjana R, Rio J, Auger C, et al. Brainstem lesions in clinically isolated syndromes. Neurology 2010 Nov; 75(21): 1933–8.

6 Lipton HL, Teasdall RD. Acute transverse myelopathy in adults. A follow-up study. Arch Neurol 1973 Apr; 28(4): 252–7.

7 Ford B, Tampieri D, Francis G. Long-term follow-up of acute partial transverse myelopathy. Neurology 1992 Jan; 42(1): 250–2.

8 Gajofatto A, Monaco S, Fiorini M, Zanusso G, Vedovello M, Rossi F, et al. Assessment of outcome predictors in first-episode acute myelitis: a retrospective study of 53 cases. Arch Neurol 2010 Jun; 67(6): 724–30.

9 Sellner J, Luthi N, Buhler R, Gebhardt A, Findling O, Greeve I, et al. Acute partial transverse myelitis: risk factors for conversion to multiple sclerosis. Eur J Neurol 2008 Apr; 15(4): 398–405.

10 Fisniku LK, Brex PA, Altmann DR, Miszkiel KA, Benton CE, Lanyon R, et al. Disability and T2 MRI lesions: a 20-year follow-up of patients with relapse onset of multiple sclerosis. Brain 2008 Mar; 131(Pt 3): 808–17.

11 Tintore M, Rovira A, Rio J, Tur C, Pelayo R, Nos C, et al. Do oligoclonal bands add information to MRI in first attacks of multiple sclerosis? Neurology 2008 Mar; 70(13 Pt 2): 1079–83.

12 Masjuan J, Alvarez-Cermeno JC, Garcia-Barragan N, Diaz-Sanchez M, Espino M, Sadaba MC, et al. Clinically isolated syndromes: a new oligoclonal band test accurately predicts conversion to MS. Neurology 2006 Feb; 66(4): 576–8.

13 Poser CM, Paty DW, Scheinberg L, McDonald WI, Davis FA, Ebers GC, et al. New diagnostic criteria for multiple sclerosis: guidelines for research protocols. Ann Neurol 1983 Mar; 13(3): 227–31.

14 McDonald WI, Compston A, Edan G, Goodkin D, Hartung HP, Lublin FD, et al. Recommended diagnostic criteria for multiple sclerosis: guidelines from the International Panel on the diagnosis of multiple sclerosis. Ann Neurol 2001 Jul; 50(1): 121–7.

15 Dalton CM, Brex PA, Miszkiel KA, Hickman SJ, MacManus DG, Plant GT, et al. Application of the new McDonald criteria to patients with clinically isolated syndromes suggestive of multiple sclerosis. Ann Neurol 2002 Jul; 52(1): 47–53.

16 Polman CH, Reingold SC, Edan G, Filippi M, Hartung HP, Kappos L, et al. Diagnostic criteria for multiple sclerosis: 2005 revisions to the "McDonald Criteria". Ann Neurol 2005 Dec; 58(6): 840–6.

17 Polman CH, Reingold SC, Banwell B, Clanet M, Cohen JA, Filippi M, et al. Diagnostic criteria for multiple sclerosis: 2010 revisions to the McDonald criteria. Ann Neurol 2011 Feb; 69(2): 292–302.

18 Lebrun C, Bensa C, Debouverie M, De Seze J, Wiertlievski S, Brochet B, et al. Unexpected multiple sclerosis: follow-up of 30 patients with magnetic resonance imaging and clinical conversion profile. J Neurol Neurosurg Psychiatry 2008 Feb; 79(2): 195–8.

19 Lebrun C, Bensa C, Debouverie M, Wiertlevski S, Brassat D, de Seze J, et al. Association between clinical conversion to multiple sclerosis in radiologically isolated syndrome and magnetic resonance imaging, cerebrospinal fluid, and visual evoked potential: follow-up of 70 patients. Arch Neurol 2009 Jul; 66(7): 841–6.

20 Okuda DT, Mowry EM, Beheshtian A, Waubant E, Baranzini SE, Goodin DS, et al. Incidental MRI anomalies suggestive of multiple sclerosis: the radiologically isolated syndrome. Neurology 2009 Mar; 72(9): 800–5.

21 Siva A, Saip S, Altintas A, Jacob A, Keegan BM, Kantarci OH. Multiple sclerosis risk in radiologically uncovered asymptomatic possible inflammatory-demyelinating disease. Mult Scler 2009 Aug; 15(8): 918–27.

22 Okuda DT, Mowry EM, Cree BA, Crabtree EC, Goodin DS, Waubant E, et al. Asymptomatic spinal cord lesions predict disease progression in radiologically isolated syndrome. Neurology 2011 Feb; 76(8): 686–92.

23 Boster A, Caon C, Perumal J, Hreha S, Zabad R, Zak I, et al. Failure to develop multiple sclerosis in patients with neurologic symptoms without objective evidence. Mult Scler 2008 Jul; 14(6): 804–8.

24 Miller DH, Weinshenker BG, Filippi M, Banwell BL, Cohen JA, Freedman MS, et al. Differential diagnosis of suspected multiple sclerosis: a consensus approach. Mult Scler 2008 Nov; 14(9): 1157–74.

25 Waters P, Vincent A. Detection of anti-aquaporin-4 antibodies in neuromyelitis optica: current status of the assays. Int MS J 2008 Sep; 15(3): 99–105.

26 Oksanen V, Gronhagen-Riska C, Fyhrquist F, Somer H. Systemic manifestations and enzyme studies in sarcoidosis with neurologic involvement. Acta Med Scand 1985; 218(1): 123–7.

27 Joseph FG, Scolding NJ. Neurosarcoidosis: a study of 30 new cases. J Neurol Neurosurg Psychiat 2009 Mar; 80(3): 297–304.

28 Marangoni S, Argentiero V, Tavolato B. Neurosarcoidosis. Clinical description of 7 cases with a proposal for a new diagnostic strategy. J Neurol 2006 Apr; 253(4): 488–95.

29 Tahmoush AJ, Amir MS, Connor WW, Farry JK, Didato S, Ulhoa-Cintra A, et al. CSF-ACE activity in probable CNS neurosarcoidosis. Sarcoidosis Vasc Diffuse Lung Dis 2002 Oct; 19(3): 191–7.

30 Pickuth D, Heywang-Kobrunner SH. Neurosarcoidosis: evaluation with MRI. J Neuroradiol 2000 Sep; 27(3): 185–8.

31 Akman-Demir G, Serdaroglu P, Tasci B. Clinical patterns of neurological involvement in Behcet's disease: evaluation of 200 patients. The Neuro-Behcet Study Group. Brain 1999 Nov; 122(Pt 11): 2171–82.

32 Joseph FG, Scolding NJ. Neuro-Behcet's disease in Caucasians: a study of 22 patients. Eur J Neurol 2007 Feb; 14(2): 174–80.

33 Kozin F, Haughton V, Bernhard GC. Neuro-Behcet disease: two cases and neuroradiologic findings. Neurology 1977 Dec; 27(12): 1148–52.

34 Roussel V, Yi F, Jauberteau MO, Couderq C, Lacombe C, Michelet V, et al. Prevalence and clinical significance of anti-phospholipid antibodies in multiple sclerosis: a study of 89 patients. J Autoimmun 2000 May; 14(3): 259–65.

35 Collard RC, Koehler RP, Mattson DH. Frequency and significance of antinuclear antibodies in multiple sclerosis. Neurology 1997 Sep; 49(3): 857–61.

36 Ferreira S, D'Cruz DP, Hughes GR. Multiple sclerosis, neuropsychiatric lupus and antiphospholipid syndrome: where do we stand? Rheumatology (Oxford) 2005 Apr; 44(4): 434–42.

37 Kovacs B, Lafferty TL, Brent LH, DeHoratius RJ. Transverse myelopathy in systemic lupus erythematosus: an analysis of 14 cases and review of the literature. Ann Rheum Dis 2000 Feb; 59(2): 120–4.

38 Alexander GE, Provost TT, Stevens MB, Alexander EL. Sjogren syndrome: central nervous system manifestations. Neurology 1981 Nov; 31(11): 1391–6.

39 Delalande S, de Seze J, Fauchais AL, Hachulla E, Stojkovic T, Ferriby D, et al. Neurologic manifestations in primary Sjogren syndrome: a study of 82 patients. Medicine (Baltimore) 2004 Sep; 83(5): 280–91.

40 de Seze J, Devos D, Castelnovo G, Labauge P, Dubucquoi S, Stojkovic T, et al. The prevalence of Sjogren syndrome in patients with primary progressive multiple sclerosis. Neurology 2001 Oct; 57(8): 1359–63.

41 de Seze J, Dubucquoi S, Fauchais AL, Hachulla E, Matthias T, Lefranc D, et al. Autoantibodies against alpha-fodrin in Sjogren's syndrome with neurological manifestations. J Rheumatol 2004 Mar; 31(3): 500–3.

42 Steere AC, McHugh G, Damle N, Sikand VK. Prospective study of serologic tests for lyme disease. Clin Infect Dis 2008 Jul; 47(2): 188–95.

43 Feder HM, Jr., Johnson BJ, O'Connell S, Shapiro ED, Steere AC, Wormser GP, et al. A critical appraisal of "chronic Lyme disease. " N Engl J Med 2007 Oct; 357(14): 1422–30.

44 Krupp LB, Hyman LG, Grimson R, Coyle PK, Melville P, Ahnn S, et al. Study and treatment of post Lyme disease (STOP-LD): a randomized double masked clinical trial. Neurology 2003 Jun; 60(12): 1923–30.

45 Kaplan RF, Trevino RP, Johnson GM, Levy L, Dornbush R, Hu LT, et al. Cognitive function in post-treatment Lyme disease: do additional antibiotics help? Neurology 2003 Jun; 60(12): 1916–22.

46 Volcy M, Toro ME, Uribe CS, Toro G. Primary angiitis of the central nervous system: report of five biopsy-confirmed cases from Colombia. J Neurol Sci 2004 Dec; 227(1): 85–9.

47 Stone JH, Pomper MG, Roubenoff R, Miller TJ, Hellmann DB. Sensitivities of noninvasive tests for central nervous system vasculitis: a comparison of lumbar puncture, computed tomography, and magnetic resonance imaging. J Rheumatol 1994 Jul; 21(7): 1277–82.

48 Liem MK, Lesnik Oberstein SA, Haan J, van der Neut IL, van den Boom R, Ferrari MD, et al. Cerebral autosomal dominant arteriopathy with subcortical infarcts and leukoencephalopathy: progression of MR abnormalities in prospective 7-year follow-up study. Radiology 2008 Dec; 249(3): 964–71.

49 Harding AE, Sweeney MG, Miller DH, Mumford CJ, Kellar-Wood H, Menard D, et al. Occurrence of a multiple sclerosis-like illness in women who have a Leber's hereditary optic neuropathy mitochondrial DNA mutation. Brain 1992 Aug; 115(Pt 4): 979–89.

50 Perez F, Anne O, Debruxelles S, Menegon P, Lambrecq V, Lacombe D, et al. Leber's optic neuropathy associated with disseminated white matter disease: a case report and review. Clin Neurol Neurosurg 2009 Jan; 111(1): 83–6.

51 Puccioni-Sohler M, Yamano Y, Rios M, Carvalho SM, Vasconcelos CC, Papais-Alvarenga R, et al. Differentiation of HAM/TSP from patients with multiple sclerosis infected with HTLV-I. Neurology 2007 Jan; 68(3): 206–13.

52 Louis ED, Lynch T, Kaufmann P, Fahn S, Odel J. Diagnostic guidelines in central nervous system Whipple's disease. Ann Neurol 1996 Oct; 40(4): 561–8.

53 Shorvon SD, Carney MW, Chanarin I, Reynolds EH. The neuropsychiatry of megaloblastic anaemia. Br Med J 1980 Oct; 281(6247): 1036–8.

54 Vrethem M, Mattsson E, Hebelka H, Leerbeck K, Osterberg A, Landtblom AM, et al. Increased plasma homocysteine levels without signs of vitamin B12 deficiency in patients with multiple sclerosis assessed by blood and cerebrospinal fluid homocysteine and methylmalonic acid. Mult Scler 2003 Jun; 9(3): 239–45.

55 Kumar N, Gross JB, Jr., Ahlskog JE. Copper deficiency myelopathy produces a clinical picture like subacute combined degeneration. Neurology 2004 Jul; 63(1): 33–9.

56 Dalmau J, Rosenfeld MR. Paraneoplastic syndromes of the CNS. Lancet Neurol 2008 Apr; 7(4): 327–40.

57 La Monaco A., L Corte R. et al. Neurological involvement in North Italian patients with Behçet disease, Rheumatol Int 2006: 26(12); 1113–19.Harding AE. Friedreich's ataxia: a clinical and genetic study of 90 families with an analysis of early diagnostic criteria and intrafamilial clustering of clinical features. Brain 1981 Sep; 104(3): 589–620.

58 Ghezzi A, Filippi M, Falini A, Zaffaroni M. Cerebral involvement in celiac disease: a serial MRI study in a patient with brainstem and cerebellar symptoms. Neurology 1997 Nov; 49(5): 1447–50.

59 Eichler F, Mahmood A, Loes D, Bezman L, Lin D, Moser HW, et al. Magnetic resonance imaging detection of lesion progression in adult patients with X-linked adrenoleuko-dystrophy. Arch Neurol 2007 May; 64(5): 659–64.

60 Rauschka H, Colsch B, Baumann N, Wevers R, Schmidbauer M, Krammer M, et al. Late-onset metachromatic leukodystrophy: genotype strongly influences phenotype. Neurology 2006 Sep; 67(5): 859–63.

CHAPTER 5

Pediatric Multiple Sclerosis and Acute Disseminated Encephalomyelitis

Tanuja Chitnis

Partners Pediatric Multiple Sclerosis Center, Department of Pediatric Neurology, Massachusetts General Hospital for Children, and Department of Neurology, Harvard Medical School Boston, MA, USA

General approach

This chapter describes immune-mediated demyelinating diseases, including acute disseminated encephalomyelitis (ADEM), clinically isolated syndromes (including transverse myelitis and optic neuritis), multiple sclerosis and neuromyelitis optica in children. Epidemiology, pathophysiology, clinical presentation, and definitions, as well as diagnostic evaluation, differential diagnosis, treatment, and outcomes are discussed. An overview of single and recurrent pediatric demyelinating disease is presented in Figure 5.1, and is referenced throughout the chapter.

Acute disseminated encephalomyelitis

ADEM is defined as a monophasic demyelinating disease associated with vaccination or a systemic viral infection, which may affect adults and children.

Epidemiology

ADEM can occur at any age, but it is generally more prevalent in children than in adults. The mean age of presentation reported in recently published pediatric cohorts was 5–8 years [1–4]. Rare cases in older adults have been reported [5].

Multiple Sclerosis: Diagnosis and Therapy, First Edition. Edited by Howard L. Weiner and James M. Stankiewicz. © 2012 John Wiley & Sons, Ltd.
Published 2012 by John Wiley and Sons, Ltd.

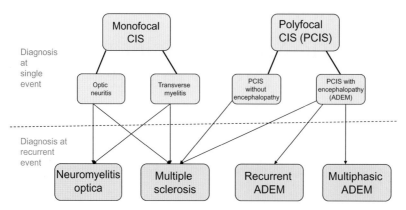

Figure 5.1 Schematic of CNS demyelinating events in children, outlining potential diagnoses at a single and recurrent event of CNS demyelination.

A recent study conducted in San Diego County, USA, found the mean incidence of ADEM as 0.4/100,000 per year among persons less than 20 years of age living in that region [6]. ADEM was more common in the winter and spring months. Five percent of these patients had received a vaccination within 1 month prior to the ADEM event, and 93% reported signs of infection in the preceding 21 days. A similar study conducted in Germany found the incidence of reported pediatric ADEM patients, defined using the International Pediatric MS Study Group criteria [7], to be 0.07/100,000 persons under the age of 16 years [8]. There was a 3-fold increased incidence in patients under the age of 10 years, compared to those 10–15 years old. In contrast, the mean incidence of multiple sclerosis (MS) in persons under the age of 16 years in this study was 0.3/100,000. Some regional cases of ADEM are linked to specific vaccines, including the Semple rabies vaccine, small-pox vaccine, and older forms of the measles vaccine. In both the San Diego and German studies, there was no gender predominance in ADEM cases. However, a male predominance has been described in other pediatric ADEM cohorts, with reported F:M ratios of 0.4 [9], 0.6 [4, 10], and 0.8 [3]. These results contrast to the 2:1 female preponderance frequently described for post-pubertal onset MS.

Pathophysiology

Post-infectious forms of ADEM typically begin within 2–21 days after an infectious event; however, longer intervals have also been described. Viral infections commonly associated with ADEM include influenza virus, enterovirus, measles, mumps, rubella, varicella-zoster, Epstein–Barr virus, cytomegalovirus, herpes simplex virus, hepatitis A, and coxsackie-virus. Bacterial triggers include mycoplasma pneumoniae, *Borrelia burgdorferi*, leptospira, and beta-hemolytic streptococcus. Acute hemorrhagic leukoencephalomyelitis (AHLE) typically follows influenza or upper respiratory infection.

The only epidemiologically and pathologically proven association between ADEM and vaccinations is with the Semple form of the antirabies vaccine [11]. Patients with serum antibodies to myelin basic protein had a higher incidence of neurological complications [11]. Other immunizations that have been temporally related to ADEM include hepatitis B, pertussis, diphtheria, measles, mumps, rubella, pneumococcus, varicella, influenza, Japanese encephalitis, and polio [3, 6, 12–17]. Vaccines produced in neural tissue culture, including the Semple form of the rabies and Japanese B encephalitis vaccines, carry a higher risk of developing ADEM, which may be related to contamination with host animal myelin antigens [18, 19]. It is important to note that vaccines with historically high rates of complications are no longer in use and have been replaced by modern formulations based on recombinant proteins [20].

Pathologically, ADEM is characterized by perivenular infiltrates of T cells and macrophages, associated with sleeves of perivenular demyelination [21]. ADEM shares common pathological features with MS, however there are no systematic studies comparing the histopathology of these two diseases. The CNS white matter typically demonstrates perivascular inflammatory infiltrates, as well as demyelination (see example in Plate 5.1a). A recent pathological study suggested that patients with demyelinating disease presenting with encephalopathy were more likely to have perivascular demyelination, compared to those without encephalopathy who typically showed diffuse demyelination [22]. Despite the sensitivity of the finding of perivenous demyelination, several cases presenting with recurrent demyelination without encephalopathy consistent with MS displayed this pattern. In addition, a distinct pattern of cortical microglial activation and aggregation without associated cortical demyelination was found among 6 perivenous demyelination patients, all of whom had encephalopathy and 4 of whom had depressed level of consciousness. Although ADEM is typically described as demyelination with relative preservation of axons, axonal damage confined to the perivenular area has been described [23, 24]. The CSF is characterized by elevated protein and white blood cells. Oligoclonal bands (OCBs) may occur in up to 30% of ADEM patients [1], and may be transient.

Acute hemorrhagic and acute necrotizing hemorrhagic leukoencephalitis (AHEM, AHL, ANHLE) of Weston Hurst shares some inflammatory histological features with ADEM; however, demyelination is often more widespread throughout the CNS and is frequently associated with a pronounced neutrophilic infiltrate. ANHLE is also characterized by the destruction of small blood vessels associated with acute and multiple small hemorrhages and fibrin deposition superimposed on demyelination.

The most likely mechanism by which ADEM occurs is molecular mimicry. Experimental evidence has shown that T cells isolated from patients with ADEM are 10 times more likely to react with myelin basic protein (MBP) than controls, likening this disease to EAE in animal models [25]. Because of the monophasic nature of the illness, it appears that the immunological response occurs acutely, but in contrast to MS further amplification of inflammation within the CNS is suppressed.

Clinical presentation

The initial symptoms and signs of ADEM usually begin within 2 days to 4 weeks after a viral infection or vaccination, and include a rapid onset of encephalopathy associated with a combination of multifocal neurological deficits, leading to hospitalization within a week. A prodromal phase with fever, malaise, headache, nausea, and vomiting may be observed shortly before the development of meningeal signs and drowsiness. The clinical course is rapidly progressive developing maximum deficits within 2–5 days [6].

ADEM can also present as a subtle disease, with nonspecific irritability, headache, or somnolence lasting more than one day. In some cases, there is rapid progression of symptoms and signs to coma and decerebrate rigidity [26]. Respiratory failure secondary to brainstem involvement or severe impaired consciousness occurs in 11–16% of cases [6, 26].

A wide variety of neurological symptoms in children has been described at clinical presentation, according to the distribution of demyelinating lesions. Unilateral or bilateral pyramidal signs (60–95%), acute hemiplegia (76%), ataxia (18–65%), cranial nerve involvement (22–45%), visual loss due to optic neuritis (7–23%), seizures (13–35%), spinal cord involvement (24%), impairment of speech (slow, slurred or aphasia) (5–21%), and hemiparesthesias (2–3%). Mental status is invariably involved, ranging from lethargy to coma [1–4, 6, 10]. Seizures are mainly seen in children younger than five years of age, usually as prolonged focal motor seizures [3].

Peripheral nervous system (PNS) involvement in ADEM patients has been reported in children [27, 28] while PNS involvement is observed in 16/36 (44%) adult patients [29].

A unique ADEM phenotype has been reported in association with group A-beta hemolytic streptococcal infection. The syndrome affected children under the age of 6, with prominent behavioral disturbances, dystonic movements and basal ganglia abnormalities on MRI [30]. The condition usually followed an acute pharyngitis infection and was associated with elevated antibasal ganglia antibodies.

Rarely, children may present with recurrent or multiphasic ADEM [3], which are defined below. These cases may be difficult to distinguish from pediatric multiple sclerosis.

Adem Definitions: To avoid misdiagnosis and to develop a uniform classification, the International Pediatric MS Study Group (Study Group) has proposed that the following three terms be applied to variations of ADEM [7].

1 ADEM: – *A first clinical event with a polysymptomatic encephalopathy, with acute or subacute onset, showing focal or multifocal hyperintense lesions predominantly affecting the CNS white matter; no evidence of previous destructive white matter changes should be present; and no history of a previous clinical episode with features of a demyelinating event. The event should be followed by improvement, either clinically, on MRI, or both, but there may be residual deficits*

   Encephalopathy is described as (i) a behavioral change, e.g. confusion, excessive irritability, or as (ii) alteration in consciousness, e.g. lethargy, coma. If a relapse takes place within 4 weeks of tapering steroid treatment or within the first 3 months from the initial event, this early relapse is considered temporally related to the same acute monophasic condition and would replace the terms "steroid dependent ADEM" or "pseudorelapsing ADEM."

2 Recurrent ADEM: – *New demyelinating event fulfilling diagnostic criteria for ADEM, occurring at least 3 months after the initial ADEM event and at least four weeks after completing steroid therapy, showing the same clinical presentation and affecting the same areas on MRI as the initial ADEM episode.*

3 Multiphasic ADEM: – *Refers to one or more ADEM relapses, including encephalopathy and multifocal deficits, but involving new areas of the CNS on MRI and neurologic exam. Relapses take place at least 3 months after initial ADEM attack and at least 4 weeks after completing steroid therapy.*

Diagnostic evaluation

Basic diagnostic evaluation for ADEM includes: neurological examination, MRI of the brain and spine, serum and CSF testing for infections in suspicious cases; standard CSF evaluation, including cell count, bacterial and fungal cultures; and oligoclonal bands and IgG Index testing. Fundoscopic examination, visual-evoked potentials and orbital MRI should be considered in cases where optic neuritis is a concern. MRI usually demonstrates multifocal white matter lesions involving the cerebrum, brainstem, cerebellum, and spinal cord, which may or may not enhance with gadolinium (Figure 5.2a). Brain lesions generally involve the subcortical and cortical white matter, and may involve cortical and deep gray matter nuclei. Several MRI patterns have been described, and include the presence of: (1) small focal punctate lesions; (2) bithalamic lesions; (3) diffuse large white matter lesions; (4) hemorrhagic, demyelinating lesions, consistent with AHLE [3]. Lesions generally resolve over time, however the clinical picture may precede MRI improvement [31].

   CSF is characterized by normal pressure, moderately elevated cell count (5–100/μL), moderately elevated protein (40–100 mg/dL), and normal

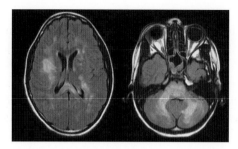

Figure 5.2a Brain FLAIR image of a 13-year-old boy with ADEM. Lesions are located in the subcortical white matter and diffusely in the pons and middle cerebellar peduncles.

glucose. The presence of red blood cells may indicate a diagnosis of hemorrhagic leukoencephalitis. CSF evaluation should include testing for infections, including viral encephalitides if suspected. Oligoclonal bands may be present and have been described in up to 29% of ADEM patients [1], and are generally transient.

Differential diagnosis

The association of an acute encephalopathy and disseminated demyelination of the CNS in a child represents a diagnostic challenge. A large number of inflammatory and noninflammatory disorders may have a similar clinical and radiological presentation and should be considered in the diagnostic evaluation. Due to the acute therapeutic implications, the exclusion of acute CNS infections should be the first and most important diagnostic step to be considered in every child with a febrile illness and neurological signs, by lumbar puncture and further microbiological laboratory tests. Serology for suspected organisms, CSF viral, fungal and bacterial cultures, as well as CSF viral polymerase chain reaction assay for HSV, CMV, EBV, enterovirus, VZV, and WNV should be performed. Mycoplasma serology may reveal an underlying infection. Neuroimaging may play a particularly helpful role in the differential diagnosis. A standard MRI scan of the brain and spinal cord, with and without gadolinium enhancement will be useful to define the regional distribution of demyelination and MRI lesion appearance.

Treatment

Acute episodes of ADEM should be treated with intravenous corticosteroids. The usual dose is 1 g/day of methylprednisolone for 5 days in adults and 20–30 mg/kg/day for 5 days for children up to 40 kg. Treatment with corticosteroids requires careful monitoring of blood pressure, urine glucose, serum potassium, and administration of gastric protection. Refractory cases have been treated with five exchanges or plasmapheresis or intravenous immune globulin (IVIg) up to 2 g/kg distributed over 2–5 days. Cases that are suspicious for MS should be followed with annual or biannual MRI studies.

Supportive care in the acute stage is critical and early antiviral treatment with acyclovir (30 mg/kg/day) is highly recommended acutely, particularly when viral encephalitis – especially herpes simplex encephalitis – is a consideration. Antibiotic prophylaxis for suspected bacterial meningitis may also be instituted in cases where this is a consideration.

Use of high-dose intravenous immunoglobulin (IVIg) for acute ADEM treatment has been reported in several case studies [32–34]. The usual total dose of IVIg is 2 g/kg, administered over 2 to 5 days. IVIg may be useful in cases refractory to intravenous steroid treatment, and we generally start treatment 2–3 days following a 5-day steroid course. IVIg may also be useful in cases of steroid-dependent demyelination, when new or fluctuating signs and symptoms occur as corticosteroids are tapered [35, 36].

The use of plasmapheresis in ADEM has been reported in a small number of severe cases, who were generally unresponsive to corticosteroid or IVIg treatment [31, 37, 38]. Three to five exchanges are generally employed, which is felt to be sufficient to reduce antibody and inflammatory factors. Moderate to severe anemia, symptomatic hypotension, hypocalcemia, and heparin-associated thrombocytopenia have been described related to plasmapheresis.

Acute hemorrhagic leukoencephalitis is often considered to be the most acute and severe form of ADEM, with a high rate of mortality within hours to days after the onset of neurologic symptoms if untreated. Survival in pediatric patients has been reported in a small number of children receiving combined high-dose IV corticosteroid therapy, IVIg, plasmapheresis, and decompressive craniotomies [6, 40, 41]. In cases of progressive deterioration due to increased uncontrolled intracranial pressure, aggressive strategies such as surgical decompression should be considered to prevent secondary injury to the brain and brainstem.

Outcomes

There is limited data regarding the natural history of ADEM. In the available case studies, there is considerable diversity with respect to antecedent infections, clinical presentation, and neuroimaging findings, further complicating outcomes analysis. Case series from Japan [42], India [43], and Russia [44] suggest that the natural history of untreated ADEM in most children is one of gradual improvement over several weeks, with 50–70% of patients experiencing full recovery. Studies from other centers in largely treated patients demonstrate similar outcomes [1, 3, 6, 8] with 8–30% experiencing residual focal neurological deficits, and 4–30% having residual behavioral or cognitive problems. Behavioral problems were most prominent in the young-onset ADEM group with poorer visuospatial/visuomotor function, even in those with fully resolved MRIs [2, 45]. In most cases, the MRI appearance improves significantly, however the continued presence of residual MRI lesions may correlate with chronic deficits.

Recovery may depend in part on antecedent infections based on serology [44]. In a cohort of patients with detailed serology, antecedent infections included rubella (33%), varicella (29%), unknown (22%). DEM cases without a defined infection had a good outcome 70% of the time, versus 54% and 43% reported for post-varicella and post-rubella ADEM, respectively. Specific recovery times were described as approximately 3 weeks for post-rubella ADEM and up to 12 weeks for multiphasic ADEM, with intermediate but more variable recovery time in the post-varicella and unknown ADEM groups. Taken together, these reports suggest that approximately two-thirds of patients make a complete recovery.

Children who have experienced an episode of ADEM are at higher risk of developing recurrent or chronic demyelination than the general population. Some children may develop recurrent or multiphasic ADEM. While others may go on to develop MS. The distinction between recurrent or multiphasic ADEM in some instances is unclear, and our policy has been to consider chronic immunosuppressive therapy in children with more than two clinical episodes.

At present, there are no clear prognostic factors that determine whether a child who has experienced an acute demyelinating event will develop MS. Clinical studies have been hampered in part by the lack of consistent definitions used across publications, and the small numbers of subjects at any one site. In available studies, the risk of developing MS after ADEM has been reported as 0% in a study from Argentina [3], 9.5% in a study from San Diego [6], and 18% to 29% in studies from France [46, 47]. Varying criteria were used to define ADEM and pediatric MS, which may have contributed to the wide range of incidence among these publications.

The KIDMUS study group from France examined pediatric patients with an acute demyelinating syndrome, including clinically isolated syndromes and ADEM events, and showed that, overall, 57% developed a second attack [47]. 86% of patients with initial optic neuritis developed MS, and 50% of those with an initial brainstem syndrome developed MS. The majority of children converted to MS within a 2-year period. Overall, positive predictive factors for the development of MS were: age at onset 10 years or older, or optic nerve lesion. A lower risk of developing MS was found in patients with mental status change at presentation, suggesting that the presence of encephalopathy may be a negative predictive factor. Of patients with an initial diagnosis of ADEM, 29% developed MS. A subsequent publication by this group stated that when the diagnosis of ADEM was redefined by the KIDSEP study to include "change in mental status" as a qualifying criterion, 18% of children were found to develop MS, as defined by the development of a second event after a mean follow-up of 5.4 years [48].

TOP TIPS 5.1

- ADEM is more common in children than adults, and occurs most commonly in children under the age of 10.
- ADEM can occur up to 4 weeks after a variety of viral and bacterial infections, and has rarely been reported following the administration of Semple rabies vaccine.
- Acute hemorrhagic leukoencephalitis (AHLE) is a form of ADEM characterized by the destruction of small blood vessels, with multiple small hemorrhages associated with demyelination.
- ADEM usually presents with acute encephalopathy and a variety of other neurological symptoms.
- Intravenous high-dose methylprednisolone for 3–7 days is the standard treatment regimen. Use of IVIg and plasmapheresis in refractory cases is anecdotal.
- Approximately 25% of ADEM cases may go on to develop pediatric multiple sclerosis.

Clinically isolated syndromes

Children may present with clinically isolated syndromes, which often are monophasic in course, however a proportion of these children may eventually develop a chronic demyelinating disease such as MS or neuromyelitis optica (NMO) (discussed in sections below). A general approach to CIS or ADEM is to evaluate the location of symptoms, the presence of mental status changes or encephalopathy at onset, and the presence of lesions along the neuro-axis (optic nerves, brain, and spinal cord) (Figure 5.1). Transverse myelitis and optic neuritis are common presentations of CIS in children and are discussed in detail here. Other presentations, including brainstem syndromes and polysymptomatic presentations, may occur.

Acute transverse myelitis

Epidemiology
The incidence of idiopathic, complete acute transverse myelitis (ATM) is approximately 1.34 persons/million per year [49]. In the United States, approximately 280 cases of ATM occur in pediatric patients annually [50, 51]. Among children, the mean age of presentation is 8 years of age [52–58]. Boys and girls are equally affected. Approximately 50% of patients report a preceding infection, typically a nonspecific upper respiratory tract infection, with an intervening symptom-free interval of 4 to 11 days [49, 50, 52, 57]. Some cases of ATM are associated with recent vaccination [59].

Pathophysiology

The pathophysiology of ATM is unclear, however, the frequent association with preceding infections and accumulating immunological data suggest that immune mechanisms, including molecular mimicry may play a role in this disorder, similar to ADEM [49, 52, 60, 61]. One report has shown increased lymphocyte responses to myelin basic protein and peripheral nerve myelin P2 protein [52]. Elevated production of interleukin-6 in the CSF of ATM patients has been described [60]. In animal models, infusion of IL-6 into the CSF results in nitric oxide-induced injury to spinal cord oligodendrocytes and axons.

Clinical presentation

The majority of patients experience motor, sensory, and bowel and bladder symptoms [50, 52–57]. Patients with ATM universally report acute to subacute bilateral leg weakness. Arm involvement is present in approximately 40% of patients. Approximately 90% of patients complain of bowel and bladder dysfunction. The majority of patients experience sensory symptoms, including paresthesias and numbness and back pain. A spinal cord sensory level is usually located in the thoracic region (80%) and less commonly in the cervical (10%) or at lumbar (10%) levels [49].

Differential diagnosis

Several disorders can mimic idiopathic ATM. Such conditions must be ruled out through a combination of history, physical examination, neuroimaging, and laboratory evaluation.

Acute compressive lesions such as tumors, spinal epidural abscesses [63], and spinal epidural hematomas [64], are neurosurgical emergencies that must be diagnosed rapidly for effective treatment. Intramedullary lesions that can mimic ATM include primary spinal cord tumors (most commonly astrocytomas and ependymomas) [65–67], radiation injury [68], spinal cord infarction, and vascular malformations [69]. Infections of the spinal cord, typically viral in etiology, can also occur, and CMV, HTLV-1 or mycoplasma infections should be considered in those at risk. ATM can also be secondary to a variety of systemic autoimmune disorders including SLE.

The initial clinical presentation of ATM can be very similar to that of Guillain–Barre syndrome. Both can present with back pain, paraparesis, and sensory abnormalities. However, the presence of a spinal cord sensory level and bowel and bladder involvement is highly suggestive of ATM. The presence of reflexes or exaggerated reflexes is suggestive of ATM, however arreflexia may be present in some cases.

ATM may occur in isolation, or in conjunction with lesions in other locations of the CNS as part of a monophasic illness such as ADEM or polyfocal CIS. In contrast, ATM may also occur as part of a chronic demyelinating disease such as MS or neuromyelitis optica (NMO). Therefore signs of multifocal demyelinating disease including optic neuritis and encephalopathy may be present.

Diagnostic evaluation

Patients with suspected ATM should undergo emergent gadolinium-enhanced MRI of the entire spine in order to confirm the diagnosis and rule out alternative diagnoses, particularly compressive lesions. All patients with ATM should also undergo gadolinium-enhanced MRI of the brain to assess for additional demyelinating lesions suggestive of ADEM or MS. Spinal MRI in ATM typically reveals T1-isointense and T2-hyperintense signal over several contiguous spinal cord segments [52], and may involve the entire spine [70]. Spinal cord swelling with effacement of the surrounding cerebrospinal fluid spaces may be present in severe cases. Contrast enhancement is present in up to 74% of patients [50]. In some patients with very suggestive clinical features, the initial spine MRI may be normal and should be repeated several days later [52, 53, 55].

Unless a specific contraindication exists, all patients with ATM should undergo lumbar puncture. Approximately 50% of pediatric patients with ATM have CSF pleocytosis ranging from mean WBC count of 136 ± 67 cells/mm^3 (range from 6 to 950 cells), typically with a lymphocytic predominance [50]. Elevated CSF protein levels, either in isolation or in conjunction with pleocytosis, are also detected in about 50% of patients [50]. Glucose is typically normal. A normal CSF profile does not rule out ATM, as this pattern is seen in approximately 25% of patients. In addition to MRI and LP, further testing should be guided by clues in the history, exam, or neuroimaging as described under "Optic neuritis" below.

Treatment

The initial treatment of ATM is intravenous high dose corticosteroids generally administered for 5–7 days. There have been no randomized, controlled trials in ATM to support this approach, however case reports have found a beneficial effect of high dose corticosteroids [54, 71, 72]. In one series of 12 children with severe ATM compared to a historical control group of 17 patients, the use of high dose intravenous methylprednisolone significantly increased the proportion of children walking independently at one month (66% compared to 18%) and with full recovery at one year (55% compared to 12%) [54]. For patients who do not adequately improve with intravenous steroids, intravenous immunoglobulins [73] or plasmapheresis may be considered. Additional treatment includes pain management, urinary bladder catheterization, bowel regimens, peptic ulcer, and deep venous thrombosis prophylaxis, physical therapy, and psychosocial support. Mechanical ventilation is required in approximately 5% of patients.

Outcomes

Although limited by variable definitions in the literature, the prognosis for pediatric patients with ATM is generally favorable [74]. Paine and Byers' recovery categories have been the most widely reported outcome scale [57]. Based on this scale, approximately 80% of pediatric patients who receive high-dose IV steroids achieve full or good recovery and 20% have a fair or poor outcome [54, 71]. Among patients not treated with high-dose IV steroids, 60% have a full or good recovery, while 40% have a fair or poor outcome [57]. Higher rostral levels and number of overall spinal segments on spine MRI predicts worse outcome [50].

A retrospective study of children with ATM treated at a quaternary-referral center studied the long-term outcome in 47 cases [50]. At a median follow-up of 3.2 years, this study found that approximately 40% of patients were nonambulatory and 50% required bladder catheterization. However, these results may have been influenced by referral bias, as well as a higher percentage of patients less than age 3 years and patients with cervical involvement compared to other studies. In this study, factors associated with a better functional outcome included older age at time of diagnosis, shorter time to diagnosis, lower sensory and anatomic levels of spinal injury, absence of T1-hypointensity on spinal MRI obtained during the acute period, lack of WBC in the CSF, and fewer affected spinal cord segments. Interestingly, neither rapid progression to maximum impairment in less than 1 day, nor any antecedent illness, immunization, or trauma was associated with a worse outcome.

During recovery, motor function returns first, with an average time to independent ambulation of 56 days in one study [52] and 25 days in a group of patients treated with high-dose IV steroids [54].

Bowel/bladder control recovers more slowly with an average time to recovery of normal urinary function of 7 months in those patients with complete recovery [52].

The overwhelming majority of pediatric patients with idiopathic, complete ATM have a monophasic course. In a series of 24 pediatric patients with complete ATM with a mean follow up of 7 years, there were no recurrences [52]. In another study of children with a variety of initial acute demyelinating events, only 2 of 29 (7%) patients with transverse myelitis experienced a subsequent demyelinating event [47, 75]. As opposed to complete ATM, partial ATM seems to carry a much higher risk of MS. Adult patients with partial ATM and additional asymptomatic brain MRI lesions have a greater than 80% of developing MS within the first few years, while those with normal brain MRI have a 10–20% chance [58]. However, patients who have complete ATM followed by subsequent attacks of optic neuritis and/or complete ATM may have NMO.

> **TOP TIPS 5.2**
>
> - The mean age of acute transverse myelitis (ATM) in children is 8 years old.
> - Boys and girls are equally affected.
> - The majority of patients experience motor, sensory, and bowel and bladder symptoms.
> - Intravenous high-dose methylprednisolone for 3–7 days is the standard treatment regimen, and has been associated with improved outcomes.
> - Isolated acute transverse myelitis in children rarely progresses to become multiple sclerosis or neuromyelitis optica.

Optic neuritis

Epidemiology

The incidence of optic neuritis in children is unclear. Data from four case series ($n = 170$) suggests a mean age of onset from 9 to 12 years of age and an approximate 1.5 to 1 female to male ratio [76–78]. In these studies approximately one-third of patients report a preceding viral infection.

Pathophysiology

Similar to the other CNS demyelinating disorders, indirect evidence suggest that autoimmune mechanisms are involved in the pathogenesis of optic neuritis. Due to the high risk of complications and the availability of noninvasive diagnostic techniques, biopsy of the optic nerve in patients with suspected optic neuritis is rarely performed. Direct pathological data is therefore limited. However, the frequent association of optic neuritis with more diffuse disorders such as ADEM or MS suggests common autoimmune mechanisms. Optic neuritis may occur as part of the NMO spectrum of disorders, which may have distinct pathophysiological mechanisms.

Clinical features

The major presenting symptom of optic neuritis is vision loss, which typically affects the central visual field more than the periphery. In children, the vision loss is usually severe, with visual acuity of 20/200 or worse in approximately 75% of patients [76–78]. Bilateral involvement has been reported in up to 50% of patients. In children, pain on eye movement is a specific, but not a sensitive, test with only 40% of pediatric patients reporting this symptom [76]. A normal fundoscopic examination is seen in 30% of patients and does not rule out the diagnosis, since many cases are due to retrobulbar inflammation. An examination may also reveal an afferent pupillary defect and color vision difficulties in patients with optic neuritis.

Diagnostic evaluation

All patients with optic neuritis should be evaluated by an ophthalmologist. Testing should include formal visual field testing, low contrast sensitivity, and color vision assessment. Additional testing should be guided by clues in the history, exam, or neuroimaging. Advanced neuro-ophthalmological techniques, including optical coherence tomography, may be considered to evaluate the extent of damage to the nerve fiber layer [79].

Orbital MRI including coronal sequences with thin cuts through the orbits should be obtained in all patients with optic neuritis. Brain and spine MRI should also be considered in all patients to define the extent of demyelination. Lumbar puncture should be performed if direct CNS infection cannot be ruled out clinically. Following appropriate neuroimaging to rule out mass lesions, lumbar puncture with measurement of opening pressure is also required if idiopathic intracranial hypertension is suspected.

Differential diagnosis

The differential diagnosis of optic neuritis includes mitochondrial disease, Vitamin B12 deficiency, adrenoleukodystrophy, optic neuropathy, and optic nerve glioma. Sarcoidosis may be present with optic neuritis or cranial nerve defects. Isolated optic neuritis can be confused with Leber hereditary optic neuropathy, especially when pain on eye movements is absent. Family history, brain MRI, and mitochondrial DNA mutation analysis can be used to distinguish these conditions. In the case of tumor, papilledema from increased intracranial pressure can appear the same as swelling of the optic discs from bilateral optic neuritis. The former typically presents more slowly, is not usually associated with severe vision loss (especially early in the course), and is not associated with an afferent pupillary defect. Optic neuritis can be isolated or associated with more widespread involvement of the CNS, as in ADEM, MS, or NMO. Optic neuritis can also be associated with a variety of systemic autoimmune disorders including SLE and Sjogren syndrome.

Treatment

Similar to other acute CNS demyelinating syndromes, patients with optic neuritis are often treated with high-dose intravenous methylprednisolone. In the Optic Neuritis Treatment Trial in adults, a 3-day course of intravenous methylprednisolone increased the rate of recovery in patients with visual acuity less than 20/40, but did not affect the long-term visual acuity outcomes [80]. However at 2 years, color vision and contrast sensitivity were better in treated patients. There is no controlled data on the effect of intravenous steroids on optic neuritis outcomes in children. Our practice is generally to administer high-dose intravenous steroids to optic neuritis cases. Limited trials in adults suggest that IVIg is not useful as monotherapy in the acute treatment of optic neuritis [81], but its role in steroid-refractory optic neuritis is unclear. One case series of 10 adult patients with steroid and/or IVIg refractory optic neuritis suggested a 70% rate of improvement with plasma exchange [82].

Prognosis

Most children recover well from optic neuritis, with approximately 50–75% demonstrating a visual acuity of 20/40 or better at follow-up [76–78, 83]. However, patients with optic neuritis frequently report subjective changes in vision, even when visual acuity returns to 20/20 and may only be detected with specialized techniques such as optical coherence tomography or visual-evoked potentials [79, 84]. In some cases, adaptive equipment and visual rehabilitation may be required.

Despite the favorable prognosis for immediate functional recovery, some patients may later develop MS or NMO. The distinguishing factor for development of MS after optic neuritis appears to be the presence of one or more MRI lesions typical for MS [77]. In this study of 36 children with optic neuritis, all of the children who developed MS presented with concomitant MRI brain lesions, and none of the patients without brain lesions developed MS. In two studies, bilateral ON was more likely to be associated with MS outcome [77, 78]. In the KIDMUS study 86% of patients with initial optic neuritis developed MS, however the presence of brain MRI lesions in this cohort was not defined [47].

TOP TIPS 5.3

- Optic neuritis in children typically presents with central vision loss.
- Up to 75% of patients may present with a visual acuity of 20/200 or worse.
- Our practice is to administer a course of intravenous high-dose methylprednisolone for 3–5 days.
- The presence of brain lesions at the time of optic neuritis presentation is a strong predictor for the development of multiple sclerosis.

Multiple sclerosis

Epidemiology

Multiple sclerosis (MS) affects approximately 400,000 persons in the United States, with an onset predominantly in early adulthood. It is increasingly recognized that MS can present in childhood or adolescence. The youngest onset of MS in the medical literature is 2 years of age, however the majority of children are diagnosed in their early teens [85]. Studies have estimated the prevalence of pediatric-onset MS, to range from 2.7 to 10.5% (i.e. 2.7% [86], 3.6% [87], 4.4% [88], 5% [89], and 10.5% [90]) of total MS populations. We have recently found that 3.06% of our adult MS population of 4399 patients with an electronic MS history record experienced a first attack under the age of 18 years [91], suggesting that these patients may represent a pediatric-onset population. Recent studies have suggested that there are significant differences in ethnic and racial characteristics of children with MS as compared to an adult MS population [92]. In our study of adults MS patients from one Center, we found a higher proportion of non-Caucasian patients in the pediatric-onset group (11.7%) when compared to an adult-onset group (6.18%; p = 0.014) [91], supporting this finding. Moreover, of patients from our pediatric MS Center, 33.3% were non-Caucasian, compared to 5.5% in the comparative adult MS cohort [93].

Pathophysiology

There are few reports of pathological changes in cases of pediatric MS and ADEM. The majority are cases of tumefactive demyelination, which may represent a bias in the tendency to biopsy these particular cases [94–98]. Those cases with detailed pathology report a dense accumulation of lymphocytes and macrophages in a prominent perivascular distribution, extending into the white matter, with rare B cells (see Plate 5.1b). Demyelination is present, while axonal damage is typically absent [94]. No systematic studies have been carried out specifically evaluating the pathology of pediatric MS, and it is unclear whether pathological changes are similar to or differ from subtypes described in adult MS [99].

T cells play a key role in the pathophysiology of MS. Current immunological models of the disease indicate that activated T cells cross the blood–brain barrier and incite an inflammatory reaction within the CNS [100]. Several groups have studied T cell responses to various antigenic stimuli in pediatric MS. A recent study of a large cohort of children with CNS inflammatory demyelination, type I diabetes (T1D) and CNS injury, demonstrated that children with CNS inflammatory demyelination, CNS injury, and T1D exhibited heightened peripheral T cell responses to a wide array of self-antigens compared to healthy controls. Children with autoimmune diseases and CNS injury also exhibited abnormal T-cell responses against multiple cow-milk proteins [101] A smaller study compared T-cell responses to myelin basic protein (MBP) and myelin oligodendrocyte glycoprotein (MOG) epitopes in adult and pediatric MS, and found similar responses predominantly to MBP 83–102, 139–153, 146–162, and MOG 1–26, 38–60, and 63–87, in both groups to the same set of peptides [102]. Interestingly, responses to fetal-MBP were minimal, and similar in both groups.

The role of circulating antimyelin antibodies have been debated extensively in adult MS studies [103, 104], and have recently been actively studied in pediatric MS. Myelin oligodendrocyte glycoprotein is an attractive target since it is expressed on the outer myelin membrane and may be easily targeted by the immune response. Using a tetramer approach, anti-MOG antibodies were higher in the serum of the younger children with MS and in children with an initial attack that was clinically indistinguishable from ADEM, whether or not they were subsequently found to have MS [105]. Using myelin-transfected cells as a detection system, 38.7% of patients less than 10 years of age at disease onset were found to have MOG Abs, compared to 14.7% of patients in the 10- to 18-year age group. Interestingly, a study examining antimyelin basic protein (MBP) antibodies in the serum and CSF found that approximately 20% of pediatric MS patients, as well as healthy controls, had high-affinity high-titer antibodies. In the pediatric MS patients, these antibodies were also found in the CSF, and the presence of antibodies was associated with an encephalopathic type of onset. These studies reiterate an emerging theme, which suggests that antimyelin antibodies may not be exclusive to pediatric MS, however their presence is associated with a more fulminant, inflammatory onset of the disease, and may be a product of an immature immune system.

Studies examining markers of axonal damage in the CSF found minimal changes in the majority of children with MS, however a subgroup with prominent clinical symptoms at the time of CSF examination exhibited elevated levels of tau protein [106], which may reflect increased CNS damage.

Clinical presentation

Children with MS overwhelmingly experience a relapsing-remitting course at onset [86, 88]. Primary progressive MS is extremely rare. We have recently shown that children with MS experience more 2–3 times as many relapses than adults with MS [93]. Moreover, recovery from relapses appears to be more rapid in children than in adult MS patients (mean time of relapse related symptoms: 4.3 weeks in pediatric MS vs. 6 to 8 weeks in adult MS [107].

Common presenting symptoms of MS in children include sensory deficits (26%), optic neuritis (21.6%), cranial nerve or brainstem symptoms (12.9%) and gait disorders (8.6%) [87]. Pediatric patients typically have a polysymptomatic presentation, although monosymptomatic presentations are not uncommon. Other features that are more common in children compared to adults with MS are encephalopathy and seizures, likely representing the overlap of acute disseminated encephalomyelitis (ADEM) and MS that is almost exclusive to children (see ADEM discussion below). In addition to physical disability, children with MS are particularly vulnerable to cognitive dysfunction and fatigue.

MRI lesions in children with MS are generally located in the periventricular and subcortical white matter. It is unknown whether cortical lesions are present, and some pre-adolescent children with MS may present with atypical MRI patterns [108]. Recent studies have shown that at the time of their MS defining attack, children meet adult MS McDonald MRI criteria only 67% of the time, suggesting a low lesion burden than adults at the time of diagnosis [109], however a formal comparison to adults has not been performed. Few studies have formally compared the extent and distribution of lesions in children with MS compared to adults with MS. One study of 58 children with CIS and adults with RRMS found that children with CIS had fewer lesions infratentorially overall, however in a subset of patients with brain lesions, children had higher volumes of infratentorial lesions [110]. Another study of 4 pediatric-onset patients found a higher frequency of large confluent T2 lesions and fewer black holes in comparison to adult-onset MS [111]. We have recently shown that children with MS demonstrate anisotropic abnormalities on diffusion tensor imaging in major white matter tracts including the corpus callosum, longitudinal association fibers and the corticospinal tracts [112], suggesting that normal appearing white matter is significantly affected in children with MS.

Pediatric MS definition: The International Pediatric MS Study group [7] agreed that the McDonald criteria for MS may be applied to patients under the age of 10 years, including dissemination in time by MRI [113, 114].

- *Neurological events should be separated by at least 3 months, and occur while off steroids for at least 1 month to prevent confusion with steroid-dependent relapses.*
- *The MRI must show three of the following four features: (1) nine or more white matter lesions or one gadolinium-enhancing lesion, (2) three or more periventricular lesions, (3) one juxtacortical lesion, (4) an infratentorial lesion. The combination of an abnormal CSF and two lesions on the MRI, of which one must be in the brain, can also meet dissemination in space criteria; the CSF must show either oligoclonal bands or an elevated IgG index.*

Although this definition stipulated that an event of ADEM cannot contribute to an MS diagnosis, several studies have since suggested that ADEM may be the presenting feature of MS in younger children [115, 116]. In addition, accompanying definitive MRI criteria for pediatric MS need to be developed.

Diagnostic evaluation

Evaluation of a child with suspected multiple sclerosis includes neurological examination, MRI of the brain and spine, fundoscopic examination and visual-evoked potentials and potentially MRI of the orbits. CSF examination may be performed, especially in younger children, or in those with progressive or atypical presentations. Serology to rule out other mimics of multiple sclerosis should include ANA, ESR, CRP, ACE level and chest x-ray, folate, B12 levels, and TSH. Testing for other disorders should be considered on a case-by-case basis as discussed in "Differential diagnosis" below. Visual-evoked potential testing or optical coherence tomography should be considered to evaluate subclinical visual changes [79, 84].

All patients with suspected MS should undergo gadolinium-enhanced MRI of the brain and spine. MRI shows discrete, ovoid T2 and FLAIR hyperintensities involving the white matter, with a predilection for the periventricular regions (Figure 5.2b). A characteristic pattern involves such lesions oriented perpendicularly to the corpus callosum called "Dawson's fingers," which is shown especially well on sagittal FLAIR sequences. When applied to children, adult MRI MS diagnostic criteria appear to be less sensitive, reflecting an overall lower disease burden in a pediatric population [109]. Younger children with MS (age < 11 years) may present with atypical MRI features, rendering diagnosis challenging, and possibly delaying the initiation of preventative therapies [108]. Brain lesions in these children may be large, with poorlydefined borders and are frequently confluent at disease onset. Such T2-bright foci in younger children may vanish on repeat scans, unlike that seen in teenagers or adults. This suggests that disease processes in the developing brain, including immune responses, may be different from those in older patients [108].

Most patients with suspected pediatric-onset MS should undergo lumbar puncture for routine studies, as well as testing for CSF oligoclonal bands and IgG index. Typically, WBC counts range from 0–50 cells/mm^3 with a lymphocytic predominance [117]. However, children under the age of 11 years have more neutrophils in the CSF than older children [118]. Protein levels may be slightly elevated, however glucose levels are normal. Oligoclonal band (OCB) testing involves a comparison of immunoglobulin patterns in the CSF to the serum. The presence of bands in the CSF, but not the serum, indicates abnormal synthesis of immunoglobulin in the CSF. Isoelectric focusing followed by immunoblot testing is preferred over agarose gel

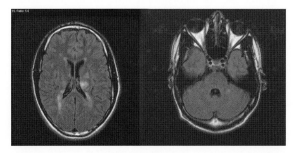

Figure 5.2b Brain FLAIR image of a 13-year-old boy with multiple sclerosis. Lesions are located in the periventricular white mater and focal lesions in the middle cerebellar peduncles.

electrophoresis for detecting oligoclonal bands as it has a higher sensitivity. The CSF profile in childhood-onset MS may vary by age. Interestingly, the absence of neutrophils in the CSF at onset is predictive of an earlier second neurological episode. Although one study reports OCB to be present in the CSF of up to 92% of children with MS [117], this may be laboratory, disease duration, and age dependent. Another study also found OCB to be less frequent in younger children (43% versus 63% in adolescents) [119]. By contrast, in ADEM, 0–29% of cases were found to have OCB. [1–3, 117].

Differential diagnosis

The differential diagnosis of pediatric multiple sclerosis includes tumor, infections, vascular disorders, metabolic disorders, mitochondrial disorders, nutritional disorders, and other autoimmune disorders (see Box 5.1). Patients presenting with white matter lesions should be subclassified into those with static versus progressive disorders. Patients with longstanding static white matter lesions should be closely evaluated for perinatal hypoxic ischemic injury. Determining whether the presentation is episodic or progressive is critical, since in most cases MS in children is an episodic disorder. Progressive presentations should be fully evaluated for other structural, vascular or metabolic defects. Evaluation should include a dermatological examination to look for stigmata of neurofibromatosis, tuberous sclerosis, Lyme disease, SLE, Fabry disease and Behcet disease. Devic disease (NMO) should be considered, particularly in cases associated with optic neuritis (see section below). Complicated migraine, antiphospholipid syndrome, CADASIL and arteriovenous malformation (AVM) should be considered in cases where headache is a prominent feature. Basal ganglia lesions may suggest Leigh disease, Wilson disease, post-streptococcal syndromes, histiocytosis, and Moya moya syndrome. Friedrich ataxia and the inherited spinocerebellar ataxias should be considered in cases with predominant cerebellar deficits. In the presence of white matter lesions with a peripheral neuropathy, adrenomyeloneuropathy (AMN), Krabbe disease, metachromatic leukodystrophy (MLD), and mitochondrial disorders should be considered.

Treatment

Acute relapse-related care for pediatric MS typically involves intravenous corticosteroids [120]. Typical dosing is methylprednisolone 20–30 mg/kg to a maximum of 1 gram daily for 3 to 7 days. Intravenous immune globulin (IVIg) at a dose of 0.4 g/kg/day for 5 days or plasma exchange (5–7 exchanges) are employed in refractory cases [31, 121].

Beta-interferons (Avonex, Betaseron, and Rebif) and glatiramer acetate (Copaxone) have been used as a prophylactic therapy with reasonable success in children [122–124]. Available studies have shown that both

BOX 5.1   Differential diagnosis of pediatric MS

Demyelinating
- Optic neuritis
- Transverse myelitis
- Devic disease (neuromyelitis optica)
- ADEM
- AHEM
- Recurrent ADEM
- Multiphasic ADEM (MDEM)

Tumor
- Llymphoma
- Astrocytoma
- Metastasis

Immunologic
- SLE
- Antiphospholipid syndrome
- Rheumatoid arthritis
- Post-streptococcal syndrome
- Behçet disease
- Sarcoidosis
- Sjogren syndrome
- Wegener granulomatosis
- Lymphomatoid granulomatosis
- Langerhan cell histiocytosis
- Hemophagocytic lymphohistiocytosis
- Hashimoto thyroiditis

Infection
- Lyme disease
- HIV
- HSV
- HTLV-1
- PML
- Neurosyphilis
- Cat scratch disease (*B. henselae*)
- Whipple disease

Vascular disorders
- Stroke
- AVM
- Sickle cell disease
- Moya moya
- CADASIL
- Complicated migraine
- Isolated angiitis of the CNS
- Susac syndrome

Nutritional
- B12 deficiency
- Folate deficiency
  - (methylenetetrahydrofolate reductase deficiency)

Metabolic
- Fabry disease
- Biotinidase deficiency
- 3-Methylglutaric acid deficiency
- Neuronal ceroid lipofuscinosis

Leukodystrophy
- Adrenoleukodystrophy or adrenomyeloneuropathy
- Metachromatic leukodystrophy
- Alexander disease
- Krabbe disease
- Pelizaeus–Merzbacher disease
- Vanishing white matter disease

Mitochondrial disease
- MELAS
- LHON
- Leigh disease

Degenerative
- Hereditary spastic paraparesis
- Friedreich ataxia
- Spinocerebellar atrophy

treatments are relatively safe, and the side effect profile is similar to that observed in adults. Typical side effects of the beta-interferons include post-injection flu-like symptoms and myalgias, headaches, depression, increased liver function tests, and (rarely) suppression of white blood cell counts. Side effects of glatiramer acetate include injection site reactions, lymphadenopathy and, rarely, immediate-post injection anxiety syndromes. Although placebo-controlled double-blind studies have not been performed in children, the majority of studies have demonstrated a reduction in relapse rate following the initiation of first-line treatments. However, some children continue to experience breakthrough disease. The definition of treatment failure is not uniform across clinicians and centers, but evidence of ongoing relapses, MRI activity, and disability accrual may suggest switching first-line treatment or escalating to second-line therapy.

There are few studies describing the use of second-line treatments in children with MS. We conducted a retrospective study of 17 children, aged 9–18 years, treated with cyclophosphamide at either pulse or induction therapy [125]. In the majority of cases the relapse frequency and EDSS improved 1 year following the initiation of cyclophosphamide therapy. There are several reports of natalizumab (Tysabri) treatment in adolescents with MS [126, 127]. Although natalizumab was effective in controlling relapse rates in these very active cases, the risks of PML and other serious side effects in children requires further assessment.

Pediatric MS is a lifelong chronic disease and, along with relapses and disease progression, patients may experience a variety of chronic symptoms including fatigue, depression, bladder urgency or retention, bowel constipation, or **dyssnergy** and neuropathic pain. Many of these symptoms may be ameliorated with symptomatic treatments. In addition, evaluation by subspecialists including urology, pain clinic, neuro-ophthalmology and rehabilitation may play an important role in the management of a pediatric patient.

Outcomes

Several studies have demonstrated that initial disease progression, as measured by the EDSS scale, is slower in patients with pediatric-onset MS (POMS) compared with geographically-region matched patients with adult-onset MS (AOMS) [87, 90, 128, 129]. This likely represents a difference in accrual of locomotor disability; however, these studies also demonstrated that at any given age a patient with pediatric-onset MS will have a higher disability score than a patient with adult-onset MS.

Cognitive dysfunction can present early in the course of pediatric multiple sclerosis [130–133]. One study of 37 children with MS found that 60% experienced cognitive difficulties in one major domain, and 35% had difficulties in two domains [131]. The areas that were most commonly affected were complex attention, naming, delayed recall, and visual memory. In contrast, verbal fluency and immediate recall were relatively intact. Another study of 61 children found that 31% of patients exhibited significant impairment in three assessed domains of cognitive functioning, and 53% failed at least two tests [133].

Longitudinal data over a 2-year period has shown that over 60% of children continue to accrue cognitive deficits [132]. Neuropsychological testing should be considered for all children with MS and related demyelinating diseases, since symptoms may occasionally be subtle. Moreover, children with identified issues may benefit from the implementation of an individualized educational plan and in some cases cognitive rehabilitation may be warranted [134]. In a subset of patients who underwent psychiatric evaluation, almost half were diagnosed with depression or an anxiety disorder. These findings underline the need for routine neuropsychological testing and psychiatric evaluation as a part of the management of childhood MS. Interaction with the school system is critical in order to ensure that a tailored educational program is implemented for each child.

TOP TIPS 5.4

- Pediatric-onset multiple sclerosis may present in 3–5% of all MS cases.
- Current data suggests a similar pathophysiology of pediatric and adult-onset MS.
- Over 95% of pediatric MS cases present with a relapsing-remitting course.
- High-dose intravenous steroids are generally used for the treatment of relapses.
- Beta-interferons or glatiramer acetate are used as first-line treatments in children with MS.
- Some children have refractory disease and require second-line treatments. There is limited information on the use of second-line treatments such as cyclophosphamide and natalizumab in children with MS.
- Cognitive dysfunction may be present at onset and may worsen over time.
- Neuropsychological testing and evaluation by an educational consultant is recommended in all cases of pediatric MS.

Neuromyelitis optica

Neuromyelitis optica (NMO), or Devic disease, is a subtype of MS characterized by clinical episodes of optic neuritis and transverse myelitis, and the demonstration of contiguous lesions in the spinal cord [135].

Epidemiology
NMO occurs rarely in children. The current literature is limited to small series or case reports of NMO in children [136–140]. The largest series from

the Mayo clinic described a cohort of 88 children who were found to be seropositive for the NMO IgG antibody [138]. Of those with available clinical information, 42 patients (73%) were non-Caucasian, and 20 (34%) had African ethnicity. Median age at symptom onset was 12 years (range 4–18); and 88% were girls. In another series of children with demyelinating disease, 7/9 of those with a relapsing NMO phenotype were seropositive for the NMO antibody. In contrast, no children with relapsing-remitting MS were NMO IgG seropositive. Additional autoantibodies were detected in 57 of 75 patients (76%), and 16 of 38 (42%) had a coexisting autoimmune disorder recorded (systemic lupus erythematosus, Sjogren syndrome, juvenile rheumatoid arthritis, Graves disease) [138].

Pathophysiology

NMO has a distinct lesion distribution compared to typical multiple sclerosis or ADEM, although there may be some overlap between the syndromes. NMO is characterized by optic neuritis and longitudinally extensive transverse myelitis (LETM). Lesions typical of MS are characteristically absent on a brain MRI, however lesions may be present in aquaporin-4 rich areas, including the periaqueductal gray area [141]. Pathologically, NMO is characterized by demyelination with extensive macrophage infiltration associated with large numbers of perivascular granulocytes and eosinophils and rare CD3(+) and CD8(+) T cells, as well as a pronounced perivascular deposition of immunoglobulins (mainly IgM) and complement C9neo antigen in active lesions [142]. A serum antibody to aquaporin-4 (a water channel present predominantly on the astroyctic foot processes of the blood–brain barrier) is observed in approximately 76% of those presenting with an NMO phenotype [143], and appears to be a sensitive and specific marker of the disease. In vitro, it has been shown that NMO-IgG binds to astrocytes and alters aquaporin-4 polarized expression and increases permeability of a human blood–brain barrier (BBB) endothelium/astrocyte barrier. In vitro models demonstrated astrocyte killing by NMO-Ab-dependent cellular cytotoxicity and complement-dependent granulocyte attraction through the BBB model [144].

Clinical presentation

NMO can present with either optic neuritis or transverse myelitis. The clinical symptoms of optic neuritis include blurred vision, pain on eye movement and loss of color vision. Typically children may complain of eye pain and frequent eye rubbing occurs. Transverse myelitis may present with lower extremity and upper extremity weakness or numbness. Gait may be affected, and bowel or bladder retention or incontinence is common. Pain in the lower extremities and a band-like sensation around the torso may be present. Lesions in the brainstem or area postrema may result in nausea, vomiting, or hiccups [145]. In children with NMO, an encephalopathic syndrome has been described, which can resemble the clinical presentation of ADEM. In the Mayo Clinic series, 45% of children had episodic cerebral symptoms (encephalopathy, ophthalmoparesis, ataxia, seizures, intractable vomiting, or hiccups) [140].

Diagnostic definition: The International Pediatric MS study group proposed the following diagnostic definition for pediatric NMO [7], adapted from the 2006 NMO adult criteria [135]:
  (i) *The presence of optic neuritis and myelitis.*
  (ii) *Spinal cord lesion extending over three or more vertebral segments or NMO antibody positive.*
  (iii) *Brain MRI relatively normal; exceptions with lesions in aquaporin-4 rich areas (hypothalamus, peri III, IV ventricles, corpus callosum).*
Supporting criteria may include seropositivity for NMO-IgG.

Diagnostic evaluation

Diagnostic evaluation of suspected NMO includes serum NMO IgG, testing for other autoimmune disorders including SLE (ANA, ESR), Sjogren syndrome, rheumatoid arthritis, and autoimmune thyroid disease. In rare cases, NMO IgG in the CSF may be positive in the absence of serum antibody [146], and testing should be considered in cases with high clinical suspicion. Standard CSF testing demonstrates elevations in WBC (5–600) with approximately equal lymphocyte and neutrophil proportions [140]. Protein may be elevated. Oligoclonal band testing is generally negative. MRI of the brain can demonstrate lesions in the subcortical white matter, periaqueductal gray, and the hypothalamus (Figure 5.2c). Spinal cord MRI typically demonstrates longitudinally extensive lesions extending over three or more segments. Optic neuritis may be diagnosed clinically and supporting studies

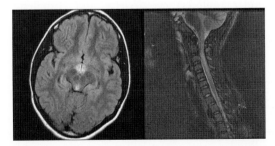

Figure 5.2c Brain FLAIR image of a 14-year-old girl with neuromyelitis optica, and T2-weighted image of a spinal cord from the same patient. Lesions are located in the peri-third and peri-fourth ventricular areas. There is a longitudinally extensive lesion from the brainstem to C7.

include fundoscopic examination, visual-evoked potential testing, and orbital MRI.

Differential diagnosis

The differential diagnosis of NMO largely includes MS and ADEM. LHON and B12 deficient may be considered in cases of chronic optic neuritis. SLE, ALD, HTLV-1 and ischemia should be considered for transverse myelitis presentations.

Treatment

There is no FDA-approved treatment for NMO. Intravenous steroids are typically used for acute relapses, and are administered at a dose of 20–30 mg/kg (up to 1 g/day) for a 3–5 day period. Plasmapheresis may be used as first- or second-line treatment for acute attacks, and five exchanges are administered every other day or as tolerated. NMO titers may be reduced following plasmapheresis, suggesting that the antibody is linked to relapses. IVIg (up to 2 g/kg divided into two to five doses) has been used as third-line therapy by some investigators [137]. Prophylatic therapies used for NMO in adults include Rituximab (anti-CD20 antibody), azathioprine, mycophenolate mofetil, and mitoxantrone. The same treatments have been used in children with NMO, and one group has described their approach with initial immunosuppression with azathioprine or mycophenolate mofetil, while refractory cases are treated with Rituximab [137].

Outcomes

In adults with NMO, disability can accrue after relapses, however the disease progression that occurs in MS is described as typically absent [147]. It is likely that this rule also applies to children. In one study of children with NMO, after resolution of the acute attacks, visual impairment persisted in 26 patients (54%) and 21 patients (44%) had residual weakness [140]. Cognitive dysfunction and long-term outcomes in children with NMO have not been systematically studied.

TOP TIPS 5.5

- Neuromyelitis optica (NMO) rarely occurs in children.
- The adult diagnostic criteria for NMO may be applied to pediatric cases.
- NMO IgG may be negative in some pediatric patients with a clinical presentation of NMO.
- Use of intravenous steroids or plasmapheresis has been reported for pediatric cases of NMO.
- Long-term prophylactic treatment can include rituximab, mycophenolate mofetil, and azathioprine.

Conclusion

This past decade has seen significant advances in pediatric immune-mediated demyelinating diseases. However, several outstanding questions remain, including the identification of optimal treatment and greater insight into the causes of these diseases in children. National and multinational studies are underway to address these questions and should lead to promising insights in the next 5 years.

References

1 Dale RC, de Sousa C, Chong WK, Cox TC, Harding B, Neville BG. Acute disseminated encephalomyelitis, multiphasic disseminated encephalomyelitis and multiple sclerosis in children. Brain 2000 Dec; 123(Pt 12): 2407–22.

2 Hynson JL, Kornberg AJ, Coleman LT, Shield L, Harvey AS, Kean MJ. Clinical and neuroradiologic features of acute disseminated encephalomyelitis in children. Neurology 2001 May 22; 56(10): 1308–12.

3 Tenembaum S, Chamoles N, Fejerman N. Acute disseminated encephalomyelitis: a long-term follow-up study of 84 pediatric patients. Neurology 2002 Oct 22; 59(8): 1224–31.

4 Anlar B, Basaran C, Kose G, Guven A, Haspolat S, Yakut A, et al. Acute disseminated encephalomyelitis in children: outcome and prognosis. Neuropediatrics 2003 Aug; 34(4): 194–9.

5 Schwarz S, Mohr A, Knauth M, Wildemann B, Storch-Hagenlocher B. Acute disseminated encephalomyelitis: a follow-up study of 40 adult patients. Neurology 2001 May 22; 56(10): 1313–18.

6 Leake JA, Albani S, Kao AS, Senac MO, Billman GF, Nespeca MP, et al. Acute disseminated encephalomyelitis in childhood: epidemiologic, clinical and laboratory features. Pediatr Infect Dis J 2004 Aug; 23(8): 756–64.

7 Krupp LB, Banwell B, Tenembaum S. Consensus definitions proposed for pediatric multiple sclerosis and related disorders. Neurology 2007 Apr 17; 68 (16 Suppl 2): S7–12.

8 Pohl D, Hennemuth I, von Kries R, Hanefeld F. Paediatric multiple sclerosis and acute disseminated encephalomyelitis in Germany: results of a nationwide survey. Eur J Pediat 2007 May; 166(5): 405–12.

9 Singhi PD, Ray M, Singhi S, Kumar Khandelwal N. Acute disseminated encephalomyelitis in North Indian children: clinical profile and follow-up. J Child Neurol 2006 Oct; 21(10): 851–7.

10 Murthy SN, Faden HS, Cohen ME, Bakshi R. Acute disseminated encephalomyelitis in children. Pediatrics 2002 Aug; 110(2 Pt 1): e21.

11 (a) Hemachudha T, Griffin DE, Giffels JJ, Johnson RT, Moser AB, Phanuphak P. Myelin basic protein as an encephalitogen in encephalomyelitis and polyneuritis following rabies vaccination. N Engl J Med 1987; 316: 369–374. (b) Hemachudha T, Phanuphak P, Johnson RT, Griffin DE, Ratanavongsiri J, Siriprasomsup W. Neurologic complications of Semple-type rabies vaccine: clinical and immunologic studies. Neurology 1987; 37: 550–556.

12 Fenichel GM. Neurological complications of immunization. Ann Neurol 1982; 12: 119–128.

13 Tourbah A, Gout O, Liblau R, et al. Encephalitis after hepatitis B vaccination: recurrent disseminated encephalitis or MS? Neurology 1999; 53: 396–401.

14 Ozawa H, Noma S, Yoshida Y, Sekine H, Hashimoto T. Acute disseminated encephalomyelitis associated with poliomyelitis vaccine. Pediatr Neurol 2000; 23: 177–179.

15 Takahashi H, Pool V, Tsai TF, Chen RT. (2000) Adverse events after Japanese enephalitis vaccination: review of post-marketing surveillance data from Japan and the United States. The VAERS Working Group. Vaccine 18: 2963–2969.

16 Karaali-Savrun F, Altintas A, Saip S, Siva A. Hepatitis B vaccine related-myelitis? Eur J Neurol 2001; 8: 711–715.

17 Sejvar JJ, Labutta RJ, Chapman LE, Grabenstein JD, Iskander J, Lane JM. Neurologic adverse events associated with smallpox vaccination in the United States, 2002–2004. JAMA 2005; 294: 2744–2750.

18 Hemachudha T, Griffin DE, Johnson RT, Giffels JJ. Immunologic studies of patients with chronic encephalitis induced by post-exposure Semple rabies vaccine. Neurology 1988; 38: 42–44.

19 Wingerchuk DM. Postinfectious encephalomyelitis. Curr Neurol Neurosci Rep 2003; 3: 256–264.

20 Menge T, Kieseier BC, Nessler S, Hemmer B, Hartung HP, Stuve O. Acute disseminated encephalomyelitis: an acute hit against the brain. Curr Opin Neurology 2007; 20: 247–254.

21 Prineas et al. 2002

22 Young MM, Kinsella TJ, Miser JS, et al. Treatment of sarcomas of the chest wall using intensive combined modality therapy. International journal of radiation oncology, biology, physics 1989; 16: 49–57.

23 DeLuca 2004.

24 Ghosh N, DeLuca GC, Esiri MM. Evidence of axonal damage in human acute demyelinating diseases. J Neurol Sci 2004; 222: 29–34.

25 Pohl-Koppe A, Burchett SK, Thiele EA, Hafler DA.Myelin basic protein reactive Th2 T cells are found in acute disseminated encephalomyelitis. J Neuroimmunol 1998 Nov 2; 91(1–2): 19–27.

26 Wingerchuk DM. Postinfectious encephalomyelitis. Curr Neurol Neurosci Rep 2003; 3: 256–264.

27 Amit R, Glick B, Itzchak Y, Dgani Y, Meyeir S. Acute severe combined demyelination. Childs Nerv Syst 1992 Sep; 8(6): 354–6.

28 Erazo-Torricelli R. [Acute disseminated encephalomyelitis in children]. Revista neurologia 2006 Apr 10; 42VIS (Suppl 3): S75–82.

29 Marchioni E, Marinou-Aktipi K, Uggetti C, Bottanelli M, Pichiecchio A, Soragna D, et al. Effectiveness of intravenous immunoglobulin treatment in adult patients with steroid-resistant monophasic or recurrent acute disseminated encephalomyelitis. J Neurol 2002 Jan; 249(1): 100–4.

30 Dale RC, Church AJ, Cardoso F, Goddard E, Cox TC, Chong WK, et al. Poststreptococcal acute disseminated encephalomyelitis with basal ganglia involvement and auto-reactive antibasal ganglia antibodies. Ann Neurol 2001 Nov; 50(5): 588–95.

31 Khurana DS, Melvin JJ, Kothare SV, Valencia I, Hardison HH, Yum S, et al. Acute disseminated encephalomyelitis in children: discordant neurologic and neuroimaging abnormalities and response to plasmapheresis. Pediatrics 2005 Aug; 116(2): 431–6.

32 Kleiman M, Brunquell P. Acute disseminated encephalomyelitis: response to intravenous immunoglobulin. J Child Neurol 1995 Nov; 10(6): 481–3.

33 Straussberg R, Schonfeld T, Weitz R, Karmazyn B, Harel L. Improvement of atypical acute disseminated encephalomyelitis with steroids and intravenous immunoglobulins. Pediatric neurology 2001 Feb; 24(2): 139–43.

34 Pittock SJ, Keir G, Alexander M, Brennan P, Hardiman O. Rapid clinical and CSF response to intravenous gamma globulin in acute disseminated encephalomyelitis. Eur J Neurol 2001 Nov; 8(6): 725.

35 Hahn JS, Siegler DJ, Enzmann D. Intravenous gammaglobulin therapy in recurrent acute disseminated encephalomyelitis. Neurology 1996 Apr; 46(4): 1173–4.

36 Revel-Vilk S, Hurvitz H, Klar A, Virozov Y, Korn-Lubetzki I. Recurrent acute disseminated encephalomyelitis associated with acute cytomegalovirus and Epstein-Barr virus infection. J Child Neurol 2000 Jun; 15(6): 421–4.

37 Balestri P, Grosso S, Acquaviva A, Bernini M. Plasmapheresis in a child affected by acute disseminated encephalomyelitis. Brain Dev 2000 Mar; 22(2): 123–6.

38 Kanter DS, Horensky D, Sperling RA, Kaplan JD, Malachowski ME, Churchill WH, Jr., Plasmapheresis in fulminant acute disseminated encephalomyelitis. Neurology 1995 Apr; 45(4): 824–7.

39 Miyazawa R, Hikima A, Takano Y, Arakawa H, Tomomasa T, Morikawa A. Plasmapheresis in fulminant acute disseminated encephalomyelitis. Brain Dev 2001 Oct; 23(6): 424–6.

40 Mader I, Wolff M, Niemann G, Kuker W. Acute haemorrhagic encephalomyelitis (AHEM): MRI findings. Neuropediatrics 2004 Apr; 35(2): 143–6.

41 Payne ET, Rutka JT, Ho TK, Halliday WC, Banwell BL. Treatment leading to dramatic recovery in acute hemorrhagic leukoencephalitis. J Child Neurol 2007 Jan; 22(1): 109–13.

42 Kimura S, Nezu A, Ohtsuki N, Kobayashi T, Osaka H, Uehara S. Serial magnetic resonance imaging in children with postinfectious encephalitis. Brain Dev 1996 Nov-Dec; 18(6): 461–5.

43 Murthy JM, Yangala R, Meena AK, Jaganmohan Reddy J. Acute disseminated encephalomyelitis: clinical and MRI study from South India. J Neurol Sci 1999 Jun 1; 165(2): 133–8.

44 Idrissova Zh R, Boldyreva MN, Dekonenko EP, Malishev NA, Leontyeva IY, Martinenko IN, et al. Acute disseminated encephalomyelitis in children: clinical features and HLA-DR linkage. Eur J Neurol 2003 Sep; 10(5): 537–46.

45 Hahn CD, Miles BS, MacGregor DL, Blaser SI, Banwell BL, Hetherington CR. Neurocognitive outcome after acute disseminated encephalomyelitis. Pediat Neurol 2003 Aug; 29(2): 117–23.

46 Mikaeloff Y, Adamsbaum C, Husson B, Vallee L, Ponsot G, Confavreux C, et al. MRI prognostic factors for relapse after acute CNS inflammatory demyelination in childhood. Brain 2004 Sep; 127(Pt 9): 1942–7.

47 Mikaeloff Y, Suissa S, Vallee L, Lubetzki C, Ponsot G, Confavreux C, et al. First episode of acute CNS inflammatory demyelination in childhood: prognostic factors for multiple sclerosis and disability. J Pediat 2004 Feb; 144(2): 246–52.

48 Mikaeloff Y, Caridade G, Husson B, Suissa S, Tardieu M. Acute disseminated encephalomyelitis cohort study: prognostic factors for relapse. Eur J Paediatr Neurol 2007 Mar; 11(2): 90–5.

49 Berman M, Feldman S, Alter M, Zilber N, Kahana E. Acute transverse myelitis: incidence and etiologic considerations. Neurology 1981 Aug; 31(8): 966–71.

50 Pidcock FS, Krishnan C, Crawford TO, Salorio CF, Trovato M, Kerr DA. Acute transverse myelitis in childhood: center-based analysis of 47 cases. Neurology 2007 May 1; 68(18): 1474–80.

51 Banwell BL. The long (-itudinally extensive) and the short of it: transverse myelitis in children. Neurology 2007 May 1; 68(18): 1447–9.

52 Defresne P, Hollenberg H, Husson B, Tabarki B, Landrieu P, Huault G, et al. Acute transverse myelitis in children: clinical course and prognostic factors. J Child Neurol 2003 Jun; 18(6): 401–6.

53 Miyazawa R, Ikeuchi Y, Tomomasa T, Ushiku H, Ogawa T, Morikawa A. Determinants of prognosis of acute transverse myelitis in children. Pediat Int 2003 Oct; 45(5): 512–16.

54 Defresne P, Meyer L, Tardieu M, Scalais E, Nuttin C, De Bont B, et al. Efficacy of high dose steroid therapy in children with severe acute transverse myelitis. J Neurol, Neurosurg, Psychiat 2001 Aug; 71(2): 272–4.

55 Knebusch M, Strassburg HM, Reiners K. Acute transverse myelitis in childhood: nine cases and review of the literature. Devel Med Child Neurol 1998 Sep; 40(9): 631–9.

56 Dunne K, Hopkins IJ, Shield LK. Acute transverse myelopathy in childhood. Devel Med Child Neurol 1986 Apr; 28(2): 198–204.

57 Paine RS, Byers RK. Transverse myelopathy in childhood. AMA 1953 Feb; 85(2): 151–63.

58 Scott TF, Kassab SL, Singh S. Acute partial transverse myelitis with normal cerebral magnetic resonance imaging: transition rate to clinically definite multiple sclerosis. Multiple Sclerosis (Houndmills, Basingstoke, England) 2005 Aug; 11(4): 373–7.

59 Matsui M, Kawano H, Matsukura M, Otani Y, Miike T. Acute transverse myelitis after Japanese B encephalitis vaccination in a 4-year-old girl. Brain Devel 2002 Apr; 24(3): 187–9.

60 Kaplin AI, Deshpande DM, Scott E, Krishnan C, Carmen JS, Shats I, et al. IL-6 induces regionally selective spinal cord injury in patients with the neuroinflammatory disorder transverse myelitis. J Clin Invest 2005 Oct; 115(10): 2731–41.

61 Minami K, Tsuda Y, Maeda H, Yanagawa T, Izumi G, Yoshikawa N. Acute transverse myelitis caused by Coxsackie virus B5 infection. J Paediat Child Health 2004 Jan–Feb; 40(1–2): 66–8.

62 Abramsky O, Teitelbaum D. The autoimmune features of acute transverse myelopathy. Ann Neurol 1977 Jul; 2(1): 36–40.

63 Auletta JJ, John CC. Spinal epidural abscesses in children: a 15-year experience and review of the literature. Clin Infect Dis 2001 Jan; 32(1): 9–16.

64 Patel H, Boaz JC, Phillips JP, Garg BP. Spontaneous spinal epidural hematoma in children. Pediat Neurol 1998 Oct; 19(4): 302–7.

65 Auguste KI, Gupta N. Pediatric intramedullary spinal cord tumors. Neurosurg Clin North Am 2006 Jan; 17(1): 51–61.

66 DeSousa AL, Kalsbeck JE, Mealey J, Jr., Campbell RL, Hockey A. Intraspinal tumors in children. A review of 81 cases. J Neurosurg 1979 Oct; 51(4): 437–45.

67 Innocenzi G, Raco A, Cantore G, Raimondi AJ. Intramedullary astrocytomas and ependymomas in the pediatric age group: a retrospective study. Childs Nerv Syst 1996 Dec; 12(12): 776–80.

68 Ullrich NJ, Marcus K, Pomeroy SL, Turner CD, Zimmerman M, Lehmann LE, et al. Transverse myelitis after therapy for primitive neuroectodermal tumors. Pediat Neurol 2006 Aug; 35(2): 122–5.

69 Sure U, Wakat JP, Gatscher S, Becker R, Bien S, Bertalanffy H. Spinal type IV arteriovenous malformations (perimedullary fistulas) in children. Childs Nerv Syst 2000 Aug; 16(8): 508–15.

70 Andronikou S, Albuquerque-Jonathan G, Wilmshurst J, Hewlett R. MRI findings in acute idiopathic transverse myelopathy in children. Pediat Radiol 2003 Sep; 33(9): 624–9.

71 Lahat E, Pillar G, Ravid S, Barzilai A, Etzioni A, Shahar E. Rapid recovery from transverse myelopathy in children treated with methylprednisolone. Pediat Neurol 1998 Oct; 19(4): 279–82.

72 Sebire G, Hollenberg H, Meyer L, Huault G, Landrieu P, Tardieu M. High dose methylprednisolone in severe acute transverse myelopathy. Arch Dis Child 1997 Feb; 76(2): 167–8.

73 Shahar E, Andraus J, Savitzki D, Pilar G, Zelnik N. Outcome of severe encephalomyelitis in children: effect of high-dose methylprednisolone and immunoglobulins. J Child Neurol. 2002 Nov; 17(11): 810–4.

74 Pittock SJ, Lucchinetti CF. Inflammatory transverse myelitis: evolving concepts. Curr Opin Neurol 2006 Aug; 19(4): 362–8.

75 Weinshenker BG, Wingerchuk DM, Vukusic S, Linbo L, Pittock SJ, Lucchinetti CF, et al. Neuromyelitis optica IgG predicts relapse after longitudinally extensive transverse myelitis. Ann Neurol 2006 Mar; 59(3): 566–9.

76 Morales DS, Siakowski RM, Howard CW, Warman R. Optic neuritis in children. J Ophthal Nurs Technol 2000 Nov–Dec; 19(6): 270–4; quiz 5–6.

77 Wilejto M, Shroff M, Buncic JR, Kennedy J, Goia C, Banwell B. The clinical features, MRI findings, and outcome of optic neuritis in children. Neurology 2006 Jul 25; 67(2): 258–62.

78 Lucchinetti CF, Kiers L, O'Duffy A, Gomez MR, Cross S, Leavitt JA, et al. Risk factors for developing multiple sclerosis after childhood optic neuritis. Neurology 1997 Nov; 49(5): 1413–8.

79 Yeh EA, Weinstock-Guttman B, Lincoff N, Reynolds J, Weinstock A, Madurai N, et al. Retinal nerve fiber thickness in inflammatory demyelinating diseases of childhood onset. Multiple Sclerosis (Houndmills, Basingstoke, England) 2009 Jul; 15(7): 802–10.

80 Beck RW, Cleary PA, Anderson MM, Jr., Keltner JL, Shults WT, Kaufman DI, et al. A randomized, controlled trial of corticosteroids in the treatment of acute optic neuritis. The Optic Neuritis Study Group. New Engl J Med 1992 Feb 27; 326(9): 581–8.

81 Roed HG, Langkilde A, Sellebjerg F, Lauritzen M, Bang P, Morup A, et al. A double-blind, randomized trial of IV immunoglobulin treatment in acute optic neuritis. Neurology 2005 Mar 8; 64(5): 804–10.

82 Ruprecht K, Klinker E, Dintelmann T, Rieckmann P, Gold R. Plasma exchange for severe optic neuritis: treatment of 10 patients. Neurology 2004 Sep 28; 63(6): 1081–3.

83 Hwang JM, Lee YJ, Kim MK. Optic neuritis in Asian children. J Pediat Ophthalmol Strabis 2002 Jan–Feb; 39(1): 26–32.

84 Pohl D, Rostasy K, Treiber-Held S, Brockmann K, Gartner J, Hanefeld F. Pediatric multiple sclerosis: detection of clinically silent lesions by multimodal evoked potentials. J Pediat 2006 Jul; 149(1): 125–7.

85 Chitnis T. Pediatric multiple sclerosis. Neurologist 2006 Nov; 12(6): 299–310.

86 Duquette P, Murray TJ, Pleines J, Ebers GC, Sadovnick D, Weldon P, et al. Multiple sclerosis in childhood: clinical profile in 125 patients. J Pediat 1987 Sep; 111(3): 359–63.

87 Boiko A, Vorobeychik G, Paty D, Devonshire V, Sadovnick D. Early onset multiple sclerosis: a longitudinal study. Neurology 2002 Oct 8; 59(7): 1006–10.

88 Ghezzi A, Deplano V, Faroni J, Grasso MG, Liguori M, Marrosu G, et al. Multiple sclerosis in childhood: clinical features of 149 cases. Multiple Sclerosis (Houndmills, Basingstoke, England) 1997 Feb; 3(1): 43–6.

89 Sindern E, Haas J, Stark E, Wurster U. Early onset MS under the age of 16: clinical and paraclinical features. Acta Neurol Scand 1992 Sep; 86(3): 280–4.

90 Simone IL, Carrara D, Tortorella C, Liguori M, Lepore V, Pellegrini F, et al. Course and prognosis in early-onset MS: comparison with adult-onset forms. Neurology 2002 Dec 24; 59(12): 1922–8.

91 Chitnis T, Glanz B, Jaffin S, Healy B. Demographics of pediatric-onset multiple sclerosis in an MS center population from the Northeastern United States. Multiple Sclerosis (Houndmills, Basingstoke, England) 2009 May; 15(5): 627–31.

92 Kennedy J, O'Connor P, Sadovnick AD, Perara M, Yee I, Banwell B. Age at onset of multiple sclerosis may be influenced by place of residence during childhood rather than ancestry. Neuroepidemiology 2006; 26(3): 162–7.

93 Gorman MP, Healy BC, Polgar-Turcsanyi M, Chitnis T. Increased relapse rate in pediatric-onset compared with adult-onset multiple sclerosis. Arch Neurol 2009 Jan; 66(1): 54–9.

94 Anderson RC, Connolly ES, Jr., Komotar RJ, Mack WJ, McKhann GM, Van Orman CB, et al. Clinicopathological review: tumefactive demyelination in a 12-year-old girl. Neurosurgery 2005 May; 56(5): 1051–7; discussion – 7.

95 Dastgir J, DiMario FJ, Jr., Acute tumefactive demyelinating lesions in a pediatric patient with known diagnosis of multiple sclerosis: review of the literature and treatment proposal. J Child Neurol 2009 Apr; 24(4): 431–7.

96 McAdam LC, Blaser SI, Banwell BL. Pediatric tumefactive demyelination: case series and review of the literature. Pediat Neurol 2002 Jan; 26(1): 18–25.

97 Riva D, Chiapparini L, Pollo B, Balestrini MR, Massimino M, Milani N. A case of pediatric tumefactive demyelinating lesion misdiagnosed and treated as glioblastoma. J Child Neurol 2008 Aug; 23(8): 944–7.

98 Vanlandingham M, Hanigan W, Vedanarayanan V, Fratkin J. An uncommon illness with a rare presentation: neurosurgical management of ADEM with tumefactive demyelination in children. Childs Nerv Syst 2009 Dec 1.

99 Lucchinetti C, Bruck W, Parisi J, Scheithauer B, Rodriguez M, Lassmann H. Heterogeneity of multiple sclerosis lesions: implications for the pathogenesis of demyelination. Ann Neurol 2000 Jun; 47(6): 707–17.

100 Chitnis T. The role of CD4 T cells in the pathogenesis of multiple sclerosis. Int Rev Neurobiol 2007; 79: 43–72.

101 Banwell B, Bar-Or A, Cheung R, Kennedy J, Krupp LB, Becker DJ, et al. Abnormal T-cell reactivities in childhood inflammatory demyelinating disease and type 1 diabetes. Ann Neurol 2008 Jan; 63(1): 98–111.

102 Correale J, Tenembaum SN. Myelin basic protein and myelin oligodendrocyte glycoprotein T-cell repertoire in childhood and juvenile multiple sclerosis. Mult Scler 2006 Aug; 12(4): 412–20.

103 Antel J, Bar-Or A. Roles of immunoglobulins and B cells in multiple sclerosis: from pathogenesis to treatment. J Neuroimmunol 2006 Nov; 180(1–2): 3–8.

104 Bar-Or A. The immunology of multiple sclerosis. Semin Neurol 2008 Feb; 28(1): 29–45.

105 O'Connor KC, McLaughlin KA, De Jager PL, Chitnis T, Bettelli E, Xu C, et al. Self-antigen tetramers discriminate between myelin autoantibodies to native or denatured protein. Nat Med 2007 Feb; 13(2): 211–17.

106 Rostasy K, Withut E, Pohl D, Lange P, Ciesielcyk B, Diem R, et al. Tau, phospho-tau, and S-100B in the cerebrospinal fluid of children with multiple sclerosis. J Child Neurol 2005 Oct; 20(10): 822–5.

107 Ruggieri M, Iannetti P, Polizzi A, Pavone L, Grimaldi LM. Multiple sclerosis in children under 10 years of age. Neurol Sci 2004 Nov; 25 (Suppl 4): S326–35.

108 Chabas D, Castillo-Trivino T, Mowry EM, Strober JB, Glenn OA, Waubant E. Vanishing MS T2-bright lesions before puberty: a distinct MRI phenotype? Neurology 2008 Sep; 71(14): 1090–3.

109 Hahn CD, Shroff MM, Blaser SI, Banwell BL. MRI criteria for multiple sclerosis: Evaluation in a pediatric cohort. Neurology 2004 Mar; 62(5): 806–8.

110 Ghassemi R, Antel SB, Narayanan S, Francis SJ, Bar-Or A, Sadovnick AD, et al. Lesion distribution in children with clinically isolated syndromes. Ann Neurol 2008 Mar; 63(3): 401–5.

111 Balassy C, Bernert G, Wober-Bingol C, Csapo B, Kornek B, Szeles J, et al. Long-term MRI observations of childhood-onset relapsing-remitting multiple sclerosis. Neuropediatrics 2001 Feb; 32(1): 28–37.

112 Vishwas MS, Chitnis T, Pienaar R, Healy BC, Grant PE. Tract-Based Analysis of Callosal, Projection, and Association Pathways in Pediatric Patients with Multiple Sclerosis: A Preliminary Study. AJNR 2009 Oct 22.

113 McDonald WI, Compston A, Edan G, Goodkin D, Hartung HP, Lublin FD, et al. Recommended diagnostic criteria for multiple sclerosis: guidelines from the International Panel on the diagnosis of multiple sclerosis. Ann Neurol 2001 Jul; 50(1): 121–7.

114 Polman CH, Reingold SC, Edan G, Filippi M, Hartung HP, Kappos L, et al. Diagnostic criteria for multiple sclerosis: 2005 revisions to the "McDonald Criteria". Ann Neurol 2005 Dec; 58(6): 840–6.

115 Pohl D, Waubant E, Banwell B, Chabas D, Chitnis T, Weinstock-Guttman B, et al. Treatment of pediatric multiple sclerosis and variants. Neurology 2007 Apr 17; 68 (16 Suppl 2): S54–65.

116 Banwell B, Krupp L, Kennedy J, Tellier R, Tenembaum S, Ness J, et al. Clinical features and viral serologies in children with multiple sclerosis: a multinational observational study. Lancet Neurol 2007 Sep; 6(9): 773–81.

117 Pohl D, Rostasy K, Reiber H, Hanefeld F. CSF characteristics in early-onset multiple sclerosis. Neurology 2004 Nov 23; 63(10): 1966–7.

118 Chabas D, Strober J, Waubant E. Pediatric multiple sclerosis. Curr Neurol Neurosci Rep 2008; 8: 434–441.

119 Chabas D, Ness J, Belman A, Yeh EA, Kuntz N, Gorman M, et al. Younger children with pediatric MS have a distinct CSF inflammatory profile at disease onset. under review 2009.

120 Banwell B. Treatment of children and adolescents with multiple sclerosis. Expert Rev Neurother 2005 May; 5(3): 391–401.

121 Keegan M, Pineda AA, McClelland RL, Darby CH, Rodriguez M, Weinshenker BG. Plasma exchange for severe attacks of CNS demyelination: predictors of response. Neurology 2002 Jan; 58(1): 143–6.

122 Banwell B, Reder AT, Krupp L, Tenembaum S, Eraksoy M, Alexey B, et al. Safety and tolerability of interferon beta-1b in pediatric multiple sclerosis. Neurology 2006 Feb; 66(4): 472–6.

123 Pohl D, Rostasy K, Gartner J, Hanefeld F. Treatment of early onset multiple sclerosis with subcutaneous interferon beta-1a. Neurology 2005 Mar; 64(5): 888–90.

124 Ghezzi A. Immunomodulatory treatment of early onset multiple sclerosis: results of an Italian Co-operative Study. Neurol Sci 2005 Dec; 26 (Suppl 4): S183–6.

125 Makhani N, Gorman MP, Branson HM, Stazzone L, Banwell BL, Chitnis T. Cyclophosphamide therapy in pediatric multiple sclerosis. Neurology 2009 Jun; 72(24): 2076–82.

126 Huppke P, Stark W, Zurcher C, Huppke B, Bruck W, Gartner J. Natalizumab use in pediatric multiple sclerosis. Arch Neurol 2008 Dec; 65(12): 1655–8.

127 Borriello G, Prosperini L, Luchetti A, Pozzilli C. Natalizumab treatment in pediatric multiple sclerosis: a case report. Eur J Paediat Neurol 2009 Jan; 13(1): 67–71.

128 Renoux C, Vukusic S, Mikaeloff Y, Edan G, Clanet M, Dubois B, et al. Natural history of multiple sclerosis with childhood onset. New Engl J Med 2007 Jun; 356(25): 2603–13.

129 Trojano M, Paolicelli D, Bellacosa A, Fuiani A, Cataldi S, Di Monte E. Atypical forms of multiple sclerosis or different phases of a same disease? Neurol Sci 2004 Nov; 25 (Suppl 4): S323–5.

130 Banwell BL, Anderson PE. The cognitive burden of multiple sclerosis in children. Neurology 2005 Mar; 64(5): 891–4.

131 MacAllister WS, Belman AL, Milazzo M, Weisbrot DM, Christodoulou C, Scherl WF, et al. Cognitive functioning in children and adolescents with multiple sclerosis. Neurology 2005 Apr; 64(8): 1422–5.

132 MacAllister WS, Christodoulou C, Milazzo M, Krupp LB. Longitudinal neuropsychological assessment in pediatric multiple sclerosis. Develop Neuropsychol 2007; 32(2): 625–44.

133 Amato MP, Goretti B, Ghezzi A, Lori S, Zipoli V, Portaccio E, et al. Cognitive and psychosocial features of childhood and juvenile MS. Neurology 2008 May; 70(20): 1891–7.

134 Portaccio E, Goretti B, Zipoli V, et al. Reliability, practice effects, and change indices for Rao's Brief Repeatable Battery. Mult Scler 2010; 16: 611–617.

135 Wingerchuk DM, Lennon VA, Pittock SJ, Lucchinetti CF, Weinshenker BG. Revised diagnostic criteria for neuromyelitis optica. Neurology 2006 May; 66(10): 1485–9.

136 Jeffery AR, Buncic Jr., Pediatric Devic's neuromyelitis optica. J Pediat Ophthalmol Strabis 1996 Sep–Oct; 33(5): 223–9.

137 Lotze TE, Northrop JL, Hutton GJ, Ross B, Schiffman JS, Hunter JV. Spectrum of pediatric neuromyelitis optica. Pediatrics 2008 Nov; 122(5): e1039–47.

138 McKeon A, Lennon VA, Lotze T, Tenenbaum S, Ness JM, Rensel M, et al. CNS aquaporin-4 autoimmunity in children. Neurology 2008 Jul; 71(2): 93–100.

139 Banwell B, Tenembaum S, Lennon VA, Ursell E, Kennedy J, Bar-Or A, et al. Neuromyelitis optica-IgG in childhood inflammatory demyelinating CNS disorders. Neurology 2008 Jan; 70(5): 344–52.

140 Bencherif MZ, Karib H, Tachfouti S, Guedira K, Mohcine Z. [Devic's neuromyelitis optica. A childhood case and review of the literature]. J francais d'ophtalmol 2000 May; 23(5): 488–90.

141 Pittock SJ, Lennon VA, Krecke K, Wingerchuk DM, Lucchinetti CF, Weinshenker BG. Brain abnormalities in neuromyelitis optica. Arch Neurol 2006 Mar; 63(3): 390–6.

142 Lucchinetti CF, Mandler RN, McGavern D, Bruck W, Gleich G, Ransohoff RM, et al. A role for humoral mechanisms in the pathogenesis of Devic's neuromyelitis optica. Brain 2002 Jul; 125 (Pt 7): 1450–61.

143 Lennon VA, Wingerchuk DM, Kryzer TJ, Pittock SJ, Lucchinetti CF, Fujihara K, et al. A serum autoantibody marker of neuromyelitis optica: distinction from multiple sclerosis. Lancet 2004 Dec; 364(9451): 2106–12.

144 Vincent T, Saikali P, Cayrol R, Roth AD, Bar-Or A, Prat A, et al. Functional consequences of neuromyelitis optica-IgG astrocyte interactions on blood-brain barrier permeability and granulocyte recruitment. J Immunol 2008 Oct; 181(8): 5730–7.

145 Misu T, Fujihara K, Nakashima I, Sato S, Itoyama Y. Intractable hiccup and nausea with periaqueductal lesions in neuromyelitis optica. Neurology 2005 Nov; 65(9): 1479–82.

146 Klawiter EC, Alvarez E, 3rd, Xu J, Paciorkowski AR, Zhu L, Parks BJ, et al. NMO-IgG detected in CSF in seronegative neuromyelitis optica. Neurology 2009 Mar; 72(12): 1101–3.

147 Wingerchuk DM, Pittock SJ, Lucchinetti CF, Lennon VA, Weinshenker BG. A secondary progressive clinical course is uncommon in neuromyelitis optica. Neurology 2007 Feb 20; 68(8): 603–5.

CHAPTER 6

Magnetic Resonance Imaging in Multiple Sclerosis

Mohit Neema, Antonia Ceccarelli, Jonathan S. Jackson, and Rohit Bakshi

Laboratory for Neuroimaging Research, Partners Multiple Sclerosis Center, Brigham, and Women's Hospital, and Department of Neurology, Harvard Medical School, Boston, MA, USA

Introduction

Magnetic resonance imaging (MRI) plays a critical role in the early diagnosis and monitoring of various neurologic disorders including multiple sclerosis (MS). MRI has emerged as a key supportive outcome measure in MS-related clinical trials [1–2]. Studies examining conventional MRI atrophy and lesion (T2-hyperintense, T1-hypointense, and gadolinium (Gd)-enhancing) measures have enabled significant progress in research and clinical care related to MS [1–2]. However, these conventional measures do not provide a complete picture of the underlying pathology and lack the sensitivity and specificity required to describe the current disease status and predict the risk of disease progression [3].

Advanced MRI measures such as magnetization transfer (MT), magnetic resonance spectroscopy (MRS), diffusion imaging, and relaxometry, are relatively more specific and sensitive for the underlying pathology [4] and are able to capture diffuse occult disease occurring throughout the central nervous system (CNS). Such techniques may help to resolve the dissociation between clinical and conventional MRI findings, with the potential to revolutionize research and clinical care in MS.

This chapter provides an overview of the array of tools currently available with MRI technology as it is applied to brain and spinal cord imaging in patients with MS.

Multiple Sclerosis: Diagnosis and Therapy, First Edition. Edited by Howard L. Weiner and James M. Stankiewicz. © 2012 John Wiley & Sons, Ltd. Published 2012 by John Wiley and Sons, Ltd.

T2-Hyperintense lesions

T2-weighted spin-echo MR images of the CNS reveal MS plaques as bright areas of signal abnormality, which are typically referred to as T2-hyperintense lesions (Figure 6.1). The pathological features of T2-hyperintense lesions are entirely nonspecific, and the underlying causes consist of varying degrees of inflammation, demyelination, gliosis, edema, Wallerian degeneration, and axonal damage [5]. T2-hyperintense lesions in the brain are typically oval to ovoid in shape and greater than 5 mm in diameter (Figure 6.1). Lesions commonly affect the periventricular white matter (WM) regions, the inner surface of the corpus callosum, the juxtacortical gray–white junction, the infratentorial brain regions, and the spinal cord. In many patients, finger-like hyperintensities perpendicular to the lateral ventricles can be appreciated. These so-called "Dawson's fingers" reflect the typical perivenular location of inflammation in MS-related WM lesions (Figure 6.1).

TOP TIPS 6.1: T2-Hyperintense lesions

- T2-hyperintense lesions are nonspecific for the underlying MS pathology and may reflect varying degrees of inflammation, demyelination, gliosis, edema, and tissue loss.
- In cross-sectional studies, T2-hyperintense lesions show unreliable correlations with clinical status.
- T2-hyperintense lesions have longitudinal predictive value for disease progression in established MS and conversion from clinically isolated syndromes to definite MS.

Various advanced MR sequences such as fluid-attenuated inversion recovery (FLAIR), and double inversion recovery (DIR) have been applied to increase the sensitivity to MS lesions [1–2]. However, while these provide

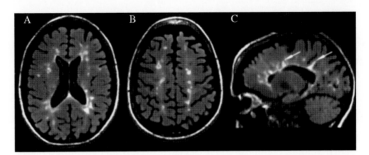

Figure 6.1 Hyperintense lesions in multiple sclerosis (MS): A to C are fluid-attenuated inversion-recovery (FLAIR) images of a patient with relapsing-remitting MS. Note the typical ovoid hyperintense lesions seen in the periventricular white matter and juxtacortical gray–white junction. Several of the periventricular lesions directly contact the ventricular ependyma. In addition, most of the lesions are 5 mm or greater in diameter. The sagittal image (C) reveals "Dawson's fingers" (arrows), which reflect the typical perivenular orientation of the inflammation seen in MS-related WM lesions

enhanced lesion detection in certain areas, conventional sequences perform better in others. For example, conventional T2-weighted images are relatively less sensitive than FLAIR and DIR in detecting periventricular and cortical–juxtacortical lesions (see section on cortical lesions) [6]. Conversely, FLAIR is relatively insensitive to lesions in the posterior fossa and spinal cord due to flow-related artifacts. High-field MRI [i.e. 3 Tesla (T) and higher] further enhances the sensitivity and yield of lesions detection than 1.5 T scanners [7–8].

Newly formed T2-hyperintense lesions have a variable course of evolution. Some lesions may resolve and wane over time [9]; most, however, chronically persist as "footprints" of damage (Figure 6.2). Brain T2-hyperintense lesions in both cross-sectional and longitudinal studies have shown unreliable correlations with clinical status as measured by the Expanded Disability Status Scale (EDSS) [3]. This so-called clinical-MRI paradox has been attributed to many factors, including the failure of T2-weighted images to characterize diffuse disease, the compensatory abilities of brain tissue, the presence of spinal cord disease, and the limitations of the clinical rating scale. Nonetheless, the degree of T2-hyperintense lesions assumes clinical significance early in the disease course of MS and has a prognostic value in predicting conversion from a clinically isolated syndrome (CIS) to clinically definite MS [10]. T2- lesion-based measures have also been used to monitor the therapeutic value of various drugs [1–2]. One of the major limitations in

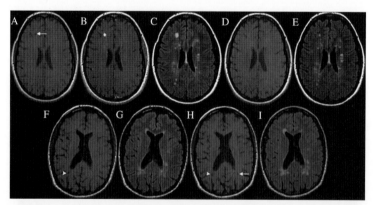

Figure 6.2 Black holes (BHs) in multiple sclerosis (MS): Transient (top panel) and chronic (lower panel). A, B, D, F, and H are T1-weighted images. B is a postcontrast (gadolinium) T1-weighted image. C, E, G, and I are fluid-attenuated inversion recovery (FLAIR) images. A to E are from a patient with relapsing-remitting MS. The baseline images (A–C) show a newly formed BH (arrow). Ten months later (D, E), the BH has resolved on the T1-weighted image with a small residual lesion remaining on the FLAIR image. F to I are from a patient with relapsing-remitting MS. The baseline images (F, G) show various BHs (arrowhead). Eleven months later (H, I), the BHs are persistent on the T1-weighted image (arrowhead) with new BHs appearing on the T1-weighted image (H: arrow).

using T2 lesion load as a longitudinal measure is the plateauing relationship between T2 lesion load and disability [11], reflecting in part the engulfing of T2-hyperintensities by the expanding cerebrospinal fluid (CSF) spaces.

T1-Hypointense lesions

A subset of MS plaques seen on conventional T2-weighted and FLAIR images in the brain may appear dark on corresponding T1-weighted images in comparison to surrounding normal appearing WM (NAWM) (Figure 6.2). These dark hypointense lesions on T1-spin-echo images are commonly referred to as "black holes" (BHs). BHs are rarely observed in the posterior fossa and spinal cord.

The pathological correlates of BHs are nonspecific in the acute phase; however, they become more specific when persisting for 6–12 months [12]. BHs initially start as Gd-enhancing lesions, and evolve into one of two categories of lesions: transient (reversible) or chronic (persistent) (Figure 6.2). About half of the newly formed BHs disappear within 6–12 months and revert back to isointensity as a result of remyelination and resolution of edema/inflammation. BHs that persist for more than 12 months are especially likely to reflect severe irreversible demyelination and axonal loss [13–15].

TOP TIPS 6.2: Hypointense lesions or black holes (BHs)

- Categorized as transient (reversible) or chronic (persistent – lasting more than 6–12 months).
- Transient BHs primarily reflect edema and partial demyelination with subsequent repair/recovery.
- Chronic BHs reflect severe irreversible demyelination and axonal loss and show better correlations with disability than T2-hyperintense lesions.

Patients with secondary progressive MS (SPMS) and primary progressive MS (PPMS) have a tendency to show a higher BH lesion load than patients with relapsing-remitting MS (RRMS) [16]. Significant correlations have been found between BHs and neurologic disability in some but not all cross-sectional and longitudinal studies. Global BH volume tends to show better correlations with clinical status than does a conventional T2 lesion load [12]. While the global BH lesion load has served as a useful marker to evaluate the treatment effect of various MS-related drugs [2, 17], the interpretation of these studies is complicated by the potential for resolution of individual BHs. Longitudinal analysis of the evolution of each newly formed BH can overcome this limitation [18–19]. The ratio of T2-hyperintense lesions that subsequently develop into black holes (T1/T2 ratio) may also be used as an alternate approach to characterize the destructive potential of individual lesions [20].

Blood–brain barrier compromise

MS is characterized by disruption of the blood–brain barrier (BBB). It is still unknown whether BBB disruption is the initial event that triggers MS lesion formation or a secondary effect of damage occurring in the CNS parenchyma. Conventional T1-spin-echo imaging before and after infusion of an intravenous Gd contrast agent is routinely used to detect damage to the BBB [21]. The contrast agent reduces the T1 relaxation time causing lesions to appear bright and enters the brain parenchyma only in areas of BBB disruption (Figure 6.3). Gd enhancement usually precedes or accompanies new T2-hyperintense lesion formation and lasts for an average of three (range 2–12) weeks [22]. Methodological improvements, for example delivering an off-resonance MT pulse, delaying the scanning by more than 5 minutes after Gd injection, increasing the Gd dose, or applying higher field MRI, have considerably enhanced the sensitivity in detecting such lesions [2]. Subtle BBB disruptions that are missed on visual inspection can also be detected using quantitative T1-relaxometry analysis [23].

TOP TIPS 6.3: Gadolinium (Gd)-enhancing lesions

- Represent blood–brain barrier disruption and passage of blood-borne lymphocytes into the central nervous system.
- Usually precedes or accompanies new T2-hyperintense lesion formation but disappears after an average of 3 weeks.
- Occur more frequently in the early stages than in the late progressive clinical stages.
- Show poor correlations with disability.
- Are more common than relapses, providing a useful marker for monitoring subclinical disease activity.

Various morphologic types of T1-lesions such as concentric ring, open ring, heterogeneous, tumor-like and homogeneous enhancing lesions (Figure 6.3) have been described in patients with MS, with the latter being most common [24–27]. Each subtype shows a diversity of pathological changes, which may include inflammation, edema, and demyelination. Open ring lesions are fairly specific for MS, but are uncommon [24]. Ring-enhancing lesions exhibit higher levels of tissue damage compared with homogeneously enhancing lesions [26], and thus tend to resolve more slowly and are at higher risk for conversion to chronic T1-hypointense lesions [27].

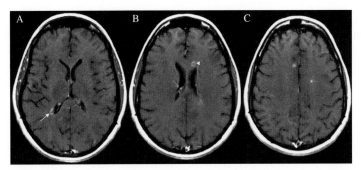

Figure 6.3 Gadolinium (Gd)-enhancing lesions in multiple sclerosis (MS): Post-Gd T1-weighted spin-echo images (A–C) of a patient with relapsing-remitting MS showing multiple-enhancing lesions. The open-ring pattern of enhancement (A: arrow) is typical of MS. Other morphologic types such as concentric ring (B: arrowhead), heterogeneous (B, C), and homogeneous (C) enhancing lesions can also be seen, with the latter being most common.

Gd enhancement typically occurs at a higher rate in the early RR stage than the late progressive SP stage in MS. While Gd-enhancing lesions serve as a useful marker for monitoring active disease and outcome measure in MS drug trials, they often are clinically inert and therefore show a poor correlation with current clinical status [28] and disability progression [29]. However, their presence reflects increased risk of continuous disease activity [30] and the short-term appearance of clinical relapses [31].

Concerns about the frequent use of Gd-based contrast agent in MRI studies have arisen as a result of its association with nephrogenic systemic fibrosis [32]. Newer, safer cell and molecule specific contrast agents for BBB disruption are being developed and tested and show promise in increasing sensitivity while reducing the risk of toxicity [33]. Recently, a new contrast agent based on ultra-small superparamagnetic particles of iron oxide (USPIO) has been used for tracking macrophage infiltration in the CNS. Such agents may provide more precise information about the pathophysiologic cascade of the inflammatory events in-vivo in MS [34–35].

T1 and T2 shortening

On noncontrast T1-weighted spin-echo images, MS plaques may show abnormal bright signal (areas of T1 shortening). Such lesions are commonly called T1-hyperintense lesions [36–37]. T1 shortening in MS lesions most likely represents iron deposition, but may also reflect of paramagnetic free radicals, abnormal accumulation of protein (albumin) secondary to blood–brain barrier disruption, or macrophage infiltration [37]. An initial study indicates that the presence of T1-hyperintense lesions is more common with advancing physical disability, brain atrophy, and a progressive disease course in patients with MS [37].

TOP TIPS 6.4: T1 and T2 shortening

- T1 shortening in WM lesions may reflect iron deposition.
- T1 shortening in lesions is associated with clinical disability and brain atrophy.
- T2 shortening (T2 hypointensity) is widespread in MS GM vs. healthy normal controls and most likely represents iron deposition.
- GM T2 hypointensity is related to brain atrophy, physical disability, disability progression and cognitive impairment.

A common finding in patients with MS on spin-echo T2-weighted images is diffuse hypointensity of the cortical and deep gray matter (GM) areas (e.g. the red nucleus, thalamus, dentate nucleus, lentiform nucleus, caudate, and rolandic cortex) compared to age-matched normal controls (Figure 6.4) [38–39]. This T2 hypointensity, reflecting T2 shortening most likely represents pathological iron deposition as shown by both animal and human histologic-MRI correlation studies [40–41], magnetic field correlation imaging at 3 T [42], phase imaging at 7 T [43] and relaxometry [44]. T2 hypointensity in the GM has been shown to be associated with brain atrophy, physical disability, disability progression, and cognitive impairment in patients with MS [39, 45]. Excessive iron deposition in the GM may contribute to the pathophysiology of MS through the Fenton reaction and the resulting generation of free radicals. However, it remains

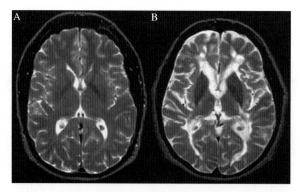

Figure 6.4 T2 hypointensity in multiple sclerosis (MS): T2-weighted fast spin-echo axial MRI scans obtained at 1.5 T of a healthy control (A) in the fifth decade and an age-matched patient with relapsing-remitting MS (B). In the patient with MS, note the bilateral hypointensity of various deep gray matter areas, including the thalamus, lentiform nucleus, and caudate compared to the healthy control. This T2 hypointensity most likely represents pathological iron deposition. The patient also has brain atrophy.

unknown whether iron deposition is purely an epiphenomenon, resulting from tissue degeneration or if it contributes directly to neurotoxicity in the GM.

Proton magnetic resonance spectroscopy

Biochemical changes in neurological disorders including MS can be investigated by proton MRS, a technique that reveals the relative concentration of key metabolites in-vivo. Altered concentrations of various CNS metabolites have been found in MS, including N-acetylaspartate *(NAA)*, creatine *(Cr)*, choline *(Cho)*, lactate *(Lac)*, lipids, myoinositol *(mI)*, and glutamate/glutamine [46]. These metabolites may be useful as indicators of specific pathological processes. For example, in patients with MS, decreased *NAA* is proposed as a marker for the loss of axonal/neuronal integrity, increased *Cho* indicates membrane turnover such as that seen with inflammation and demyelination/remyelination, increased *Lac* indicates energy failure, increased lipid represents myelin breakdown or necrosis, increased *Cr* and *mI* reflects gliosis, and increased glutamate/glutamine levels reflects excitotoxicity [46]. Other metabolites such as glutathione, ascorbic acid, gamma-aminobutyric acid and macromolecules related to myelin (valine, alanine, leucine, isoleucine, and threonine) can be detected with special post-processing techniques at high field strength MRI (3 T or higher) [4]. Thus, MRS measures can be useful to characterize the involvement of processes such as inflammation, demyelination, neuroaxonal injury, oxidative stress, and neurodegeneration in the different subtypes and stages of MS. They can also be used to study the therapeutic effect of immunotherapy [47].

> ### TOP TIPS 6.5: Proton magnetic resonance spectroscopy
>
> - MRS reveals the concentration of key metabolites in vivo, which are thought to reflect specific aspects of the underlying pathology.
> - Decreased NAA reflects axonal/neuronal loss or injury and correlates with clinical disability.
> - Increased choline reflects demyelination and inflammation.
> - Increased myoinositol reflects gliosis.

MRS has added much to our understanding of the natural evolution of MS lesions and microscopic changes occurring in normal appearing brain tissue. Newly formed Gd-enhancing lesions often show elevated *Cho, Lac, Cr, mI,* glutamate and lipids and reduced *NAA* [48–49]. The extent of recovery of these metabolites is highly variable during the course of the disease. While

Lac, Cho, Cr, and lipids levels appear normal in most lesions after an initial surge, suggestive of remyelination and the resolution of edema [50], *NAA* tends to remain persistently low or shows only partial recovery [51], which is indicative of irreversible axonal injury/loss. Both NAWM and normal appearing GM (NAGM) show altered levels of these metabolites. Regional and whole-brain MRS studies show that occult changes in normal appearing brain tissue may appear early in the disease course [52] and months before the development of T2-hyperintense lesions [51], indicating that intrinsic brain parenchymal changes may precede the development of visible MS plaques. There is evidence from both cross-sectional and longitudinal studies that MRS measures, in particular *NAA*, in WM and GM show relatively better correlations with clinical measures of disability (i.e. cognitive dysfunction and physical disability) than conventional MRI measures suggesting that MRS measures can be employed to monitor disease progression and predict the development of disability. MRS has also been applied to the study of spinal cord disease in MS [46].

While MRS may not be practical for routine clinical use in the near future, MRS research continues to increase sensitivity to new metabolites and yields valuable new information about MS disease processes and progression.

Magnetization transfer imaging

MTI is a technique utilizing the exchange of protons between the free water pool and the macromolecular-bound water pool. The loss of macromolecules associated with demyelination and axonal damage in MS leads to a reduced water (proton) exchange between these two pools. MTI is able to capture these subtle tissue changes in the form of a decreased magnetization transfer ratio (MTR) [53]. Inflammation, gliosis, and edema can also contribute to decreased MTR [53]. A recovery of MTR is thought to primarily reflect remyelination and repair [54]. Quantitative MTI techniques have been developed to increase the specificity and sensitivity for myelin detection [55–56].

Serial MTI studies have yielded useful information on the development of new MS lesions and the extent of damage during their evolution over time. A new Gd-enhancing lesion initially shows a decreased MTR, which over time can either return to normal or remain low [53]. While a transient recovery in the MTR signal is suggestive of partial remyelination and reduced inflammation [53, 56], a substantial reduction of MTR in such lesions is indicative of severe tissue damage (axonal loss and demyelination) and is associated with an increased risk of conversion to chronic BHs [12]. MTR reduction in lesions is more apparent in the progressive stages of MS and is more closely related to physical disability than overt T2 lesion load [53]. Advanced approaches to MTI analysis including voxel wise analysis, which is used to track demyelination and remyelination in individual lesions, and atlas-based analysis, which classifies lesions in chronological order [57–58] have been developed to further characterize changes in lesions. These developments may improve our understanding of the correlates of disability and help to improve the monitor efficacy of neuroprotective agents MS [53].

TOP TIPS 6.6: Magnetization transfer imaging (MTI)

- MS-related demyelination and axonal damage leads to a decreased magnetization transfer ratio (MTR).
- Decreased MTR in lesions and normal appearing brain parenchyma (WM and GM) shows significant correlations with clinical disability.
- MTI can detect subtle pathology, preceding by several months, the appearance of overt lesions.

MTI is particularly useful in capturing diffuse abnormalities in normal appearing brain tissue that escape detection by conventional MRI. NAWM and NAGM MTR decreases have been observed in all MS phenotypic subtypes, with more pronounced reductions in the advanced stages [53]. Regional NAGM MTR reductions have been observed in some but not all studies [59]. Nonetheless, diffuse MTR changes can be detected early in the disease course [60], and can precede the formation of overt lesions by several months [61]. NAWM adjacent to T2-hyperintese lesions shows significantly lower MTR than regions distant to lesions, suggesting that the extent of damage in MS lesions is greater than shown by conventional MRI [53].

Numerous MTI studies have revealed that the degree of MTR reduction in lesions, NAWM and NAGM, is associated with disability and cognitive impairment [53]. Longitudinal studies suggest that MTR may be a sensitive marker for predicting subsequent disability and monitoring disease progression [62–63]. Advanced voxel-based MTI analyses may clarify the relationship between the location of damage and its functional impact (disability and cognitive function), which thus far has proved elusive [64]. MTI has also been used to characterize spinal cord disease [53, 65].

MTI has advantages over conventional MRI, in particular it is useful for monitoring the evolution of lesion damage, normal appearing parenchymal changes, and testing experimental treatment in MS. However, despite efforts to standardize MTI acquisition, MTI is currently more widely used in research settings than in MS clinical trials [66]. Hopefully, with better MRI technology and post-processing software, MTI can become a common modality in drug trials and clinical settings.

Diffusion imaging

Water diffusion in brain tissue can be estimated using diffusion-weighted imaging (DWI), while diffusion tensor imaging (DTI) [67] allows characterization of the preferential diffusion of water along WM tracts. The apparent diffusion coefficient (ADC), derived from DWI, is increased in pathological conditions including MS and reflects nonspecific tissue changes such as demyelination, gliosis, inflammation, and axonal damage [68]. In addition to mapping water diffusion, as the mean diffusivity (MD), DTI provides the fractional anisotropy (FA), a measure of preferential diffusion of water along one spatial direction [67]. Furthermore, DTI forms the basis for tractography, which can be used to define WM tracts and assess connectivity between regions (Plate 6.1). Both MD and FA are altered in MS [69] and principally reflect axonal and myelin damage [70]. However, other factors such as gliosis, edema, and inflammation also contribute to diffusivity changes. Improved pathological specificity can be obtained by investigating the axial and radial diffusivity from DTI images, which are proposed markers of axonal integrity and myelin content respectively [71].

Diffusion imaging has been a valuable tool for examining the biophysical nature of focal and diffuse brain parenchymal changes in MS. In general, T2-hyperintense MS lesions are characterized by increased ADC and MD, with decreased FA compared to adjacent NAWM. Lesions that appear as BHs on T1-weighted images show pronounced diffusivity changes indicating irreversible tissue loss, axonal damage, and gliosis. However, with enhancing lesions, inconsistent results have been reported regarding diffusivity changes and the underlying pathological substrates [72]. Outside visible MS lesions, DTI is extremely sensitive for detecting occult diffuse tissue damage in MS. DTI changes in NAWM (increased MD with decreased FA) and NAGM (increased MD) have been found in the early phases of the disease [73–74] with more pronounced changes in the advanced phases of MS [69].

TOP TIPS 6.7: Diffusion imaging

- MR diffusion imaging, maps the diffusion of water movement in tissue, and includes scalar diffusion-weighted imaging (DWI) and three-dimensional diffusion tensor imaging (DTI)

- Diffusion abnormalities (increased MD and ADC with reduced FA) have been described in focal lesions as well as normal appearing parenchymal tissue throughout the central nervous system

- Occurring in the early stages, diffusion abnormalities are believed to reflect primarily axonal and myelin damage but are also influenced by gliosis, edema, and inflammation

Various studies have looked at the clinical relevance of DTI measures in patients with MS and have shown better correlations with neurological dysfunction than conventional MRI measures in both cross-sectional and longitudinal studies [69]. Regional DTI analyses have provided additional insights into the structural changes associated with disability and cognitive dysfunction in MS [75–77]. The integrity of WM tracts in specific neuronal circuits, such as the motor or cognitive networks, can be evaluated using DTI-based tractography [78]. Diffusivity changes in the corticospinal tract [79–80] and corpus callosum [81] have correlated with motor and cognitive impairment better than T2 lesion burden and global diffusivity changes suggesting that damage in clinically eloquent brain regions contributes significantly to clinical dysfunctions in MS. Due to its ability to detect longitudinal changes [66], DTI has been proposed, but not formally tested in clinical trials for the evaluation of therapies [82] and monitoring of disease progression in MS [69]. In addition, DTI has been used to evaluate spinal cord damage in MS [69, 83].

Diffusion imaging has the potential to contribute to the understanding of MS pathological processes, particularly in the longitudinal evaluation of axonal damage in MS lesions and in normal appearing brain tissue. While diffusion imaging has made significant advances, its current use is restricted to research settings in MS. Like other advanced techniques (MRS and MTR), questions on the best methodology and interpretation of diffusion imaging data still remain before it can be widely applied to clinical trials and in individual patients [69, 84].

T1 and T2 relaxometry

Pathological changes in lesions on T1- and T2-weighted conventional MRI can be quantified using MR T1 and T2 relaxometry. Furthermore, diffuse changes not apparent with conventional imaging can be measured precisely using these techniques. These relaxation times differ between tissue types, providing the principal source of image contrast in conventional imaging. Owing to the sensitivity of T2 and T1 to changes in water content (e.g. reflecting inflammation and macromolecular density) and iron deposition, relaxometry is a powerful means of assessing MS pathology [85].

T1 relaxometry maps the longitudinal relaxation time, T1, reflecting the time taken for the magnetization to recover following a radio frequency pulse. The inversion-recovery sequence remains the gold standard for T1 measurement, by fitting a mono-exponential curve to data acquired at a range of different inversion times [86]. Other faster techniques such as the saturation-recovery method (data acquired for a range of different repetition times) [86] and Look-Locker [87] sequences are widely used for whole-brain T1 measurements. T1 relaxation changes are widespread in MS including lesions, NAWM, and NAGM areas. These changes are non-specific however, with diverse processes including edema, axonal loss, demyelination and gliosis contributing to T1 prolongation [85]. Globally, NAWM and NAGM T1 relaxation times are higher in MS than controls, and higher in SPMS compared to RRMS and PPMS [88]. Normal appearing GM and WM T1 increases have been found over time in all subtypes of MS (RR, SP, and PP). Some studies have indicated a link between global T1 measures and clinical disability [88–89], while others found no association [90].

TOP TIPS 6.8: T1 and T2 relaxometry

- Focal and diffuse changes are observed throughout the brain with T1 and T2 relaxometry, increasing with disease duration.
- While axonal loss is the primary correlate, T1 prolongation can reflect a variety of pathological changes.
- Myelin water mapping using multicomponent T2 may allow the monitoring of myelination status in MS.

T2 relaxometry maps the transverse relaxation time, T2, which reflects the time for the signal to dephase following a radio frequency pulse. To measure T2, an exponential function is fitted to the MRI signal measured at a number of different echo times. While T1 is well represented by a single exponential component in brain tissues, T2 in general follows a multi-exponential decay, reflecting different tissue water pools relaxing at different rates [85]. The short T2 component of the multi-exponential decay indicates myelin water (Plate 6.2) [91–92], while the intermediate component reflects intra- and extracellular water, and the longer component reflects CSF. Estimating the intermediate component from images at two different echo times [91] reveals global T2 prolongation in NAWM as well as lesions [91, 93]. Acquiring more echoes allows separation of the different components for increased specificity to pathological substrates. Myelin water mapping – a technique estimating the short T2 component – has shown reductions in myelin water fraction in both MS lesions and NAWM [94], and can allow longitudinal monitoring of demyelination and remyelination in MS [95]. The emergence of a long T2 component has been observed in areas of BBB breakdown and edema [96]. Presently, studies of NAWM have failed to find an association between disability (EDSS) and the intermediate component of T2 [93, 97], however a moderate association has been found with the myelin water fraction [98].

T1 and T2 relaxometry allow a more objective assessment of disease burden, both in visible lesions and in the normal brain parenchymal tissue, compared to conventional estimates of lesion load that are somewhat subjective. These measures can provide a good assessment of disease burden, however the unreliable association with concurrent disability and disability progression indicates that the clinical relevance of these techniques requires further investigation. Although sensitive, relaxation time measurements are not specific to pathology, for example while increased water content causes T2 and T1 prolongation, increased iron deposition results in T1 and T2 shortening [39]. Increased specificity to pathological substrates has been demonstrated by multi-component techniques such as myelin water mapping, which has potential for the investigation and monitoring of MS disease processes in-vivo [85].

Brain atrophy

Brain atrophy is a well-established and a clinically relevant component of MS pathology. It reflects irreversible tissue loss and is likely a pathologically nonspecific by-product of diverse underlying mechanisms. Measures of global and regional atrophy are suitable biomarkers of disease severity and progression in clinical research and therapeutic trials [1, 2, 99].

On MRI images, brain atrophy manifests as the enlargement of cerebro-spinal fluid (CSF) spaces, including sulci, cisterns, fissures, and the ventricular system, combined with reduced size of parenchymal structures, in comparison with age-matched healthy controls (Figure 6.5). In addition to visual inspection, the ventricular width (lateral and third), intercaudate distance and area of the corpus callosum on a sagittal section are quantitative markers for atrophy that can be implemented readily in a clinical setting [99].

Global brain atrophy is thought to occur as a consequence of focal and diffuse parenchymal damage. Evidence suggests a link between atrophy and diffuse changes in the normal appearing brain tissue, seen as decreased NAA [100], decreased MTR [101], and increased diffusivity [102]. Atrophy is also moderately associated with both T2 WM lesions [103] and cortical GM lesions [104]. The relative contribution of focal and diffuse pathology however remains unclear.

TOP TIPS 6.9: Brain atrophy

- Brain atrophy is a consequence of focal and diffuse damage in MS.
- It begins in the early stages and continues throughout the disease.
- Moderate correlations are found with disability and cognitive processes.
- Gray matter loss, in particular in subcortical structures, may be a better marker of disease progression than whole brain or white matter fractions.

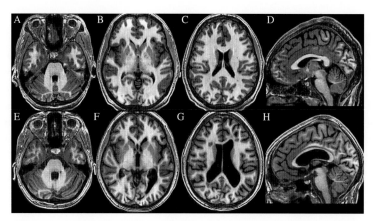

Figure 6.5 Brain atrophy in multiple sclerosis (MS): Qualitative comparison of a noncontrast T1-weighted modified driven equilibrium Fourier transform (MDEFT) MRI scans performed at 3 T in our center of a healthy control in the fourth decade (A–D) versus an age-matched patient with relapsing-remitting MS (E–H). Note the widespread enlargement ventricular cerebrospinal fluid (CSF) spaces and callosum thinning in the patient with MS compared to the healthy control.

Atrophy can be seen using MRI from the earliest stages of the disease in CIS patients prior to conversion to clinically definitive MS [99]. The annual rate of brain parenchymal volume loss is estimated to be in the range 0.5–1.4% in all stages of MS, compared to 0–0.3% for control subjects, with slight variations seen between populations and measurement methods [105]. Brain volume loss is associated with disease duration, and SPMS patients have smaller brain volumes than RRMS and PPMS patients. Whole brain atrophy correlates better with clinical status (including both physical disability and cognitive impairment) than conventional T2 lesion measures, and early atrophy appears related to future disability [99].

While focal WM damage is more apparent on conventional MRI as described above, GM pathology is also known to play a significant role in the clinical status of patients with MS. Many recent studies have used automated image segmentation tools to independently assess the relationship between GM and WM atrophy, and clinical variables [99]. Reduced GM and WM volume compared to healthy controls is a consistent finding in cross-sectional studies, however longitudinal studies in general observe a reduction of GM volume without an accompanying WM volume loss [106]. This may indicate that GM volume change is the more sensitive marker for disease progression. GM loss follows a different pattern of regional distribution according to clinical subtype [107]. GM atrophy is more strongly associated with both disability and cognitive dysfunction than whole brain or WM atrophy [108–109]. Measurement of CNS volume can also be affected by nonpathological factors such as medication effects and hydration status, and WM volume in particular may fluctuate due to the inflammation and gliosis that occur to a greater extent in WM compared to GM lesions in MS [99].

While the association with disability and cognitive function shown by whole brain and GM volume measures is moderate at best, regional volumetric analyses have revealed stronger relationships between specific functional domains and the associated GM areas [110]. For example, thalamic atrophy consistently shows a stronger association with cognitive deficits than cortical GM volume [111]. The degree of atrophy in the deep gray nuclei is also proportionately higher than cerebral GM or the whole brain [112–113]. Cortical thickness analyses [114] (Plate 6.3) are also a valuable tool to investigate GM pathology in-vivo, with cortical thinning observed in many areas including frontal and temporal lobes [99], in agreement with the distribution of demyelination in the cortex observed in histopathological studies [115]. These advanced measures have the potential to further increase the sensitivity and specificity of atrophy measures as a surrogate maker of disease progression in clinical research and therapeutic trials.

Cortical lesions

Cortical lesions are some of the principal manifestations of GM disease in MS. Postmortem studies indicate that focal demyelinating lesions in the cortical GM involve a higher fraction of tissue than lesions affecting WM. Cortical lesions show a variety of pathological changes including demyelination, microglial activation, and neuronal apoptosis [116], and have been subdivided into morphologic subtypes based on histologic characteristics and location [117]. They are thought to be less inflammatory as compared to WM lesions [106], and the extent and distribution to which cortical demyelination is believed to be independent of WM pathology [118].

TOP TIPS 6.10: Cortical lesions

- Cortical demyelination can be widespread in multiple sclerosis.
- Cortical lesions are rarely visible on conventional MRI.
- The double inversion recovery (DIR) sequence allows visualization of these lesions by suppressing the signal from white matter and cerebrospinal fluid.
- Cortical lesions appear progressively throughout the disease course and are associated with gray matter atrophy, cognitive impairment, and disability.

FLAIR and T2-weighted imaging at clinical field strengths has a limited ability to detect cortical lesions [119]. This is due to the poor contrast resolution between GM lesion and normal-appearing GM, and contamination with the CSF and WM signal (partial-volume effects). Significant improvement in cortical lesion detection can be achieved by using the double inversion recovery (DIR) sequence, which suppresses the signal from CSF and WM, at the higher field strength of 3 T [6, 7, 120]. An accompanying high-resolution T1-weighted structural scan [121] can aid in the differentiation between purely cortical and mixed GM–WM lesions, which is challenging using DIR or FLAIR images alone (Figure 6.6).

Cortical lesions appear early in the disease, and are present in all subtypes. Initial studies indicate that the accrual rate of new MR-visible cortical lesions is similar in both RRMS and SPMS [104]. The presence and accumulation of cortical lesions is associated with GM atrophy, disease duration, cognitive impairment, and physical disability [104, 122]. Furthermore, the cortical lesion load correlates more strongly with disability than the WM lesion load [123].

The detection of cortical lesions and classification into juxtacortical, intracortical and subpial subtypes remains challenging with MRI. Imaging at ultra-high field strengths (>3 T) allows better visualization of the relationship between lesions and the vasculature, and reveals iron deposition around cortical lesions, thought to be associated with macrophage activity [124]. While postmortem studies indicate that not all cortical lesions are MR visible, even with ultra-high field imaging [125], it is hoped that

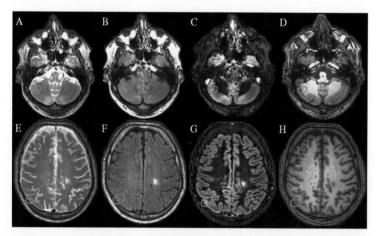

Figure 6.6 Gray matter (GM) lesions in multiple sclerosis (MS). GM MS lesions in cerebellum (A-D) and cerebral cortex (E-F) are poorly visualized on T2-weighted (A, E) and fluid-attenuated inversion recovery (FLAIR) (B, F) images. Bright regions (gray outline) in the cortical surface on a double inversion recovery (DIR) sequence are suggestive of GM lesions (C, G), with precise localization provided by the high-resolution T1-weighted fast gradient echo sequence (D, H). All scans were performed on a 3 T MRI system. Figure courtesy of Dr. Massimo Filippi.

techniques developed at ultra-high field will ultimately increase the sensitivity to cortical lesions possible with clinical scanners in the future [123].

Spinal cord imaging

Conventional T2-weighted imaging of the spinal cord can play an important role in the diagnosis of MS, with MR visible cord lesions found in the majority (>80%) of newly diagnosed MS patients [126]. In general, cord lesions are more likely to be symptomatic than brain lesions [127] but are also less common than brain lesions [128].

Imaging the spinal cord is challenging due to the relatively small size of the cord and the occurrence of imaging artifacts from CSF pulsation and cardiovascular and respiratory motion. Fast spin-echo PD/T2 imaging is widely used clinically for its specificity to lesions in the cord [129]. Greater lesion sensitivity can be achieved by the addition of STIR (short tau inversion recovery) or PSIR (phase-sensitive inversion recovery) sequences [130]. Active T2-cord lesions can be identified with Gd-enhanced T1-weighted imaging, however they occur less frequently than Gd-enhancing brain lesions.

Focal and diffuse abnormalities are both seen on T2 MRI in MS. In the RRMS stage, patients tend to have focal cord lesions. Later, in the SPMS stage, there is an increasing frequency of confluent lesions and diffuse abnormality, accompanied by cord atrophy [131]. In PPMS, cord abnormalities are extensive compared to brain abnormalities [132] and diffuse abnormalities are more common than in the other MS phenotypes [133]. Most focal lesions are found in the cervical cord, typically in the lateral and posterior columns including GM areas [134]. Despite the higher incidence of symptomatic lesions in the cord, physical disability correlates poorly with the total T2-hyperintense lesion volume seen with 1.5 T or 3 T MRI [135]. This is in agreement with the histopathological observation that axonal damage in the cord is largely independent of T2 lesions [136].

TOP TIPS 6.11: Spinal cord imaging

- Spinal cord imaging can be valuable in the diagnosis of MS.
- Cord abnormalities are associated with disease duration in all subtypes of MS, but are most extensive in primary progressive MS.
- Atrophy of the cervical cord is a useful surrogate of disease progression, while T2 cord lesions show a poor correlation with clinical status.
- Focal cord damage appears to occur mostly independently of WM lesions in the brain.

Measuring cord atrophy is challenging, but can yield strong correlations with clinical disability (EDSS) [137–138]. While early methods involved manual cord outlining, new techniques such as active-surface based contouring [138] promise to reduce analysis time and increase reproducibility. Still the changes seen in MS are small compared to the variability in the normal population, which limits the utility of this technique in the clinic. The cervical cord is often chosen as the region of interest as much of the disease effect is reflected here. In the absence of cord images, the medulla oblongata volume has been found to be a suitable biomarker for cord damage, correlating strongly with the upper cervical cord volume [139].

High-resolution quantitative MRI mapping of the cord in-vivo is an active area of research, promising to provide greater specificity and sensitivity to specific cord pathology [140]. Quantitative measures such as: T1 mapping, MTR, and diffusion anisotropy (in lesions, NAWM and DAWM) show strong correlation with both myelin content and axonal density in a histopathological postmortem study at 7 T [141]. It should be noted, however, that other studies at 4.7 T suggest that MR visible changes reflect demyelination rather than axonal loss [142]. In-vivo, diffuse T1 changes have been found in the cervical cord, with T1 significantly increased in patients compared to controls, and in SPMS compared to RRMS. These T1 changes correlate with cervical cord area, brain NAWM T1, and physical disability [143]. This suggests that a relationship may exist between diffuse changes in the brain and spinal cord, where no similar relationship is apparent for focal abnormalities. Similarly, DTI [83] and MTI [65] measures in the cervical cord have shown a significant relationship with clinical disability.

Acknowledgments

This work was supported by research grants from the National Institutes of Health (NIH-NINDS K23 NS42379-01 and R01 NS055083-01) and National Multiple Sclerosis Society (RG3705A1; RG3798A2). We would like to thank Drs Massimo Filippi and Daniel Goldberg-Zimring for use of their figures. We also thank all the members of the Laboratory for Neuroimaging Research and the clinical staff at the Partners MS Center who have made all of our work possible.

References

1 Bakshi R, Minagar A, Jaisani Z, Wolinsky JS. Imaging of multiple sclerosis: role in neurotherapeutics. NeuroRx 2005; 2: 277–303.
2 Neema M, Stankiewicz J, Arora A, Guss ZD, Bakshi R. MRI in multiple sclerosis: what's inside the toolbox? Neurotherapeutics 2007; 4: 602–17.
3 Filippi M, Rocca MA. Conventional MRI in multiple sclerosis. J Neuroimag 2007; 17: 3S–9S.

4 Bakshi R, Thompson AJ, Rocca MA, Pelletier D, Dousset V, Barkhof F, et al. MRI in multiple sclerosis: current status and future prospects. Lancet Neurol 2008; 7: 615–25.

5 Bruck W, Bitsch A, Kolenda H, Brück Y, Stiefel M, Lassmann H. Inflammatory central nervous system demyelination: correlation of magnetic resonance imaging findings with lesion pathology. Ann Neurol 1997; 42: 783–93.

6 Geurts JJ, Pouwels PJ, Uitdehaag BM, Polman CH, Barkhof F, Castelijns JA. Intracortical lesions in multiple sclerosis: improved detection with 3D double inversion-recovery MR imaging. Radiology 2005; 236: 254–60.

7 Wattjes MP, Barkhof F. High field MRI in the diagnosis of multiple sclerosis: high field-high yield? Neuroradiology 2009; 51: 279–22.

8 Stankiewicz JM, Glanz BI, Healy BC, Arora A, Neema M, Benedict RH, et al. Brain MRI lesion load at 1.5T and 3T versus clinical status in multiple sclerosis. J Neuroimag 2011; 21(2): e50–6.

9 Meier DS, Weiner HL, Guttmann CR. Time-series modeling of multiple sclerosis disease activity: a promising window on disease progression and repair potential? Neurotherapeutics 2007; 4: 485–98.

10 Brex PA, Ciccarelli O, O'Riordan JI, Sailer M, Thompson AJ, Miller DH. A longitudinal study of abnormalities on MRI and disability from multiple sclerosis. N Engl J Med 2002; 346: 158–64.

11 Li DK, Held U, Petkau J, Daumer M, Barkhof F, Fazekas F, et al. MRI T2 lesion burden in multiple sclerosis: a plateauing relationship with clinical disability. Neurology 2006; 66: 1384–9.

12 Sahraian MA, Radue EW, Haller S, Kappos L. Black holes in multiple sclerosis: definition, evolution, and clinical correlations. Acta Neurol Scand 2010; 122: 1–8.

13 Truyen L, van Waesberghe JH, van Walderveen MA, van Oosten BW, Polman CH, Hommes OR, et al. Accumulation of hypointense lesions ("black holes") on T1 spin-echo MRI correlates with disease progression in multiple sclerosis. Neurology 1996; 47: 1469–76.

14 Bitsch A, Kuhlmann T, Stadelmann C, Lassmann H, Lucchinetti C, Brueck W. A longitudinal MRI study of histopathologically defined hypointense multiple sclerosis lesions. Ann Neurol 2001; 49: 793–6.

15 Fisher E, Chang A, Fox RJ, Tkach JA, Svarovsky T, Nakamura K, et al. Imaging correlates of axonal swelling in chronic multiple sclerosis brains. Ann Neurol 2007; 62: 219–28.

16 van Walderveen MA, Lycklama ANijeholt GJ, Adèr HJ, Jongen PJ, Polman CH, Castelijns JA, et al. Hypointense lesions on T1-weighted spin-echo magnetic resonance imaging: relation to clinical characteristics in subgroups of patients with multiple sclerosis. Arch Neurol 2001; 58: 76–81.

17 Molyneux PD, Brex PA, Fogg C, Lewis S, Middleditch C, Barkhof F, et al. The precision of T1 hypointense lesion volume quantification in multiple sclerosis treatment trials: a multicenter study. Mult Scler 2000; 6: 237–40.

18 Filippi M, Rovaris M, Rocca MA, Sormani MP, Wolinsky JS, Comi G. Glatiramer acetate reduces the proportion of new MS lesions evolving into "black holes". Neurology 2001; 57: 731–3.

19 Dalton CM, Miszkiel KA, Barker GJ, MacManus DG, Pepple TI, Panzara M, et al. Effect of natalizumab on conversion of gadolinium enhancing lesions to T1 hypointense lesions in relapsing multiple sclerosis. J Neurol 2004; 251: 407–13.

20 Bakshi R, Neema M, Healy BC, Liptak Z, Betensky RA, Buckle GJ, et al. Predicting clinical progression in multiple sclerosis with the magnetic resonance disease severity scale. Arch Neurol 2008; 65: 1449–53.

21 Waubant E. Biomarkers indicative of blood-brain barrier disruption in multiple sclerosis. Dis Markers 2006; 22: 235–44.

22 Cotton F, Weiner HL, Jolesz FA, Guttmann CR. MRI contrast uptake in new lesions in relapsing-remitting MS followed at weekly intervals. Neurology 2003; 60: 640–6.

23 Soon D, Tozer DJ, Altmann DR, Tofts PS, Miller DH. Quantification of subtle blood-brain barrier disruption in nonenhancing lesions in multiple sclerosis: a study of disease and lesion subtypes. Mult Scler 2007; 13: 884–94.

24 Masdeu JC, Moreira J, Trasi S, Visintainer P, Cavaliere R, Grundman M. The open ring: a new imaging sign in demyelinating disease. J Neuroimag 1996; 6: 104–7.

25 Bakshi R, Glass J, Louis DN, Hochberg FH. Magnetic resonance imaging features of solitary inflammatory brain masses. J Neuroimag 1998; 8: 8–14.

26 Rovira A, Alonso J, Cucurella G, Nos C, Tintoré M, Pedraza S, et al. Evolution of multiple sclerosis lesions on serial contrast-enhanced T1-weighted and magnetization-transfer MR images. AJNR Am J Neuroradiol 1999; 20: 1939–45.

27 Minneboo A, Uitdehaag BM, Ader HJ, Barkhof F, Polman CH, Castelijns JA. Patterns of enhancing lesion evolution in multiple sclerosis are uniform within patients. Neurology 2005; 65: 56–61.

28 McFarland HF, Stone LA, Calabresi PA, Maloni H, Bash CN, Frank JA. MRI studies of multiple sclerosis: implications for the natural history of the disease and for monitoring effectiveness of experimental therapies. Mult Scler 1996; 2: 198–205.

29 Kappos L, Moeri D, Radue EW, Schoetzau A, Schweikert K, Barkhof F, et al. Predictive value of gadolinium-enhanced magnetic resonance imaging for relapse rate and changes in disability or impairment in multiple sclerosis: a meta-analysis. Lancet 1999; 353: 964–9.

30 Molyneux PD, Filippi M, Barkhof F, Gasperini C, Yousry TA, Truyen L, et al. Correlations between monthly enhanced MRI lesion rate and changes in T2 lesion volume in multiple sclerosis. Ann Neurol 1998; 43: 332–9.

31 Smith ME, Stone LA, Albert PS, Frank JA, Martin R, Armstrong M, et al. Clinical worsening in multiple sclerosis is associated with increased frequency and area of gadopentetate dimenglumine-enhancing magnetic resonance imaging lesions. Ann Neurol 1993; 33: 480–9.

32 Broome DR, Girguis MS, Baron PW, Cottrell AC, Kjellin I, Kirk GA. Gadodiamide-associated nephrogenic systemic fibrosis: why radiologists should be concerned. Am J Roentgenol 2007; 188: 586–92.

33 Lövblad KO, Anzalone N, Dörfler A, Essig M, Hurwitz B, Kappos L, et al. MR imaging in multiple sclerosis: review and recommendations for current practice. Am J Neuroradiol 2010; 31: 983–9.

34 Dousset V, Brochet B, Deloire MS, Lagoarde L, Barroso B, Caille JM, et al. MR imaging of relapsing multiple sclerosis patients using ultra-small-particle iron oxide and compared with gadolinium. Am J Neuroradiol 2006; 27: 1000–5.

35 Vellinga MM, Oude Engberink RD, Seewann A, Pouwels PJ, Wattjes MP, van der Pol SM, et al. Pluriformity of inflammation in multiple sclerosis shown by ultra-small iron oxide particle enhancement. Brain 2008; 131: 800–7.

36 Drayer BP. Magnetic resonance imaging of multiple sclerosis. BNI Q 1987; 3: 65–73.

37 Janardhan V, Suri S, Bakshi R. Hyperintense lesions in the brain on noncontrast T1-weighted MR scans (T1 shortening) in multiple sclerosis. Radiology 2007; 244: 823–31.

38 Stankiewicz J, Panter SS, Neema M, Arora A, Batt CE, Bakshi R. Iron in chronic brain disorders: imaging and neurotherapeutic implications. Neurotherapeutics 2007; 4: 371–86.

39 Neema M, Stankiewicz J, Arora A, Dandamudi VS, Batt CE, Guss ZD, et al. T1- and
    T2-based MRI measures of diffuse gray matter and white matter damage in patients
    with multiple sclerosis. J Neuroimag 2007; 17: 16S–21S.

40 Smith MA, Castellani R, Napoli S, Perry G, Guttmann CRG, De Girolami U, et al. Gray
    matter iron deposition in patients with multiple sclerosis: a histochemical study.
    Neurology 2007; 68: A118.

41 Williams R, Wang WT, Choi IY, Lee SP, Berman NEJ, Lynch SG, et al. Cerebral vascular
    changes in an experimental model of multiple sclerosis. Mult Scler 2010; 6: 1010.

42 Ge Y, Jensen JH, Lu H, Helpern JA, Miles L, Inglese M, et al. Quantitative assessment
    of iron accumulation in the deep gray matter of multiple sclerosis by magnetic field
    correlation imaging. Am J Neuroradiol 2007; 28: 1639–44.

43 Hammond KE, Metcalf M, Carvajal L, Okuda DT, Srinivasan R, Vigneron D, et al.
    Quantitative in vivo magnetic resonance imaging of multiple sclerosis at 7 Tesla with
    sensitivity to iron. Ann Neurol 2008; 64: 707–13.

44 Khalil M, Enzinger C, Langkammer C, Tscherner M, Wallner-Blazek M, Jehna M,
    et al. Quantitative assessment of brain iron by R(2)* relaxometry in patients with
    clinically isolated syndrome and relapsing-remitting multiple sclerosis. Mult Scler
    2009; 15: 1048–54.

45 Neema M, Arora A, Healy BC, Guss ZD, Brass SD, Duan Y, et al. Deep gray matter
    involvement on brain MRI scans is associated with clinical progression in multiple
    sclerosis. J Neuroimag 2009; 19: 3–8.

46 Sajja BR, Wolinsky JS, Narayana PA. Proton magnetic resonance spectroscopy in
    multiple sclerosis. Neuroimaging Clin N Am 2009; 19: 45–58.

47 De Stefano N, Filippi M, Miller D, Pouwels PJ, Rovira A, Gass A, et al. Guidelines for
    using proton MR spectroscopy in multicenter clinical MS studies. Neurology 2007; 69:
    1942–52.

48 Davie CA, Hawkins CP, Barker GJ, Brennan A, Tofts PS, Miller DH, et al. Serial proton
    magnetic resonance spectroscopy in acute multiple sclerosis lesions. Brain 1994; 117:
    49–58.

49 Husted CA, Goodin DS, Hugg JW, Maudsley AA, Tsuruda JS, de Bie SH, et al.
    Biochemical alterations in multiple sclerosis lesions and normal-appearing white
    matter detected by in vivo 31P and 1H spectroscopic imaging. Ann Neurol 1994; 36:
    157–65.

50 Narayana PA. Magnetic resonance spectroscopy in the monitoring of multiple
    sclerosis. J Neuroimag 2005; 15: 46S–57S.

51 De Stefano N, Matthews PM, Antel JP, Preul M, Francis G, Arnold DL. Chemical
    pathology of acute demyelinating lesions and its correlation with disability. Ann
    Neurol 1995; 38: 901–9.

52 Wattjes MP, Harzheim M, Lutterbey GG, Bogdanow M, Schild HH, Träber F. High field
    MR imaging and 1H-MR spectroscopy in clinically isolated syndromes suggestive of
    multiple sclerosis: correlation between metabolic alterations and diagnostic MR
    imaging criteria. J Neurol 2008; 255: 56–63.

53 Ropele S, Fazekas F. Magnetization transfer MR imaging in multiple sclerosis.
    Neuroimaging Clin N Am 2009; 19: 27–36.

54 Schmierer K, Scaravilli F, Altmann DR, Barker GJ, Miller DH. Magnetization transfer
    ratio and myelin in postmortem multiple sclerosis brain. Ann Neurol 2004; 56:
    407–15.

55 Schmierer K, Tozer DJ, Scaravilli F, Altmann DR, Barker GJ, Tofts PS, et al. Quan-
    titative magnetization transfer imaging in postmortem multiple sclerosis brain.
    J Magnet Reson Imaging 2007; 26: 41–51.

56 Levesque IR, Giacomini PS, Narayanan S, Ribeiro LT, Sled JG, Arnold DL, et al. Quantitative magnetization transfer and myelin water imaging of the evolution of acute multiple sclerosis lesions. Magnet Reson Med 2010; 63: 633–40.

57 Chen JT, Collins DL, Freedman MS, Atkins HL, Arnold DL; Canadian MS/BMT Study Group. Local magnetization transfer ratio signal inhomogeneity is related to subsequent change in MTR in lesions and normal-appearing white-matter of multiple sclerosis patients. Neuroimage 2005; 25: 1272–8.

58 Chen JT, Kuhlmann T, Jansen GH, Collins DL, Atkins HL, Freedman MS, et al. Voxel-based analysis of the evolution of magnetization transfer ratio to quantify remyelination and demyelination with histopathological validation in a multiple sclerosis lesion. Neuroimage 2007; 36: 1152–8.

59 Sharma J, Zivadinov R, Jaisani Z, Fabiano AJ, Singh B, Horsfield MA, et al. A magnetization transfer MRI study of deep gray matter involvement in multiple sclerosis. J Neuroimag 2006; 16: 302–10.

60 Rocca MA, Agosta F, Sormani MP, Fernando K, Tintorè M, Korteweg T, et al. A three-year, multi-parametric MRI study in patients at presentation with CIS. J Neurol 2008; 255: 683–91.

61 Filippi M, Rocca MA, Martino G, Horsfield MA, Comi G. Magnetization transfer changes in the normal appearing white matter precede the appearance of enhancing lesions in patients with multiple sclerosis. Ann Neurol 1998; 43: 809–14.

62 Agosta F, Rovaris M, Pagani E, Sormani MP, Comi G, Filippi M. Magnetization transfer MRI metrics predict the accumulation of disability 8 years later in patients with multiple sclerosis. Brain 2006; 129: 2620–7.

63 Fisniku LK, Altmann DR, Cercignani M, Tozer DJ, Chard DT, Jackson JS, et al. Magnetization transfer ratio abnormalities reflect clinically relevant grey matter damage in multiple sclerosis. Mult Scler 2009; 15: 668–77.

64 Khaleeli Z, Cercignani M, Audoin B, Ciccarelli O, Miller DH, Thompson AJ. Localized grey matter damage in early primary progressive multiple sclerosis contributes to disability. Neuroimage 2007; 37: 253–61.

65 Agosta F, Pagani E, Caputo D, Filippi M. Associations between cervical cord gray matter damage and disability in patients with multiple sclerosis. Arch Neurol 2007; 64: 1302–5.

66 Bermel RA, Fisher E, Cohen JA. The use of MR imaging as an outcome measure in multiple sclerosis clinical trials. Neuroimaging Clin N Am 2008; 18: 687–701.

67 Basser PJ, Pierpaoli C. Microstructural and physiological features of tissues elucidated by quantitative-diffusion-tensor MRI. J Magnet Reson B 1996; 111: 209–19.

68 Goldberg-Zimring D, Mewes AU, Maddah M, Warfield SK. Diffusion tensor magnetic resonance imaging in multiple sclerosis. J Neuroimag 2005; 15: 68S–81S.

69 Rovaris M, Agosta F, Pagani E, Filippi M. Diffusion tensor MR imaging. Neuroimaging Clin N Am 2009; 19: 37–43.

70 Schmierer K, Wheeler-Kingshott CA, Boulby PA, Scaravilli F, Altmann DR, Barker GJ, et al. Diffusion tensor imaging of post mortem multiple sclerosis brain. Neuroimage 2007; 35: 467–77.

71 Alexander AL, Lee JE, Lazar M, Field AS. Diffusion tensor imaging of the brain. Neurotherapeutics 2007; 4: 316–29.

72 Rovaris M, Gass A, Bammer R, Hickman SJ, Ciccarelli O, Miller DH, et al. Diffusion MRI in multiple sclerosis. Neurology 2005; 65: 1526–32.

73 Yu CS, Lin FC, Liu Y, Duan Y, Lei H, Li KC. Histogram analysis of diffusion measures in clinically isolated syndromes and relapsing-remitting multiple sclerosis. Eur J Radiol 2008; 68: 328–34.

74 Rovaris M, Judica E, Ceccarelli A, Ghezzi A, Martinelli V, Comi G, et al. A 3–year diffusion tensor MRI study of grey matter damage progression during the earliest clinical stage of MS. J Neurol 2008; 255: 1209–14.

75 Ceccarelli A, Rocca MA, Valsasina P, Rodegher M, Pagani E, Falini A, et al. A multiparametric evaluation of regional brain damage in patients with primary progressive multiple sclerosis. Hum Brain Mapp 2009; 30: 3009–19.

76 Hecke WV, Nagels G, Leemans A, Vandervliet E, Sijbers J, Parizel PM. Correlation of cognitive dysfunction and diffusion tensor MRI measures in patients with mild and moderate multiple sclerosis. J Magnet Reson Imaging 2010; 31: 1492–8.

77 Bodini B, Khaleeli Z, Cercignani M, Miller DH, Thompson AJ, Ciccarelli O. Exploring the relationship between white matter and gray matter damage in early primary progressive multiple sclerosis: an in vivo study with TBSS and VBM. Hum Brain Mapp 2009; 30: 2852–61.

78 Ciccarelli O, Catani M, Johansen-Berg H, Clark C, Thompson A. Diffusion-based tractography in neurological disorders: concepts, applications, and future developments. Lancet Neurol 2008; 7: 715–27.

79 Lin X, Tench CR, Morgan PS, Niepel G, Constantinescu CS. 'Importance sampling' in MS: use of diffusion tensor tractography to quantify pathology related to specific impairment. J Neurol Sci 2005; 237: 13–19.

80 Lin F, Yu C, Jiang T, Li K, Chan P. Diffusion tensor tractography based group mapping of the pyramidal tract in relapsing-remitting multiple sclerosis patients. Am J Neuroradiol 2007; 28: 278–82.

81 Ozturk A, Smith SA, Gordon-Lipkin EM, Harrison DM, Shiee N, Pham DL, et al. MRI of the corpus callosum in multiple sclerosis: association with disability. Mult Scler 2010; 16: 166–77.

82 Fox RJ. Picturing multiple sclerosis: conventional and diffusion tensor imaging. Semin Neurol. 2008; 28: 453–66.

83 Agosta F, Absinta M, Sormani MP, Ghezzi A, Bertolotto A, Montanari E, et al. In vivo assessment of cervical cord damage in MS patients: a longitudinal diffusion tensor MRI study. Brain 2007; 130: 2211–19.

84 Pagani E, Hirsch JG, Pouwels PJ, Horsfield MA, Perego E, Gass A, et al. Intercenter differences in diffusion tensor MRI acquisition. J Magnet Reson Imaging 2010; 31: 1458–68.

85 MacKay AL, Vavasour IM, Rauscher A, Kolind SH, Mädler B, Moore GRW, et al. MR relaxation in multiple sclerosis. Neuroimaging Clin N Am 2009; 19: 1–26.

86 Haacke ME, Brown RW, Thompson ME, Venkatesan R. Magnetic Resonance Imaging, Physical Principles and Sequence Design. John Wiley & Sons: New York, 1999.

87 Look DC, Locker DR. Time saving in measurement of NMR and EPR relaxation times. Rev Sci Instrum 1970; 41: 250–1.

88 Vrenken H, Geurts JJG, Knol DL, van Dijk LN, Dattola V, Jasperse B, et al. Whole-brain T1 mapping in multiple sclerosis: global changes of normal-appearing gray and white matter. Radiology 2006; 240: 811–20.

89 Parry A, Clare S, Jenkinson M, Smith S, Palace J, Matthews PM. White matter and lesion T1 relaxation times increase in parallel and correlate with disability in multiple sclerosis. J Neurol 2002; 249: 1279–86.

90 Parry A, Clare S, Jenkinson M, Smith S, Palace J, Matthews PM. MRI brain T1 relaxation time changes in MS patients increase over time in both the white matter and the cortex. J Neuroimag 2003; 13: 234–9.

91 Whittall KP, MacKay AL, Li DK. Are mono-exponential fits to a few echoes sufficient to determine T2 relaxation for in vivo human brain? Magnet Reson Med 1999; 41: 1255–7.

92 Laule C, Kozlowski P, Leung E, Li DKB, Mackay AL, Moore GRW. Myelin water imaging of multiple sclerosis at 7 T: correlations with histopathology. Neuroimage 2008; 40: 1575–80.

93 Neema M, Goldberg-Zimring D, Guss ZD, Healy BC, Guttmann CR, Houtchens MK, et al. 3 T MRI relaxometry detects T2 prolongation in the cerebral normal-appearing white matter in multiple sclerosis. Neuroimage 2009; 46: 633–41.

94 Laule C, Vavasour IM, Moore GR, Oger J, Li DK, Paty DW, et al. Water content and myelin water fraction in multiple sclerosis. A T2 relaxation study. J Neurol 2004; 251: 284–93.

95 Vavasour IM, Laule C, Li DK, Oger J, Moore GR, Traboulsee A, et al. Longitudinal changes in myelin water fraction in two MS patients with active disease. J Neurol Sci 2009; 276: 49–53.

96 Armspach JP, Gounot D, Rumbach L, Chambron J. In vivo determination of multi-exponential T2 relaxation in the brain of patients with multiple sclerosis. Magnet Reson Imaging 1991; 9: 107–13.

97 Stevenson VL, Parker GJ, Barker GJ, Birnie K, Tofts PS, Miller DH, et al. Variations in T1 and T2 relaxation times of normal appearing white matter and lesions in multiple sclerosis. J Neurol Sci 2000; 178: 81–7.

98 Oh J, Han ET, Lee MC, Nelson SJ, Pelletier D. Multislice brain myelin water fractions at 3T in multiple sclerosis. J Neuroimag 2007; 17: 156–63.

99 Bermel RA, Bakshi R. The measurement and clinical relevance of brain atrophy in multiple sclerosis. Lancet Neurol 2006; 5: 158–70.

100 Ge Y, Gonen O, Inglese M, Babb JS, Markowitz CE, Grossman RI. Neuronal cell injury precedes brain atrophy in multiple sclerosis. Neurology 2004; 62: 624–7.

101 Davies GR, Altmann DR, Hadjiprocopis A, Rashid W, Chard DT, Griffin CM, et al. Increasing normal-appearing grey and white matter magnetisation transfer ratio abnormality in early relapsing-remitting multiple sclerosis. J Neurol 2005; 252: 1037–44.

102 De Stefano N, Iannucci G, Sormani MP, Guidi L, Bartolozzi ML, Comi G, Federico A, et al. MR correlates of cerebral atrophy in patients with multiple sclerosis. J Neurol 2002; 249: 1072–7.

103 Chard DT, Brex PA, Ciccarelli O, Griffin CM, Parker GJ, Dalton C, et al. The longitudinal relation between brain lesion load and atrophy in multiple sclerosis: a 14 year follow up study. J Neurol Neurosurg Psychiat 2003; 74: 1551–4.

104 Calabrese M, Rocca MA, Atzori M, Mattisi I, Favaretto A, Perini P, et al. A 3-year magnetic resonance imaging study of cortical lesions in relapse-onset multiple sclerosis. Ann Neurol 2010; 67: 376–83.

105 Bakshi R, Dandamudi VSR, Neema M, De C, Bermel RA. Measurement of brain and spinal cord atrophy by magnetic resonance imaging as a tool to monitor multiple sclerosis. J Neuroimag 2005; 15: 30S–45S.

106 Pirko I, Lucchinetti CF, Sriram S, Bakshi R. Gray matter involvement in multiple sclerosis. Neurology 2007; 68: 634–42.

107 Ceccarelli A, Rocca MA, Pagani E, Colombo B, Martinelli V, Comi G. et al. A voxel-based morphometry study of grey matter loss in MS patients with different clinical phenotypes. Neuroimage 2008; 42: 315–22.

108 Sanfilipo MP, Benedict RHB, Sharma J, Weinstock-Guttman B, Bakshi R. The relationship between whole brain volume and disability in multiple sclerosis: a

comparison of normalized gray vs. white matter with misclassification correction. Neuroimage 2005; 26: 1068–77.

109 Fisher E, Lee JC, Nakamura K, Rudick RA. Gray matter atrophy in multiple sclerosis: a longitudinal study. Ann Neurol 2008; 64: 255–65.

110 Grassiot B, Desgranges B, Eustache F, Defer G. Quantification and clinical relevance of brain atrophy in multiple sclerosis: a review. J Neurol 2009; 256: 1397–1412.

111 Wylezinska M, Cifelli A, Jezzard P, Palace J, Alecci M, Matthews PM. Thalamic neurodegeneration in relapsing-remitting multiple sclerosis. Neurology 2003; 60: 1949–54.

112 Bermel RA, Innus MD, Tjoa CW, Bakshi R. Selective caudate atrophy in multiple sclerosis: a 3D MRI parcellation study. Neuroreport 2003; 14: 335–9.

113 Houtchens MK, Benedict RHB, Killiany R, Sharma J, Jaisani Z, Singh B, et al. Thalamic atrophy and cognition in multiple sclerosis. Neurology 2007; 69: 1213–23.

114 Fischl B, Dale AM. Measuring the thickness of the human cerebral cortex from magnetic resonance images. Proc Natl Acad Sci USA 2000; 97: 11050–5.

115 Geurts JJ, Barkhof F. Grey matter pathology in multiple sclerosis. Lancet Neurol 2008; 7: 841–51.

116 Peterson JW, Bö L, Mörk S, Chang A, Trapp BD. Transected neurites, apoptotic neurons, and reduced inflammation in cortical multiple sclerosis lesions. Ann Neurol 2001; 50: 389–400.

117 Bø L, Vedeler CA, Nyland HI, Trapp BD, Mørk SJ. Subpial demyelination in the cerebral cortex of multiple sclerosis patients. J Neuropathol Exp Neurol 2003; 62: 723–32.

118 Bö L, Geurts JJG, van der Valk P, Polman C, Barkhof F. Lack of correlation between cortical demyelination and white matter pathologic changes in multiple sclerosis. Arch Neurol 2007; 64: 76–80.

119 Bakshi R, Ariyaratana S, Benedict RH, Jacobs L. Fluid-attenuated inversion recovery magnetic resonance imaging detects cortical and juxtacortical multiple sclerosis lesions. Arch Neurol 2001; 58: 742–8.

120 Simon B, Schmidt S, Lukas C, Gieseke J, Träber F, Knol DL, et al. Improved in vivo detection of cortical lesions in multiple sclerosis using double inversion recovery MR imaging at 3 Tesla. Eur Radiol 2010; 20: 1675–83.

121 Nelson F, Poonawalla A, Hou P, Wolinsky JS, Narayana PA. 3D MPRAGE improves classification of cortical lesions in multiple sclerosis. Mult Scler 2008; 14: 1214–19.

122 Calabrese M, Agosta F, Rinaldi F, Mattisi I, Grossi P, Favaretto A, et al. Cortical lesions and atrophy associated with cognitive impairment in relapsing-remitting multiple sclerosis. Arch Neurol 2009; 66: 1144–50.

123 Chard DT, Miller DH. What you see depends on how you look: Gray matter lesions in multiple sclerosis. Neurology 2009; 73: 918–19.

124 Mainero C, Benner T, Radding A, van der Kouwe A, Jensen R, Rosen BR, et al. In vivo imaging of cortical pathology in multiple sclerosis using ultra-high field MRI. Neurology 2009; 73: 941–8.

125 Schmierer K, Parkes HG, So P, An SF, Brandner S, Ordidge RJ, et al. High field (9.4 Tesla) magnetic resonance imaging of cortical grey matter lesions in multiple sclerosis. Brain 2010; 133: 858–67.

126 Bot JC, Barkhof F, Polman CH, Lycklama à Nijeholt GJ, de Groot V, et al. Spinal cord abnormalities in recently diagnosed MS patients: added value of spinal MRI examination. Neurology 2004; 62: 226–33.

127 Thorpe JW, Kidd D, Moseley IF, Kenndall BE, Thompson AJ, MacManus DG, et al. Serial gadolinium-enhanced MRI of the brain and spinal cord in early relapsing-remitting multiple sclerosis. Neurology 1996; 46: 373–8.

128 Thorpe JW, Kidd D, Kendall BE, Tofts PS, Barker GJ, Thompson AJ, et al. Spinal cord MRI using multi-array coils and fast spin echo. I. Technical aspects and findings in healthy adults. Neurology 1993; 43: 2625–31.

129 Bot JC, Barkhof F. Spinal-cord MRI in multiple sclerosis: conventional and nonconventional MR techniques. Neuroimag Clin N Am 2009; 19: 81–99.

130 Poonawalla AH, Hou P, Nelson FA, Wolinsky JS, Narayana PA. Cervical spinal cord lesions in multiple sclerosis: T1-weighted inversion-recovery MR imaging with phase-sensitive reconstruction. Radiology 2008; 246: 258–64.

131 Nijeholt GJ, van Walderveen MA, Castelijns JA, van Waesberghe JH, Polman C, Scheltens P, et al. Brain and spinal cord abnormalities in multiple sclerosis. Correlation between MRI parameters, clinical subtypes and symptoms. Brain 1998; 121: 687–97.

132 Kidd D, Thorpe JW, Thompson AJ, Kendall BE, Moseley IF, MacManus DG, et al. Spinal cord MRI using multi-array coils and fast spin echo. II. Findings in multiple sclerosis. Neurology 1993; 43: 2632–7.

133 Nijeholt GJ, Barkhof F, Scheltens P, Castelijns JA, Adèr H, van Waesberghe JH, et al. MR of the spinal cord in multiple sclerosis: relation to clinical subtype and disability. AJNR Am J Neuroradiol 1997; 18: 1041–8.

134 Gilmore CP, Bö L, Owens T, Lowe J, Esiri MM, Evangelou N. Spinal cord gray matter demyelination in multiple sclerosis – a novel pattern of residual plaque morphology. Brain Pathol 2006; 16: 202–8.

135 Stankiewicz JM, Neema M, Alsop DC, Healy BC, Arora A, Buckle GJ, et al. Spinal cord lesions and clinical status in multiple sclerosis: A 1.5 T and 3 T MRI study. J Neurol Sci 2009; 279: 99–105.

136 Bergers E, Bot JC, De Groot CJ, Polman CH, Lycklama à Nijeholt GJ, Castelijns JA, et al. Axonal damage in the spinal cord of MS patients occurs largely independent of T2 MRI lesions. Neurology 2002; 59: 1766–71.

137 Losseff NA, Webb SL, O'Riordan JI, Page R, Wang L, Barker GJ, et al. Spinal cord atrophy and disability in multiple sclerosis. A new reproducible and sensitive MRI method with potential to monitor disease progression. Brain 1996; 119: 701–8.

138 Horsfield MA, Sala S, Neema M, Absinta M, Bakshi A, Sormani MP, et al. Rapid semi-automatic segmentation of the spinal cord from magnetic resonance images: application in multiple sclerosis. Neuroimage 2010; 50: 446–55.

139 Liptak Z, Berger AM, Sampat MP, Charil A, Felsovalyi O, Healy BC, et al. Medulla oblongata volume: a biomarker of spinal cord damage and disability in multiple sclerosis. AJNR Am J Neuroradiol 2008; 29: 1465–70.

140 Zackowski KM, Smith SA, Reich DS, Gordon-Lipkin E, Chodkowski BA, Sambandan DR, et al. Sensorimotor dysfunction in multiple sclerosis and column-specific magnetization transfer-imaging abnormalities in the spinal cord. Brain 2009; 132: 1200–9.

141 Mottershead JP, Schmierer K, Clemence M, Thornton JS, Scaravilli F, Barker GJ, et al. High field MRI correlates of myelin content and axonal density in multiple sclerosis – a post-mortem study of the spinal cord. J Neurol 2003; 250: 1293–1301.

142 Bot JC, Blezer EL, Kamphorst W, Lycklama A Nijeholt GJ, Ader HJ, Castelijns JA, et al. The spinal cord in multiple sclerosis: relationship of high-spatial-resolution quantitative MR imaging findings to histopathologic results. Radiology 2004; 233: 531–40.

143 Vaithianathar L, Tench CR, Morgan PS, Constantinescu CS. Magnetic resonance imaging of the cervical spinal cord in multiple sclerosis – a quantitative T1 relaxation time mapping approach. J Neurol 2003; 250: 307–15.

CHAPTER 7

Predicting Clinical Course

Brian Healy[1] and Maria Liguori[1,2]

[1]Partners Multiple Sclerosis Center, Brigham and Women's Hospital, Boston, MA, USA
[2]National Research Council, Institute of Neurological Sciences, Mangone, Italy

Introduction

As described in previous chapters, multiple sclerosis (MS) affects roughly 1 out of 1000 adults in the United States and other countries, and it is the most common neurological disorder among young adults [1]. Over the past 50 years, several longitudinal follow-up studies have described the natural history of MS prior to the availability of first-line disease modifying therapy [2–4], and these studies have shown the population characteristics of the disease as well as the patient-to-patient heterogeneity. Additional studies of both treated and untreated patients have further investigated the natural history of MS [5–7]. Although the amount of heterogeneity in the disease course has been questioned recently [8], MS has been broken into four disease categories based on consensus definitions: relapsing-remitting (RRMS), secondary progressive (SPMS), primary progressive (PPMS), and progressive relapsing (PRMS) (Figure 7.1) [9]. These four disease categories can be combined into two main types of disease: relapsing-onset and progressive-onset.

The relapsing-onset disease encompasses approximately 85% of MS patients, and this disease course follows a relatively consistent pattern (Figure 7.2). In relapsing-onset patients, the disease course starts with an initial clinical episode called a clinically isolated syndrome (CIS). Although all patients who have RRMS start with a CIS by definition, not all patients with a CIS will develop RRMS, and predictors of conversion to RRMS are discussed below. Once the relapsing-remitting phase begins, the patient experiences intermittent episodes of neurological symptoms that are followed by either complete recovery or residual deficit. One study estimated that 42% of patients who experience a relapse have residual deficit 6 months after the relapse [10]. After the initial relapsing course, around 65% of RRMS patients will convert to SPMS [11]. SPMS is characterized by a steady

Multiple Sclerosis: Diagnosis and Therapy, First Edition. Edited by Howard L. Weiner and James M. Stankiewicz.   © 2012 John Wiley & Sons, Ltd.
Published 2012 by John Wiley and Sons, Ltd.

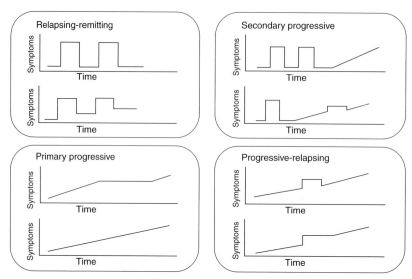

Figure 7.1 Disease course types: relapsing-remitting **(a)**, secondary progressive **(b)**, primary progressive **(c)**, and progressive-relapsing **(d)**. (Adapted from Lublin and Reingold [9] with permission from Lippincott Williams & Wilkins.)

worsening, with or without accompanying relapses, possibly because the disease changes from a predominantly inflammatory to a degenerative phase. The conversion to SPMS signals that the patient will no longer fully recover their neurological functioning, and predictors of this conversion are particularly important.

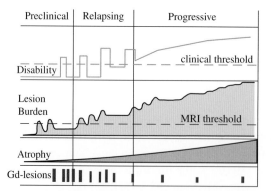

Figure 7.2 Clinical and MRI features of relapsing-onset MS. At early stages of the disease, patients experience more inflammatory events as evidenced by relapses and Gd-enhancing lesions. As the disease process continues, the inflammatory events decrease, but the degenerative process begins to dominate. (Adapted from Meier et al. [83] with permission from Oxford University Press.)

The two other main disease categories are classified as progressive-onset MS, which accounts for the remaining 15% of MS patients. In these patients, the disease course is predominantly degenerative from the onset. Most progressive-onset MS patients are classified as PPMS, which is characterized as disease progression from disease onset with no relapses. Conversely, PRMS patients have disease progression with superimposed relapses as well. Some question the need for a distinction between PPMS and PRMS [8, 12], but both categories are prevalent in the literature and clinical practice.

In this chapter, we will discuss predictors of the clinical course, focusing on predictors in three main areas. First, we will identify the characteristics of relapsing-onset vs. progressive-onset disease because the initial course is the best determinant of disability progression, especially early in the disease course. Second, we will focus on two important transitions for patients with relapsing onset: conversion from CIS to RRMS and conversion from RRMS to SPMS. Finally, we will describe the characteristics of patients who develop a special form of MS called benign MS.

Measures of disease course

Throughout this chapter, predictors of the disease course will be described, and in order to have a predictor, measures of the disease course are required. The most commonly used measure of disease severity is the Expanded Disability Status Scale (EDSS) [13] which is a combination of seven functional system scales (pyramidal, cerebellar, brainstem, sensory, bowel/bladder, visual, mental) as well as an other symptom indicator. The time to various EDSS landmarks has been proposed as the optimal approach to study predictors of long-term progression in MS, and the use of survival analysis techniques has been advocated [1]. The most common landmark in long-term studies is the development of an EDSS of 6, which corresponds to requiring unilateral support for walking 100 yards. The advantages of this EDSS level are that it is measured very accurately in a clinical examination, has limited interrater variability, and can be ascertained retrospectively, even though the accuracy of retrospective ascertainment has been questioned recently [14]. Other scales, including the multiple sclerosis functional composite (MSFC) [15], have been developed and shown to have desirable properties compared to the EDSS, but the EDSS remains the most commonly used measure of disability.

For short-term disease progression, sustained progression on the EDSS has been utilized in most studies, and the most common definition is a 1 unit increase on the EDSS sustained for 3 or 6 months for patients with an initial EDSS less than 5.5 or a 0.5 unit increase on the EDSS sustained for

3 or 6 months for patients with an initial EDSS of 5.5 or greater [16]. Although this is commonly used in the literature and clinical trials, one important limitation of this measure is that it does not guarantee that patients have truly progressed [16, 17]. Alternatives, including a Markov model for transitions between EDSS states, have been used to model short-term disease progression [18, 19], but these approaches are not popular in general. Given these difficulties related to short-term disease progression, our focus will be studies that have identified predictors of long-term disease progression since these are the most reliable.

Relapsing-onset/progressive-onset MS

The most important determinant of a patient's disease course is the type of disease onset. Patients with progressive onset reach higher levels of disability significantly faster than patients with relapsing onset [7]. Although similarities between the two types of onset in terms of age at progression and time from mild disability to moderate or severe disability have been noticed [7, 12], the time from disease onset to all levels of disability are significantly faster in progressive-onset MS. In several longitudinal studies of treated (disease-modifying therapy, DMT) and/or untreated patients, the median time from disease on set to EDSS 6 has been estimated to be approximately 8 years in progressive-onset patients and approximately 20 years in relapsing-onset patients [7, 20, 21]. Some more recent studies have estimated the time to EDSS 6 as longer than previous studies [5], but the differences between relapsing-onset and progressive-onset remain highly significant. No other predictor discussed in this chapter has as dramatic an effect on the time from disease-onset to disability landmarks as the patient's disease course.

Many studies have investigated the demographic/clinical characteristics of patients following each disease course. In particular, patients with relapsing-onset MS are more likely to be female and younger at first symptom than patients with progressive-onset MS. The gender ratio (F:M) has been estimated as 2–3 to 1 in relapsing-onset patients compared to 1–1.5 to 1 in progressive-onset, and the mean age at onset has been estimated as 25–35 years in relapsing-onset compared to 35–45 in progressive-onset [6, 8, 20, 21]. The often stated axiom that males and patients with later disease onset have worse clinical courses is driven in part by the over-representation of these patients in the progressive-onset group. The effect of these factors in just relapsing-onset patients will be discussed in more detail below. Beyond the basic demographic differences, progressive-onset and relapsing-onset patients also differ in terms of the initial symptom of the disease. Relapsing-onset patients are more likely to have an optic neuritis or sensory first symptom, while progressive-onset patients more frequently experience motor deficits or cerebellar symptoms [22].

From a conventional MRI perspective, the major differences between progressive-onset and relapsing-onset patients are related to the amount of disease activity observed on brain scans and the amount of spinal cord disease. The most common MRI measures of inflammation/disease activity in MS patients are the volume of lesions on a T2-weighted image and the presence of gadolinium enhanced lesions on a T1-weighted image. Relapsing-onset patient have a greater cerebral T2 lesion volume over the disease course and more gadolinium-enhanced lesions over the first 5 years of the disease compared to progressive-onset patients [23, 24]. These results demonstrate the predominance of the inflammatory process in early relapsing-onset MS (Figure 7.2). Conversely, the presence of spinal cord atrophy on MRI has been shown to be more prevalent in progressive-onset patients, especially early in the disease [25]. This finding is not surprising given the predominance of motor symptoms in progressive-onset patients.

The differences between relapsing-onset and progressive-onset MS persist in terms of response to FDA-approved DMT as well. The four most common first-line DMTs (three forms of interferon-β (IFN-β) and glatiramer acetate (GA)) have demonstrated a reduction in the relapse rate for RRMS patients [26–28], but none of these treatments has shown efficacy in progressive-onset patients [29, 30]. Although these results are somewhat unsurprising given the immunomodulatory mechanism of action of these treatments, the results also potentially point to differences in the disease process in these two groups.

Although this section has focused on the differences between patients with relapsing-onset and progressive-onset disease, similarities between the progressive phase of both initial courses (SPMS for relapsing onset and PPMS/PRMS for progressive onset) have been observed more recently [7]. First, although the time from disease onset to the progressive phase is clearly different in relapsing-onset and progressive-onset disease, the age at entering the progressive phase is actually quite similar [6, 31]. This demonstrates that the presence of early relapses may not be particularly important in terms of the age at disease progression in both disease courses. In addition, patients with SPMS have a similar time from progression onset or lower EDSS landmarks (EDSS 3 or 4) to higher EDSS landmarks (EDSS 6 or 8) compared to PPMS and PRMS [12]. Finally, the presence of superimposed relapses after the onset of progression has been shown to have limited effect on the time to disability landmarks [32]. These observations show that disability accrues similarly regardless of initial disease course once the process of disease progression has begun. In addition to the clinical similarities between SPMS and PPMS, and despite previous evaluations, the rate of brain atrophy in the two forms of progressive disease has also been recently shown to be similar [33].

TOP TIPS 7.1

- Type of disease onset for a patient is the most important predictor of clinical course.
- Relapsing-onset patients are more likely to be female, younger at onset, have optic neuritis or sensory initial symptoms, have inflammation markers of the brain on MRI, and respond to FDA-approved DMT.
- Progressive-onset patients are more likely to be male, older at onset, have initial motor (pyramidal or cerebellar) symptoms, have spinal cord abnormalities on MRI, and fail to respond to DMT.
- The two groups behave very differently at the initial presentation, but a convergence of disease course has been observed once the disease course enters the progressive phase.

Conversion from CIS to RRMS

All patients with relapsing-onset MS have an initial episode or a CIS. Considerable research has investigated predictors of conversion from CIS to clinically definite RRMS, including identification of MRI predictors with good sensitivity and specificity. In fact, the predictive accuracy of certain MRI phenotypes was sufficiently good to cause a change in the diagnostic criteria for MS to include dissemination in space and time by MRI in the McDonald criteria of MS, as opposed to the traditional clinically definite MS (CDMS) as defined by Poser [34–37]. In this section, the MRI, clinical, demographic, and other measures associated with conversion from CIS to RRMS are described.

For the conversion from CIS to RRMS, MRI measures are considered the best predictors. The simplest, but quite effective predictor of conversion is the presence of an abnormal brain MRI, defined as the presence of lesions on T2-weighted image. In fact, patients with an abnormal brain MRI convert to RRMS approximately 60% of the time after 5 years [38] and at even higher rates as the follow-up increases [39, 40]. Conversely, patients with a normal brain MRI in the same studies convert to RRMS approximately 8% of the time after 5 years, and the amount increases to approximately 20% after 20 years of follow-up [38, 40]. Given the predictive ability of an abnormal brain MRI, several groups have identified more clearly the MRI phenotype associated with conversion. Barkhof et al. [41] and Tintorè et al. [42] provided the criteria used for dissemination in space in the first two versions of the McDonald criteria for MS [35, 36] (see Box (7.1)). These criteria focus on gadolinium-enhancing lesions and areas that are commonly affected in MS patients (spinal cord, infratentorial, juxtacortical, or periventricular regions of the brain). Compared to patients with no Barkhof criteria, the presence of 1-2 Barkhof criteria increased the hazard of conversion to RRMS

BOX 7.1   Barkhof/Tintorè Criteria

- At least one gadolinium-enhancing lesion or nine T2-hyperintense lesions if no gadolinium-enhancing lesion.
- At least one infratentorial lesion.
- At least one juxtacortical lesion.
- At least three periventricular lesions.

Criteria adopted by international panel regarding MS diagnosis using data from Barkhof et al. and Tintorè et al. [41, 42]

---

by 6.1 and the presence of 3-4 Barkhof criteria increased the hazard of conversion by 17.0 in one study [38], with similar results in others [43, 44]. The sensitivity and specificity of dissemination in space for conversion over the short term has also been shown to be good (>65%) in several studies [45, 46]. Further work demonstrated that simplified criteria based solely on the presence of at least one lesion in two of the four mentioned areas can lead to improved sensitivity without reducing specificity or accuracy [45, 47], and these criteria have now been adopted for dissemination in space for the revised McDonald criteria for MS diagnosis [37]. Additionally, mean brain atrophy over the first year is significantly higher in patients who develop CDMS compared to those who do not, and brain atrophy rate and baseline T2LV are independent risk factors for MS diagnosis in multivariate analysis [48].

In terms of clinical predictors, the symptom at onset has been shown to have varying ability to predict conversion. In the Queen's Square cohort with over 20 years of follow-up, the proportion of patients who naturally converted to clinically definite MS after 20 years was approximately the same (around 60%) regardless of first symptom [40]. In contrast, other studies have found that patients with optic neuritis have a lower than average chance of conversion over the short term, leading to the conclusion that an optic neuritis onset is the one most likely to be an isolated syndrome [49]. Interestingly, in the same study, when only patients with an abnormal MRI were considered, the proportion who converted to CDMS was similar regardless of first symptom type. Demographic predictors such as gender and age have shown an association with conversion in some studies, but the results are not conclusive across studies or in multivariate analyses [43–45].

The impact of the presence of CSF oligoclonal bands (OCBs) and the abnormality of evoked potentials (EPs) on a CIS to RRMS conversion has also been considered. Given the prevalence of MRI in clinical practice, an OCB is unlikely to replace MRI completely in the diagnosis of MS even if the predictive accuracy was excellent, so our focus is studies regarding the information that OCBs provide in addition to the MRI. Several studies have found that the presence of OCBs can improve the predictive accuracy of the MRI [43, 46, 50], and the addition of OCBs to the MRI for diagnosis has been advocated [51]. In addition, OCBs have been found to be an independent risk factor of conversion in the presence of Barkhof criteria, increasing by almost twofold the risk of a second attack [43]. On the contrary, individual abnormal EPs did not appear to significantly change the risk of conversion, but the presence of three abnormal EPs at baseline increased the risk of developing moderate subsequent disability independently from baseline MRI [52].

Beyond the clinical/MRI predictors of conversion, several clinical trials in recent years have demonstrated the ability of DMTs approved for RRMS to also delay the conversion from CIS to CDMS/RRMS. A statistically significant delay in the time to CDMS conversion and the cumulative probability of conversion over the duration of the clinical trial has been observed for all types of IFN-β and GA in separate randomized clinical trials [53–56]. Since patients can develop RRMS at any time after the initial CIS, no trial can demonstrate that conversion is prevented over the course of a lifetime. At the same time, the strong effect of DMTs has led to the recommendation of early treatment in patients with a CIS.

TOP TIPS 7.2

- MRI features have proven to reliably and accurately predict conversion from CIS to RRMS.
- Clinical/demographic measures provide limited additional information regarding the chance of conversion.
- Among the other paraclinical predictors, the presence OCB in CSF improves predictive accuracy.
- Early treatment in patients with CIS delays time to conversion to CDMS.

Conversion from RRMS to SPMS

Once a patient has converted to RRMS, the next disease landmark is the conversion from RRMS to SPMS as this signals the beginning of continued worsening for the remainder of the disease (Figure 7.2). Interestingly, after conversion to SPMS, patients begin to accrue disability at a very similar rate regardless of their previous disease course [6]. The disease trajectory changes after this transition, making this landmark a critical point in the clinical course (Figure 7.3). As with the predictors of conversion from CIS to RRMS, both clinical/demographic and MRI measures have been investigated. The most valuable predictors of long-term disease course are characteristics measured within the first 5 years of the disease. After this initial period, the predictors appear to become less useful.

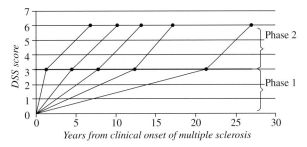

Figure 7.3 Demonstration of variability in time from disease onset of MS to moderate disability (Phase I) and the relative similarity in time from moderate to severe disability (Phase 2).

Unlike conversion from CIS to RRMS, demographic/clinical measures identified from natural history studies remain the most reliable predictors of time to conversion from RRMS to SPMS. Older patients convert to SPMS (or achieve an EDSS of 6) significantly faster than younger patients, and this result has been verified in several studies on treated and untreated patients [4, 6, 14, 57]. At the same time, older patients still convert to SPMS at an older age than patients with a younger disease onset, demonstrating the importance of the time metric in understanding disease progression. Beyond age at onset, patients with a motor symptom as the initial attack also have a faster time to SPMS compared to patients with optic neuritis or sensory symptom at onset [4, 14, 57]. The effect of gender is more variable across studies, with some showing an effect and others showing no effect [4, 6, 14, 57].

Characteristics of the initial disease course, including recovery from the initial relapse, time until the second relapse, and number of relapses in the first 2 or 5 years, have also been investigated as potential predictors. Poor recovery from initial relapse has been shown to be associated with a shorter time to SPMS [4, 58], which may indicate that either the repair potential for the patient is reduced or the patient may be prone to more severe attacks [59]. The duration between subsequent relapses is also associated with time until secondary progression in several studies [60], but not all [4]. It is unclear if part of the benefit of the increased time between the first two attacks is simply due to a longer latent period of the disease. In particular, if a patient has 5 months between the first two attacks, the patient's disease can change again anytime after the 5-month period. Conversely, if a patient has 5 years between the first two attacks, the patient likely had no clinically active disease over the period. The effect of the number of relapses during the relapsing-remitting phase on the time to progression is variable across several studies. A recent investigation showed that a higher number of relapses in the first 2 years was associated with faster disease progression, but there was no significant effect of the total number of relapses in the first

5 years [60]. Another recent study found that relapses within the first 5 years had a significant impact on time to disease progression, but the importance of later relapses was lower [61]. In total, the amount and severity of disease activity have been shown to have an effect on the time until disease progression across several cohorts, but the level of activity early in the disease course seems to be most important. The combined impact of these traits are part of the rationale behind treating patients aggressively early in the disease course, even after just a CIS.

Only a small number of studies have sufficient longitudinal follow-up to ascertain the impact of MRI features on conversion from RRMS to SPMS. Clear associations between early T2 lesion volume and long-term disability have been shown, and the rate of lesion accumulation, even within the first 5 years of disease, was higher in patients who developed SPMS compared to those with RRMS [40]. Interestingly, this study further showed that early changes in T2 lesion volume were associated with long-term disability, but late changes in T2 lesion volume had a slightly smaller impact. The limited predictive value of T2 lesion volume later in the disease course may be related to the plateau effect at high disability levels [62], but such a plateau effect has become controversial more recently [63]. Brain atrophy has also been considered a significant radiological marker of disease progression. In longitudinal evaluation, RRMS patients who converted to SPMS showed greater changes in MRI measures of brain atrophy than those who did not progress, and the largest changes were observed in the gray matter fraction (GMF) [64].

Several studies have also investigated the impact of the presence of OCB on long-term disease severity/progression, but the results remain controversial. OCB-negative patients have been found to have a longer time to both EDSS 4 and 6 in one case-control study, [65], but other studies have found no effect of OCB status on disease progression or the development of SPMS. [66, 67]. In terms of evoked potentials, although it was confirmed that they correlate with function of visual, somatosensory and motor pathways at almost every stage of the disease [68], few longitudinal studies investigated their predictive value for future disease progression. One of these investigations [69] showed that MS patients with a more severe involvement at baseline (global evoked potential score >=13) had a higher risk for disability progression than those with lower baseline score (72.5% vs 36.3%).

Finally, the impact of treatment on the conversion from RRMS to SPMS is less certain than the impact of treatment on other clinical measures due to the difficulty in completing a randomized trial. In fact, given the requirement for very long-term follow-up and the approval of DMT based on short-term outcomes, no randomized trial has investigated the effect of DMT on time to SPMS. Therefore, the data regarding a treatment effect on this conversion is based on observational data, and analysis of these data requires controlling for potential confounders. Two reports have found that treatment with IFN-β leads to slower disease progression either measured by change in the EDSS or time to EDSS landmarks [70, 71]. Long-term follow-up studies of patients in the early clinical trials have demonstrated the safety of the four first-line therapies, and the patients in the original treated arms have shown improvement in terms of disease progression or mortality in preliminary analyses even though the differences are not always statistically significant [72–74]. The lack of statistical significance is likely due, at least in part, to the similar treatment profiles after the initial trial period, but future work is required to address the methodological challenges related to estimating the treatment effect from long-term observational data.

TOP TIPS 7.3

- Age at onset and pattern of early relapses are most predictive of time to development of progression.
- Predictive value of relapses decreases as disease course continues.
- Increased burden of disease on MRI is also associated with faster disease progression.

Benign MS

Two extreme forms of multiple sclerosis are called benign MS and malignant MS. As the names indicate, patients in each group either have a long clinical course with limited development of disability (benign MS) or a large amount of disability developed over a short period of time (malignant MS). Benign MS has been studied extensively since these patients are easily identified in clinical populations. Unfortunately, little is known about malignant MS so this disease course is not described.

Since patients can develop disability at any time during the disease course, the best definition of benign MS remains controversial. One common definition is having an EDSS of 3 or less with disease duration of at least 15 years [75], but others have used different EDSS or disease duration cutoffs. The prevalence of benign MS has been estimated to be between 6 and 64%, and the wide range is due to the variety of definitions and patient populations across studies [76, 77]. In addition, a significant proportion of patients who are classified as benign at one point in the disease course fail to remain benign over longer follow-up periods [78], demonstrating that benign MS acts more as a temporary description of the patient rather than a clinical classification.

The clinical characteristics of benign MS have been studied extensively, but the varying definitions used for benign MS complicate the generalizability of the findings. Clinical/demographic features associated with benign disease include the same set of features associated with milder disease course in general, such as female gender, younger age at onset, and optic neuritis/sensory first symptom, but these traits have not been associated with benign disease in all studies [79].

One potential complicating factor for benign MS is the prevalence of cognitive impairment, which has been observed in 45% of patients with benign MS in one cohort [75]. Since the definition of benign MS uses the EDSS as the sole measure of disability and cognitive impairment is measured only through the mental functional system scale for the EDSS, patients can be classified as benign even if significant cognitive deficits are present. The question becomes whether these patients are truly benign or if the definition of benign MS should include some measure of cognitive impairment.

Recently, a panel of experts reviewed the MRI studies performed on benign MS patients in order to better understand the radiological features of benign MS and contribute to guidelines for a new definition of this condition. The radiological features of particular interest were focal tissue damage, tissue loss, intrinsic lesion damage/diffuse tissue injury, and cortical reorganization [80]. The results of this analysis showed that benign MS did not differ from RRMS in terms of T2 lesion volume or global brain atrophy, but benign patients had greater tissue preservation of clinically eloquent regions like the cerebellum and spinal cord, less severity of tissue damage within and outside MS lesions and greater presence of effective compensatory mechanisms. The analysis also showed that all these features were less pronounced in benign patients with cognitive abnormalities, further demonstrating the potential importance of including cognitive impairment as an additional criterion for future definitions of benign MS.

The exact prevalence of benign MS is likely underestimated due to patients who have demyelinating disease based on brain MRI but lack any clinical symptoms. In the past, these patients were only identified after death, but with the advent of routine brain MRI performed for other neurological symptoms, patients are sometimes discovered to have radiological evidence of disease prior to clinical symptoms. Recently, this type of patient has become of interest and has been labeled as having a radiologically isolated syndrome (RIS) [81]. Whether these patients will develop CIS or CDMS is uncertain. In a mean 5.2-years observation of 70 subjects with RIS [82], the rate of clinical conversion to CIS was estimated 33%. Of these patients, 8/23 (35%) experienced a second clinical relapse during the observational period, whereas 67% of the patients presented MRI dissemination in time at the end of the study. However, a larger cohort of individuals with RIS is needed to assess the risk of conversion. The impact of this patient group on the characteristics of benign MS is also uncertain.

TOP TIPS 7.4

- Benign MS patients have mild disease severity even after long disease duration, but many patients with benign MS do not remain benign after additional follow-up.
- Cognitive impairment has been observed frequently in benign MS patients.
- MRI features of benign MS were less severe focal tissue damage, less tissue loss, less intrinsic lesion damage/diffuse tissue injury, and greater cortical reorganization.

Conclusion

MS is a complex disease with many possible disease courses. Extensive research has identified clinical, demographic, MRI, and other characteristics associated with clinical course, especially the type of disease-onset. Predictors of conversion from CIS to RRMS have also been identified. These have led to an earlier diagnosis of the disease through new definitions of MS and to treatment protocols that delay the onset of RRMS. Even though the early parts of the disease process are generally well understood, prediction of the disease course over the long term remains challenging. Future work must identify better predictors of long-term disease course so that clinical care and treatment choices can be tailored to match each patient.

References

1 Compston A. McAlpine's Multiple Sclerosis. 4th edn. Philadelphia: Churchill Livingstone Elsevier, 2005.
2 Weinshenker BG, Bass B, Rice GP, Noseworthy J, Carriere W, Baskerville J, et al. The natural history of multiple sclerosis: a geographically based study. I. Clinical course and disability. Brain 1989; 112(Pt 1): 133–46.
3 Confavreux C, Aimard G, Devic M. Course and prognosis of multiple sclerosis assessed by the computerized data processing of 349 patients. Brain 1980; 103(2): 281–300.
4 Runmarker B, Andersen O. Prognostic factors in a multiple sclerosis incidence cohort with twenty-five years of follow-up. Brain 1993; 116(Pt 1): 117–34.
5 Tremlett H, Paty D, Devonshire V. Disability progression in multiple sclerosis is slower than previously reported. Neurology 2006; 66(2): 172–7.
6 Leray E, Yaouanq J, Le Page E, Coustans M, Laplaud D, Oger J, et al. Evidence for a two-stage disability progression in multiple sclerosis. Brain 2010; 133(7): 1900–13.
7 Confavreux C, Vukusic S, Moreau T, Adeleine P. Relapses and progression of disability in multiple sclerosis. N Engl J Med 2000; 343(20): 1430–8.
8 Confavreux C, Vukusic S. Natural history of multiple sclerosis: a unifying concept. Brain 2006; 129(Pt 3): 606–16.

9 Lublin FD, Reingold SC. Defining the clinical course of multiple sclerosis: results of an international survey. National Multiple Sclerosis Society (USA) Advisory Committee on Clinical Trials of New Agents in Multiple Sclerosis. Neurology 1996; 46(4): 907–11.

10 Lublin FD, Baier M, Cutter G. Effect of relapses on development of residual deficit in multiple sclerosis. Neurology 2003; 61(11): 1528–32.

11 Compston A, Coles A. Multiple sclerosis. Lancet 2008; 372(9648): 1502–17.

12 Kremenchutzky M, Rice GP, Baskerville J, Wingerchuk DM, Ebers GC. The natural history of multiple sclerosis: a geographically based study 9: observations on the progressive phase of the disease. Brain 2006; 129 (Pt 3): 584–94.

13 Kurtzke JF. Rating neurologic impairment in multiple sclerosis: an expanded disability status scale (EDSS). Neurology 1983; 33(11): 1444–52.

14 Tremlett H, Zhao Y, Rieckmann P, Hutchinson M. New perspectives in the natural history of multiple sclerosis. Neurology 2010; 74(24): 2004–15.

15 Cutter GR, Baier ML, Rudick RA, Cookfair DL, Fischer JS, Petkau J, et al. Development of a multiple sclerosis functional composite as a clinical trial outcome measure. Brain 1999; 122(Pt 5): 871–82.

16 Ebers GC, Heigenhauser L, Daumer M, Lederer C, Noseworthy JH. Disability as an outcome in MS clinical trials. Neurology 2008; 71(9): 624–31.

17 Liu C, Blumhardt LD. Disability outcome measures in therapeutic trials of relapsing-remitting multiple sclerosis: effects of heterogeneity of disease course in placebo cohorts. J Neurol Neurosurg Psychiatry 2000; 68(4): 450–7.

18 Wolfson C, Confavreux C. Improvements to a simple Markov model of the natural history of multiple sclerosis. I. Short-term prognosis. Neuroepidemiology 1987; 6(3): 101–15.

19 Gauthier SA, Mandel M, Guttmann CR, Glanz BI, Khoury SJ, Betensky RA, et al. Predicting short-term disability in multiple sclerosis. Neurology 2007; 68(24): 2059–65.

20 Cottrell DA, Kremenchutzky M, Rice GP, Koopman WJ, Hader W, Baskerville J, et al. The natural history of multiple sclerosis: a geographically based study. 5. The clinical features and natural history of primary progressive multiple sclerosis. Brain 1999; 122(Pt 4): 625–39.

21 Scalfari A, Neuhaus A, Degenhardt A, Rice GP, Muraro PA, Daumer M, et al. The natural history of multiple sclerosis: a geographically based study 10: relapses and long-term disability. Brain 2010; 133(Pt 7): 1914–29.

22 Miller DH, Leary SM. Primary-progressive multiple sclerosis. Lancet Neurol 2007; 6(10): 903–12.

23 Khaleeli Z, Ciccarelli O, Mizskiel K, Altmann D, Miller DH, Thompson AJ. Lesion enhancement diminishes with time in primary progressive multiple sclerosis. Mult Scler 2010; 16(3): 317–24.

24 Thompson AJ, Kermode AG, MacManus DG, Kendall BE, Kingsley DP, Moseley IF, et al. Patterns of disease activity in multiple sclerosis: clinical and magnetic resonance imaging study. BMJ 1990; 300(6725): 631–4.

25 Bieniek M, Altmann DR, Davies GR, Ingle GT, Rashid W, Sastre-Garriga J, et al. Cord atrophy separates early primary progressive and relapsing remitting multiple sclerosis. J Neurol Neurosurg Psychiatry 2006; 77(9): 1036–9.

26 Johnson KP, Brooks BR, Cohen JA, Ford CC, Goldstein J, Lisak RP, et al. Copolymer 1 reduces relapse rate and improves disability in relapsing-remitting multiple sclerosis: results of a phase III multicenter, double-blind placebo-controlled trial. The Copolymer 1 Multiple Sclerosis Study Group. Neurology 1995; 45(7): 1268–76.

27 Interferon beta-1b is effective in relapsing-remitting multiple sclerosis. I. Clinical results of a multicenter, randomized, double-blind, placebo-controlled trial. The IFNB Multiple Sclerosis Study Group. Neurology 1993; 43(4): 655–61.

28 Jacobs LD, Cookfair DL, Rudick RA, Herndon RM, Richert JR, Salazar AM, et al. Intramuscular interferon beta-1a for disease progression in relapsing multiple sclerosis. The Multiple Sclerosis Collaborative Research Group (MSCRG). Ann Neurol 1996; 39(3): 285–94.

29 Wolinsky JS, Narayana PA, O'Connor P, Coyle PK, Ford C, Johnson K, et al. Glatiramer acetate in primary progressive multiple sclerosis: results of a multinational, multicenter, double-blind, placebo-controlled trial. Ann Neurol 2007; 61(1): 14–24.

30 Leary SM, Miller DH, Stevenson VL, Brex PA, Chard DT, Thompson AJ. Interferon beta-1a in primary progressive MS: an exploratory, randomized, controlled trial. Neurology 2003; 60(1): 44–51.

31 Confavreux C, Vukusic S. Age at disability milestones in multiple sclerosis. Brain 2006; 129(Pt 3): 595–605.

32 Kremenchutzky M, Cottrell D, Rice G, Hader W, Baskerville J, Koopman W, et al. The natural history of multiple sclerosis: a geographically based study. 7. Progressive-relapsing and relapsing-progressive multiple sclerosis: a re-evaluation. Brain 1999; 122(Pt 10): 1941–50.

33 De Stefano N, Giorgio A, Battaglini M, Rovaris M, Sormani MP, Barkhof F, et al. Assessing brain atrophy rates in a large population of untreated multiple sclerosis subtypes. Neurology 2010; 74(23): 1868–76.

34 Poser CM, Paty DW, Scheinberg L, McDonald WI, Davis FA, Ebers GC, et al. New diagnostic criteria for multiple sclerosis: guidelines for research protocols. Ann Neurol 1983; 13(3): 227–31.

35 McDonald WI, Compston A, Edan G, Goodkin D, Hartung HP, Lublin FD, et al. Recommended diagnostic criteria for multiple sclerosis: guidelines from the International Panel on the diagnosis of multiple sclerosis. Ann Neurol 2001; 50(1): 121–7.

36 Polman CH, Reingold SC, Edan G, Filippi M, Hartung HP, Kappos L, et al. Diagnostic criteria for multiple sclerosis: 2005 revisions to the "McDonald Criteria". Ann Neurol 2005; 58(6): 840–6.

37 Polman CH, Reingold SC, Banwell B, Clanet M, Cohen JA, Filippi M, et al. Diagnostic criteria for multiple sclerosis: 2010 Revisions to the McDonald criteria. Ann Neurol 2011; 69(2): 292–302.

38 Tintorè M, Rovira A, Rio J, Nos C, Grive E, Tellez N, et al. Baseline MRI predicts future attacks and disability in clinically isolated syndromes. Neurology 2006; 67(6): 968–72.

39 Brex PA, Ciccarelli O, O'Riordan JI, Sailer M, Thompson AJ, Miller DH. A longitudinal study of abnormalities on MRI and disability from multiple sclerosis. N Engl J Med 2002; 346(3): 158–64.

40 Fisniku LK, Brex PA, Altmann DR, Miszkiel KA, Benton CE, Lanyon R, et al. Disability and T2 MRI lesions: a 20–year follow-up of patients with relapse onset of multiple sclerosis. Brain 2008; 131(Pt 3): 808–17.

41 Barkhof F, Filippi M, Miller DH, Scheltens P, Campi A, Polman CH, et al. Comparison of MRI criteria at first presentation to predict conversion to clinically definite multiple sclerosis. Brain 1997; 120(Pt 11): 2059–69.

42 Tintorè M, Rovira A, Martinez MJ, Rio J, Diaz-Villoslada P, Brieva L, et al. Isolated demyelinating syndromes: comparison of different MR imaging criteria to predict conversion to clinically definite multiple sclerosis. Am J Neuroradiol 2000; 21(4): 702–6.

43 Tintorè M, Rovira A, Rio J, Tur C, Pelayo R, Nos C, et al. Do oligoclonal bands add information to MRI in first attacks of multiple sclerosis? Neurology 2008; 70(13 Pt 2): 1079–83.

44 Moraal B, Pohl C, Uitdehaag BM, Polman CH, Edan G, Freedman MS, et al. Magnetic resonance imaging predictors of conversion to multiple sclerosis in the BENEFIT study. Arch Neurol 2009; 66(11): 1345–52.

45 Swanton JK, Rovira A, Tintorè M, Altmann DR, Barkhof F, Filippi M, et al. MRI criteria for multiple sclerosis in patients presenting with clinically isolated syndromes: a multicentre retrospective study. Lancet Neurol 2007; 6(8): 677–86.

46 Masjuan J, Alvarez-Cermeno JC, Garcia-Barragan N, Diaz-Sanchez M, Espino M, Sadaba MC, et al. Clinically isolated syndromes: a new oligoclonal band test accurately predicts conversion to MS. Neurology 2006; 66(4): 576–8.

47 Swanton JK, Fernando K, Dalton CM, Miszkiel KA, Thompson AJ, Plant GT, et al. Modification of MRI criteria for multiple sclerosis in patients with clinically isolated syndromes. J Neurol Neurosurg Psychiatry 2006; 77(7): 830–3.

48 Di Filippo M, Anderson VM, Altmann DR, Swanton JK, Plant GT, Thompson AJ, et al. Brain atrophy and lesion load measures over 1 year relate to clinical status after 6 years in patients with clinically isolated syndromes. J Neurol Neurosurg Psychiatry 2010; 81(2): 204–8.

49 Tintorè M, Rovira A, Rio J, Nos C, Grive E, Tellez N, et al. Is optic neuritis more benign than other first attacks in multiple sclerosis? Ann Neurol 2005; 57(2): 210–15.

50 Zipoli V, Hakiki B, Portaccio E, Lolli F, Siracusa G, Giannini M, et al. The contribution of cerebrospinal fluid oligoclonal bands to the early diagnosis of multiple sclerosis. Mult Scler 2009; 15(4): 472–8.

51 Tintorè M, Sastre-Garriga J. Role of MRI criteria and OB for diagnosing multiple sclerosis in patients presenting with clinically isolated syndromes. Mult Scler 2009; 15(4): 407–8.

52 Pelayo R, Montalban X, Minoves T, Moncho D, Rio J, Nos C, et al. Do multimodal evoked potentials add information to MRI in clinically isolated syndromes? Mult Scler 2010; 16(1): 55–61.

53 Jacobs LD, Beck RW, Simon JH, Kinkel RP, Brownscheidle CM, Murray TJ, et al. Intramuscular interferon beta-1a therapy initiated during a first demyelinating event in multiple sclerosis. CHAMPS Study Group. N Engl J Med 2000; 343(13): 898–904.

54 Kappos L, Polman CH, Freedman MS, Edan G, Hartung HP, Miller DH, et al. Treatment with interferon beta-1b delays conversion to clinically definite and McDonald MS in patients with clinically isolated syndromes. Neurology 2006; 67(7): 1242–9.

55 Comi G, Filippi M, Barkhof F, Durelli L, Edan G, Fernandez O, et al. Effect of early interferon treatment on conversion to definite multiple sclerosis: a randomised study. Lancet 2001; 357(9268): 1576–82.

56 Comi G, Martinelli V, Rodegher M, Moiola L, Bajenaru O, Carra A, et al. Effect of glatiramer acetate on conversion to clinically definite multiple sclerosis in patients with clinically isolated syndrome (PreCISe study): a randomised, double-blind, placebo-controlled trial. Lancet 2009; 374(9700): 1503–11.

57 Weinshenker BG, Rice GP, Noseworthy JH, Carriere W, Baskerville J, Ebers GC. The natural history of multiple sclerosis: a geographically based study. 3. Multivariate analysis of predictive factors and models of outcome. Brain 1991; 114(Pt 2): 1045–56.

58 Confavreux C, Vukusic S, Adeleine P. Early clinical predictors and progression of irreversible disability in multiple sclerosis: an amnesic process. Brain 2003; 126(Pt 4): 770–82.

59 Mowry EM, Pesic M, Grimes B, Deen S, Bacchetti P, Waubant E. Demyelinating events in early multiple sclerosis have inherent severity and recovery. Neurology 2009; 72(7): 602–8.

60 Scalfari A, Neuhaus A, Degenhardt A, Rice GP, Muraro PA, Daumer M, et al. The natural history of multiple sclerosis, a geographically based study 10: relapses and long-term disability. Brain 2010; 133(7): 1914–29.

61 Tremlett H, Yousefi M, Devonshire V, Rieckmann P, Zhao Y. Impact of multiple sclerosis relapses on progression diminishes with time. Neurology 2009; 73(20): 1616–23.

62 Li DK, Held U, Petkau J, Daumer M, Barkhof F, Fazekas F, et al. MRI T2 lesion burden in multiple sclerosis: a plateauing relationship with clinical disability. Neurology 2006; 66(9): 1384–9.

63 Sormani MP, Rovaris M, Comi G, Filippi M. A reassessment of the plateauing relationship between T2 lesion load and disability in MS. Neurology 2009; 73(19): 1538–42.

64 Fisher E, Lee JC, Nakamura K, Rudick RA. Gray matter atrophy in multiple sclerosis: a longitudinal study. Ann Neurol 2008; 64(3): 255–65.

65 Joseph FG, Hirst CL, Pickersgill TP, Ben-Shlomo Y, Robertson NP, Scolding NJ. CSF oligoclonal band status informs prognosis in multiple sclerosis: a case control study of 100 patients. J Neurol Neurosurg Psychiatry 2009; 80(3): 292–6.

66 Koch M, Heersema D, Mostert J, Teelken A, De Keyser J. Cerebrospinal fluid oligoclonal bands and progression of disability in multiple sclerosis. Eur J Neurol 2007; 14(7): 797–800.

67 Imrell K, Landtblom AM, Hillert J, Masterman T. Multiple sclerosis with and without CSF bands: clinically indistinguishable but immunogenetically distinct. Neurology 2006; 67(6): 1062–4.

68 Fuhr P, Borggrefe-Chappuis A, Schindler C, Kappos L. Visual and motor evoked potentials in the course of multiple sclerosis. Brain 2001; 124(Pt 11): 2162–8.

69 Leocani L, Rovaris M, Boneschi FM, Medaglini S, Rossi P, Martinelli V, et al. Multimodal evoked potentials to assess the evolution of multiple sclerosis: a longitudinal study. J Neurol Neurosurg Psychiatry 2006; 77(9): 1030–5.

70 Brown MG, Kirby S, Skedgel C, Fisk JD, Murray TJ, Bhan V, et al. How effective are disease-modifying drugs in delaying progression in relapsing-onset MS? Neurology 2007; 69(15): 1498–507.

71 Trojano M, Pellegrini F, Fuiani A, Paolicelli D, Zipoli V, Zimatore GB, et al. New natural history of interferon-beta-treated relapsing multiple sclerosis. Ann Neurol 2007; 61(4): 300–6.

72 Ebers GC, Traboulsee A, Li D, Langdon D, Reder AT, Goodin DS, et al. Analysis of clinical outcomes according to original treatment groups 16 years after the pivotal IFNB-1b trial. J Neurol Neurosurg Psychiatry 2010; 81(8): 907–12.

73 Kappos L, Traboulsee A, Constantinescu C, Eralinna JP, Forrestal F, Jongen P, et al. Long-term subcutaneous interferon beta-1a therapy in patients with relapsing-remitting MS. Neurology 2006; 67(6): 944–53.

74 Ford CC, Johnson KP, Lisak RP, Panitch HS, Shifronis G, Wolinsky JS. A prospective open-label study of glatiramer acetate: over a decade of continuous use in multiple sclerosis patients. Mult Scler 2006; 12(3): 309–20.

75 Amato MP, Zipoli V, Goretti B, Portaccio E, De Caro MF, Ricchiuti L, et al. Benign multiple sclerosis: cognitive, psychological and social aspects in a clinical cohort. J Neurol 2006; 253(8): 1054–9.

76 Perini P, Tagliaferri C, Belloni M, Biasi G, Gallo P. The HLA-DR13 haplotype is associated with "benign" multiple sclerosis in northeast Italy. Neurology 2001; 57(1): 158–9.

77 Benedikz J, Stefansson M, Guomundsson J, Jonasdottir A, Fossdal R, Gulcher J, et al. The natural history of untreated multiple sclerosis in Iceland. A total population-based 50 year prospective study. Clin Neurol Neurosurg 2002; 104(3): 208–10.

78 Hawkins SA, McDonnell GV. Benign multiple sclerosis? Clinical course, long term follow up, and assessment of prognostic factors. J Neurol Neurosurg Psychiatry 1999; 67(2): 148–52.

79 Ramsaransing GS, De Keyser J. Benign course in multiple sclerosis: a review. Acta Neurol Scand 2006; 113(6): 359–69.

80 Rovaris M, Barkhof F, Calabrese M, De Stefano N, Fazekas F, Miller DH, et al. MRI features of benign multiple sclerosis: toward a new definition of this disease phenotype. Neurology 2009; 72(19): 1693–701.

81 Okuda DT, Mowry EM, Beheshtian A, Waubant E, Baranzini SE, Goodin DS, et al. Incidental MRI anomalies suggestive of multiple sclerosis: the radiologically isolated syndrome. Neurology 2009; 72(9): 800–5.

82 Lebrun C, Bensa C, Debouverie M, Wiertlevski S, Brassat D, de Seze J, et al. Association between clinical conversion to multiple sclerosis in radiologically isolated syndrome and magnetic resonance imaging, cerebrospinal fluid, and visual evoked potential: follow-up of 70 patients. Arch Neurol 2009; 66(7): 841–6.

83 Meier DS, Weiner HL, Guttmann CR. Time-series modeling of multiple sclerosis disease activity: a promising window on disease progression and repair potential? Neurotherapeutics 2007; 4(3): 485–98.

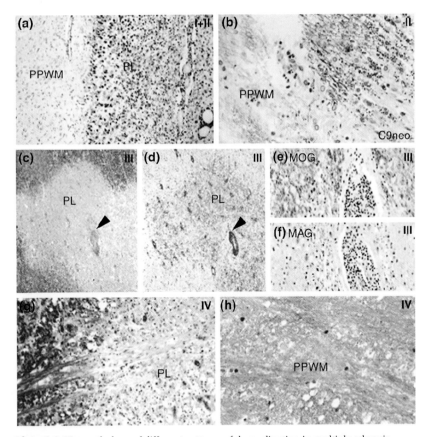

Plate 1.1 Histopathology of different patterns of demyelination in multiple sclerosis.
(a) Actively demyelinating lesion following patterns I and II. The active plaque (PL) is filled
with activated macrophages and microglia. There is a sharp demarcation between the actively
demyelinating lesions and the periplaque white matter (PPWM). Immunocytochemistry
for CD68 (to identify activated macrophages/microglia). (Magnification ×200.) (b) Actively
demyelinating plaque of pattern II that shows massive deposition of complement C9neo-
antigen (brown staining) on degenerating myelin sheaths and in myelin degradation products
taken up by macrophages in the zone of active demyelination (ADM). There is faint C9neo
reactivity on myelin sheaths in the PPWM. Immunocytochemistry for C9neo-antigen.
(Magnification ×500.) (c) Actively demyelinating lesion following pattern III. Myelin staining
using Luxol fast blue shows an ill-demarcated demyelinated plaque (PL). In the centre of the
lesion is an inflamed blood vessel surrounded by a small rim of preserved myelin (arrow).
(Magnification ×30.) (d) The same lesion as shown in (c) stained with the leukocyte marker
CD45. Myelin around the central vessel has a lower density of inflammatory cells compared to
the rest of the lesion (arrow). In addition, this lesion has an indistinct boundary compared with
the lesion in panel (a). Immunocytochemistry for CD45. (Magnification ×30.) (e) Higher
magnification of the area indicated by the arrow in panels (c) and (d) stained for myelin-
oligodendrocyte glycoprotein (MOG, brown staining). There are numerous MOG-reactive
fibers preserved in the lesion. (Magnification ×300.) (f) Higher magnification of the area
indicated by the arrow in panels (c) and (d) stained for myelin associated glycoprotein (MAG).
There is very little MAG immunoreactivity. (Magnification ×300.) (g) Actively demyelinating
lesion following pattern IV. The plaque contains numerous macrophages containing myelin
degradation products (stained blue with the Luxol fast blue myelin stain) and has a sharply
demarcated edge. (Magnification ×300.) (h) The periplaque white matter of the lesion in (g).
The myelin appears vacuolated and contains numerous oligodendrocytes with fragmented
DNA (black nuclei) identified using an in situ tailing reaction for DNA fragmentation.
(Magnification ×400.) (Reproduced from Lassman et al. [148] with permission from Elsevier.)

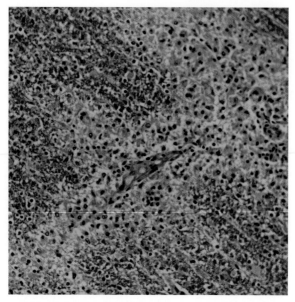

Plate 5.1a Luxol fast blue and cresyl violet stained autopsy section from the subcortical white matter of a 17-year-old boy with a diagnosis of ADEM (×10). Note the perivascular pattern of myelin loss and inflammatory cell infiltration. (Courtesy of Department of Pathology, Children's Hospital, Boston.)

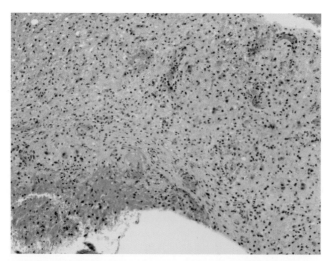

Plate 5.1b Luxol fast blue and cresyl violet stained biopsy section from the subcortical white matter of a 17-year-old girl with a diagnosis of pediatric multiple sclerosis (×10). Note the diffuse patttern of myelin loss and nodular inflammatory cell infiltration. (Courtesy of Department of Pathology, Children's Hospital, Boston.)

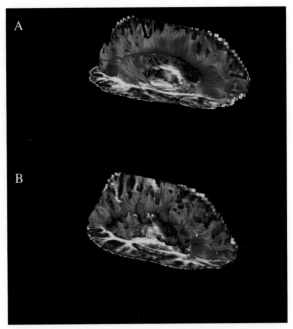

Plate 6.1 Three-dimensional visualization of the corpus callosum by diffusion tensor imaging-based tractography performed at 3 T: Individual tractography reconstruction of the corpus callosum is shown in blue from an age matched healthy subject (A) and a patient with MS (B). T2 hyperintense lesions are superimposed in red for the patient with MS. Note the clearly disrupted tracts of the corpus callosum observed with tractography (B). Analysis was performed in our laboratory using Trackvis software (www.trackvis.org).

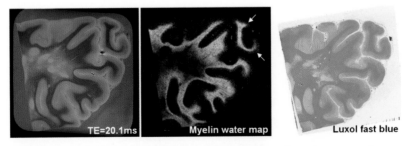

TE=20.1ms Myelin water map Luxol fast blue

Plate 6.2 Example of a 7 T multiple sclerosis image and myelin water map, and corresponding luxol fast blue histology image of the parieto-occipital region of an MS patient. A good qualitative correspondence is observed between the myelin water map and histology stain for myelin. The normal prominent myelination of the deeper cortical layers (arrows) is also visible on the myelin water image. From Laule et al. [92], with permission.

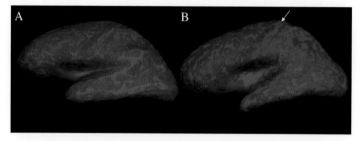

Plate 6.3 Cortical atrophy in multiple sclerosis (MS). Comparison of the reconstructed brain cortical surface from modified driven equilibrium fourier transform (MDEFT) MRI scans performed at 3 T of a healthy control (A) versus a patient with secondary progressive MS (B). Areas of significant thinning (< 2 mm) are shown in green, while red represents cortical areas thicker than 2 mm. Marked cortical thinning is seen in various areas including the sensorimotor cortex (arrow) in the patient with MS (B) as compared to the healthy control (A). Analysis was performed in our laboratory using Freesurfer software [114]. Figure courtesy of Dr. Daniel Goldberg-Zimring.

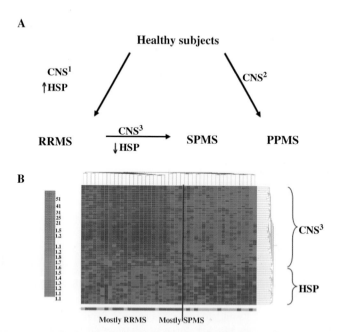

Plate 12.1 Autoantibody immune signatures of MS in the peripheral blood as revealed by antigen arrays. A: Schematic depiction of immune signatures associated with RRMS, SPMS, and PPMS. B: Heatmap depicting antibody reactivities against myelin antigens and heat shock proteins in SPMS vs RRMS.

PART II
Management

CHAPTER 8

Medication Treatment in Multiple Sclerosis

James M. Stankiewicz and Samia J. Khoury

Partners Multiple Sclerosis Center, Brigham and Women's Hospital, and Department of Neurology, Harvard Medical School, Boston, MA, USA

Introduction

In many patients, neurologists and MS specialists are now able to favorably alter the course of multiple sclerosis with disease-modifying medicines. Because of these advances, patients are doing better today than ever before. Despite these successes challenges remain. We lack robust treatments for progressive disease and remain faced with concerns related to drug route of administration, side effects, or safety. Expectations are that over the next 4 years no fewer than five new drugs may receive regulatory approval for MS, which holds further promise for patients. This chapter reviews the current understanding of available and soon-to-be-available disease-modifying agents with attention to drug mechanism of action, efficacy, and side effect profile.

FDA-approved medications

Currently there are seven FDA-approved medications for MS. IFN-β-1a subcutaneous (Betaseron) was the first to gain regulatory approval in 2001. Other injectables in order of approval are: IFN-β-1a intramuscular (Avonex), glatiramer acetate (Copaxone), and IFN-β-1a subcutaneous (Rebif). Two intravenous preparations are FDA approved: mitoxantrone (Novantrone) and natalizumab (Tysabri). The first oral agent, fingolimod (Gilenya), was approved at the end of 2010. In the United States mitoxantrone currently finds limited use due to concerns about post-treatment acute leukemias and cardiotoxicity. Tysabri, when originally released in 2004, was quite popular but its use has been limited by a recognized risk of progressive multifocal

Multiple Sclerosis: Diagnosis and Therapy, First Edition. Edited by Howard L. Weiner and James M. Stankiewicz.   © 2012 John Wiley & Sons, Ltd.
Published 2012 by John Wiley and Sons, Ltd.

leukoencephalopathy. For the purposes of convenience and to avoid confusion, injectables will be referred to by their trade names.

Injectables

Beta interferon medications

Beta interferons (IFNs) are the mainstay of MS treatment. Though IFNs have many downstream effects, the major mechanism of action is thought to be by shifting the immune cytokine profile from a proinflammatory stance (Th1) to a less harmful (Th2, Th3) response. IFN is thought to reduce T cell activation, proliferation, and blood–brain barrier migration; lessen antigen presentation; reduce IFN-γ MHC class II upregulation; and inhibit monocytes [1]. A recent report suggesting that relapsing-remitting MS patients (RRMS) with higher IL-1 secretion respond well to IFN while patients with a high IL-17 and IFN-β secretion do not. This finding, while intriguing, needs further confirmation [2].

Multiple trials with IFN have demonstrated the efficacy of these medicines in both RRMS and clinically isolated syndrome (CIS). Initial phase III trials vary in enrollment criteria, outcome measures, and length, but show benefit when compared with placebo (Table 8.1). It has become apparent that enrollment criteria affect trial outcome. Recently enrolled trials have included less affected populations, resulting in reductions in relapse rates in both placebo and treated arms. In the PRISMS placebo-controlled trial a relapse rate reduction of roughly one-third and reduction of gadolinium enhancement by 78% [3] was seen, while more recently enrolled trials have shown a relapse rate reduction compared to baseline approaching 80% [4, 5] and reduction of gadolinium enhancement up to 84% [6].

High-dose IFN treatments generally have not shown an effect on brain volume [7]. In the first year it is common to see pseudoatrophy that may be related to decreased inflammation. In its pivotal trial Avonex showed a 55% reduction in the rate of brain volume loss compared to placebo in the second year of treatment, but lack of effect in the first year led the overall result to be nonsignificant [8]. Better trials need to be done to establish whether, once accounting for potential atrophy, Avonex does preserve brain and to test whether this effect extends to the high-dose IFNs [9].

Small studies of all three IFNs have suggested that they may help to reduce cognitive impairment [10–12]. Fatigue probably benefits from IFN treatment [13]. Two randomized-controlled trials of IFN in primary progressive disease did not show an effect on disability [14]. Though four randomized controlled trials have been performed with IFN in secondary progressive MS, only the European multi-center trial of IFN-β-1b in SPMS [15] demonstrated a favorable effect on EDSS. A second larger Betaseron trial was

Table 8.1 Pivotal studies of injectable agents

Drug	Patient #	Admission Criteria	Length	Outcome Measure
Betaseron [113–115]	372	RRMS, EDSS <5.5, 2 or more relapses prior 2 years	2 years	↓ Relapse rate 34% (p < 0.0001)* ↓ MRI median T2 active lesions 83% (p = 0.009) ↓ MRI median T2 volume 17.3% (p = 0.001) ↓ Confirmed 1 point EDSS progression 29% (NS)
Avonex [116–118]	301	RRMS, EDSS 1–3.5, 2 attacks prior 3 years	2 years	↓ Confirmed 1 point EDSS progression* 37% (p = 0.02) ↓ Relapse rate 18% (p < 0.04) ↓ MRI gd + lesions 33%, (p = 0.05)
Rebif [3, 119]	560	RRMS, EDSS <5, 2 or more relapses prior 2 years	2 years	↓ Relapse rate* 32% (p<0.005) ↓ MRI median T2 active lesions 78% (p = 0.0001) ↓ Confirmed 1 point EDSS progression 30% (0.05)
Copaxone [23, 120]	251	RRMS, EDSS<5, 2 or more relapses prior 2 years	3 years	↓ Relapse rate* 29% (p < 0.007) ↓ Confirmed 1 point EDSS progression 12% (NS)
Copaxone [121]	249	RRMS, EDSS<5, 1 relapse prior 2 years, gd + on screening brain MRI	9 months	↓ MRI gd + lesions* 35%, (p = 0.001)

*Denotes primary outcome measure, EDSS = expanded disability status scale, gd = gadolinium, NS = nonsignificant.

aborted early due to a lack of efficacy [16]. Given these results it is reasonable to conclude that IFN treatment probably does not markedly influence disease progression once a patient transitions to a secondary progressive phase. It is worth noting, however, that IFN still had an effect on relapse rate and MRI activity. Though debate continues on how antibodies impact IFN efficacy, it is probably fair to conclude that sustained high titer neutralizing antibodies significantly impair the IFN effect. Different rates of antibody formation have been published for each IFN, but Betaseron consistently has the highest rates, with Rebif being second, and Avonex the lowest [17]. We do not routinely monitor antibody titers, and are more apt to switch a medicine that appears ineffective than check titers, especially because patients end up paying out-of-pocket for these tests.

IFNs are generally well tolerated. Flu-like symptoms are common but improve with time. We have found that 500 mg of naproxen taken 30 minutes prior to injection ameliorates these symptoms better than Tylenol or ibuprofen. Counter-intuitively we also observe that IFNs administered more frequently (Rebif, Betaseron) actually cause less severe flu-like symptoms. A pegylated Avonex is in development, which will be administered either every 2 or 4 weeks depending on trial results. Whether this preparation will enhance IFN tolerability remains to be seen. IFN should be used with caution in patients with a premorbid history of depression. The FDA recommends LFT testing for patients on IFN. Post-marketing cases of hepatic failure requiring liver transplantation in patients on high-dose IFN in conjunction with other potentially hepatotoxic medications have been reported. High-dose IFN cause LFT abnormalities more frequently than Avonex [18], though our experience suggests that Rebif tends to elevate LFTs more frequently than Betaseron. Because liver biopsy is infrequently obtained and serious liver toxicity related to IFN is rare, the significance of these elevations is unclear. Another controversial topic is the relative efficacies of low-dose vs high-dose IFN. Two trials suggest that high-dose IFN may have superior efficacy [19, 20], for both clinical and MRI outcomes, though some argue that these results should not be over-interpreted due to a lack of clinician blinding in the EVIDENCE trial, and a 6-month outcome measure in the INCOMIN study. The American Academy of Neurology has determined that, at least in the short term, there is good evidence to support a short-term dose-response effect [21].

Glatiramer acetate (Copaxone)

Glatiramer acetate (Copaxone) is currently the most prescribed single drug for multiple sclerosis, although IFNs in aggregate are prescribed more frequently. This daily subcutaneous injection is random polymer of four amino acids (L-glutamic acid, L-lysine, L-alanine, and L-tyrosine). Though glatiramer has many downstream immunologic effects it might work by causing a shift from a Th1 to Th2 immune profile [22]. Like IFN, Copaxone reduced relapse rate by one-third in its original trials (Table 8.1), though more recent trials show relapse rate reductions in the order of 75% compared to baseline [6]. In the original phase III Copaxone trial [23], no difference could be found in the proportion of patients with sustained progression at 90 days between Copaxone and placebo, though favorable effects were seen on other disability outcomes. The authors argued that the placebo group did especially well in the trial, perhaps limiting the trial's power to detect an effect. Extension trials have shown a favorable effect on disability in patients receiving Copaxone over the long term, though perhaps this is a self-fulfilling prophesy [24, 25]. On balance Copaxone treatment seems to prevent brain atrophy [7], but a 2-year study of glatiramer acetate was unable to demonstrate an effect on cognition [26]. A large study of Copaxone in PPMS did not demonstrate an effect on disability though a post-hoc analysis showed that Copaxone had a significantly delayed time to sustained disability progression in men [27]. An earlier trial of Copaxone in chronic progressive MS patients found a trend (p = 0.08) toward higher progression rates in the placebo group at 1 and 2 years, although the difference was nonsignificant [28].

Copaxone is generally well tolerated, with injection site reactions being the most common side effect. A self-resolving vasodilatory reaction with flushing, shortness of breath, and palpitations can occur. Lymphadenopathy can also occur, though persistently enlarged lymph nodes should be biopsied to exclude lymphoma. A small study found that patients on Copaxone may be less fatigued than those on IFN [13], but reported fatigue was similar in a head-to-head trial between Copaxone and Betaseron [4]. Better designed trials need to be performed before any definitive conclusions are made. Recent work [29] suggests that in patients stable for at least a year, Copaxone twice weekly may be equivalent to daily, though a randomized-controlled trial needs to be conducted to validate this result.

IFN vs Copaxone

Three recent trials have explored the efficacy of Copaxone vs high-dose IFN. The BEYOND trial enrolled over 2000 patients and directly compared Betaseron with Copaxone. It found no difference between the treatments on clinical measures including EDSS and relapse rate [4]. Some MRI metrics favored Betaseron, some Copaxone. Betaseron showed a larger reduction in T2 lesion volume than Copaxone at 1 year, though at years 2–3 no differences were found. Betaseron-treated patients had lower gadolinium enhancing lesion volume, though the actual number of enhancing lesions did not differ between groups. Brain atrophy was greater in the Betaseron group at year 1 but this effect was not sustained in years 2–3. The authors rightly suggest that this discrepancy might be related to early IFN effects on inflammation causing pseudoatrophy. T1-hypointense "black holes" volume did not differ between groups. In the BECOME study monthly triple gadolinium dose MRIs were obtained in 75 RRMS or CIS patients randomized to either Copaxone or Betaseron. At 2 years, no differences between treatment group could be found for relapse rate, combined active lesions, or new lesions [5]. Additional analysis revealed that the rate of conversion of new enhancing lesions to chronic T1-hypointense "black holes" was higher with Copaxone (15%) than with Betaseron (10%) (p = 0.02) [30]. The REGARD study randomized 764 patients to either Copaxone or 44 mcg of Rebif [6]. After 96 weeks, there was no significant difference between groups in time to first relapse, number and change in volume of T2 active lesions or for change in gadolinium-enhancing lesions volume, although patients treated with Rebif had significantly fewer gadolinium-enhancing lesions (0.24 vs 0.41 lesions per patient per scan, p = 0.0002). There was no difference in the mean number of new T1-hypointense lesions per patient per scan between treatment groups throughout 96 weeks. Brain volume was less in the Rebif-treated group at 96 weeks, but again this effect might potentially be attributed to pseudoatrophy. Though T1-hypointensities in the BECOME trial favor Betaseron, these results were not reproduced in the other two trials. Even if we accept this finding at face value it is difficult to attribute a clinical significance to this, given the overall [12%] low rate of T1- hypointensity formation. Similarly, volume measures over the length of the REGARD and BEYOND trials might appear to favor Copaxone, but when one considers the question of pseudoatrophy it is difficult to draw any definite conclusions.

An NIH-sponsored multicenter trial comparing Avonex and Copaxone head-to-head is ongoing, with initial results expected in the near future. Though one could quibble over trial design and specific metrics, it is our opinion that, taken together, these three randomized trials suggest a similar efficacy between high-dose IFN and Copaxone. It is also worth noting that, in these trials, the rate of discontinuation between medicines is the same, broadly suggesting a similar tolerability.

TOP TIPS 8.1: Injectable multiple sclerosis medicines

- The most prominent interferon side effect is flu-like symptoms.
- The most prominent glatiramer acetate side effect is localized injection site reactions.
- Injectables have a long-term safety track record.
- Glatiramer acetate and high-dose interferon (Rebif, Betaseron, Extavia) have comparable efficacies.
- High-dose interferon may be more effective than low-dose (Avonex).

Others

Natalizumab (Tysabri)

Natalizumab was approved for patients with RRMS in 2004. It works by inhibiting α-4 integrin on the surface of lymphocytes. This in turn prevents lymphocyte adherence to vascular cell adhesion molecule-1 (VCAM-1) impeding trafficking of T cells across the blood–brain barrier. The initial release of natulizumab garnered much attention because currently approved MS medications at that time could be expected to offer no more than a reduction in relapse rate of about a third. In the AFFIRM trial the annualized relapse rate in the natalizumab monotherapy group was 0.27, compared to 0.78 in placebo, conferring a 68% reduction in relapse rate ($p < 0.001$) [31]. MRI metrics were also favorable to natalizumab, demonstrating an 83% reduction in new and enlarging T2 lesions compared to placebo ($p < 0.001$).

It is unclear whether natalizumab may be effective in a secondary progressive population. The phase II trial [32], which included patients with secondary progressive disease, only lasted 6 months and was not powered to assess change in EDSS, though gadolinium-enhancing lesions were less frequent in the natalizumab SPMS group than in the placebo group. Mattioli et al. [33] examined the effect of natalizumab on cognition in multiple sclerosis. They found an improvement on cognitive testing at one year, while the control group remained unchanged. An effect has been shown with natalizumab treatment on brain atrophy during the second year of treatment [34], a metric that correlates with motor and cognitive disability.

In the clinical trials, natalizumab was well tolerated, though anxiety, pharyngitis, sinus congestion, peripheral edema, fatigue, and hypersensitivity reactions were seen more commonly in the Tysabri-treated group than in the placebo group. In the AFFIRM trial 6% of patients developed persistent antibodies to natalizumab, resulting in a loss of drug efficacy.

In 2005 reports of development of progressive multifocal leukoencephalopathy (PML) surfaced [35, 36], an illness historically only seen in immunocompromised patients. Natalizumab was pulled from the market, and eventually reintroduced. Original PML risk estimates were 1:1000 treated patients. More recent estimates have placed the risk at about 1:500. To this point, no MS patient has developed PML in under 1 year of treatment. More recent estimates indicate that the risk of PML increases with longer duration of treatment. Recent reviews of patients developing PML indicate that over half have been treated with a prior immunosuppressive therapy such as mitoxantrone, cyclophosphamide, or azathioprine. This proportion is not reflective of the general MS population, suggesting that prior immunosuppression may increase the risk of developing PML. Attempts to mitigate PML risk have been made. More recent research is beginning to converge on the idea that a "drug holiday" may be ill advised, potentially leading patients to incur more disability with drug discontinuation [37–39]. A potentially more effective risk mitigation strategy may be the development of a serum anti-JC virus antibody test. Recent work suggests that about half of the general population is infected with JC virus. Because JC virus infection is a required precursor to the development of PML presumably patients not infected could not develop it. All pre-PML serum samples retrospectively tested with this assay returned positive for JC virus prior to developing PML [40]. This data, of course, needs to be prospectively validated, but hope remains that we will be able to more effectively screen patients prior to treatment and by doing so significantly attenuate the risk of this potentially devastating disease.

It is worth noting that while natalizumab is generally well tolerated and in the future we may be able to better stratify risk for PML, other opportunistic infections have been reported. Because patients were generally on concomitant immunosuppressives in these cases, it is difficult to know how much of these complications can be attributed to natalizumab.

Fingolimod (Gilenya)

Recently approved by the FDA, Fingolimod is a sphingosine-1 phosphate receptor modulator that prevents lymphocytes from receiving a signal to exit lymphoid tissue, effectively blocking lymphocyte egress from lymph nodes. An important exception to this is that memory T lymphocytes do not have this receptor, and continue to circulate. Fingolimod is lipophyllic and crosses the blood–brain barrier. Two large phase III trials have been conducted. TRANSFORMS [41] was a 1-year double-blind double-dummy study, with 426 patients completing treatment with fingolimod 1.25 mg, 431 patients fingolimod 0.5 mg, and 435 patients 30 mcg IFN-β-1a. FREEDOMS [42] a 2-year double-blind randomized study of 429 completing treatment with 1.25 mg fingolimod, 425 at 0.5 mg fingolimod, and 418 placebo. In the TRANSFORMS trial an annualized relapse rate (ARR) of 0.16 was seen at 0.5 mg, which compared favorably with 0.33 seen in the IFN-β-1a group ($p < 0.001$), a 52% relative reduction. No significant differences were seen among the study groups with respect to progression of disability, although the trial was not adequately powered for this endpoint. In the FREEDOMS trial an annualized relapse rate of 0.18 was seen compared to 0.4 with placebo ($p < 0.001$), a 54% relative reduction. EDSS score change at 2 years was significantly better at both fingolimod doses compared to placebo ($p = 0.002$). MRI measures also favored fingolimod in both trials. A reduced 1-year percentage change from baseline brain volume with 0.5 mg fingolimod –0.31 vs Avonex –0.45 ($p < 0.001$) was observed in the TRANSFORMS trial. In other words, the brain atrophied about one-third less over 1 year in the fingolimod group. It has not been determined whether a lower dose of fingolimod than 0.5 mg could be effective, but plans are ongoing to conduct such a trial.

S1P1 is expressed predominantly on lymphocytes but can also be found on cardiovascular and central nervous system tissue. Because of the ubiquitous nature of the S1P1 receptor in the body, side effects were broad, though not especially common (see Box 8.1). There were two deaths in the TRANS-FORMS trial, one from herpes simplex encephalitis, another from disseminated primary varicella zoster. Both deaths occurred at the high (unapproved) dose. The patient with disseminated primary varicella zoster infection was exposed to a child with chickenpox while receiving steroids. The patient who died from herpes simplex encephalitis also received a course of steroids, and was not treated with retrovirals until a week after initial disease presentation. Both patients had been treated with fingolimod for nearly a year. Patients receiving fingolimod do develop lower respiratory tract infections more commonly. When averaging the two trials at the approved dosage, herpes zoster was seen less frequently than with placebo. Opportunistic infections were not seen. At the time of this writing, over 20,000 patients worldwide have received fingolimod, with no opportunistic infections readily attributable to the medicine occurring. Patients were excluded from trial if they had ever received cladribine or cytoxan in the past, or mitoxantrone within the past 5 years. Patients who had previously received azathioprine or rituximab were included if they had not received these medicines 6 months prior to trial enrollment. Steroids can be employed concomitantly with fingolimod treatment, as this was done in the trials. Lymphocytes returned to normal range about 3 months after drug discontinuation.

Bradycardia is commonly seen after the first dose of fingolimod, with an average decrease in the phase III trials of 8 beats per minute, peaking at 4 to 5 hours after administration seen in both trials. Symptomatic bradycardia was seen in $\leq 0.7\%$ of patients in the trials at the FDA-approved dose, with 0.2% of patients having a second-degree AV block in both trials. Serious heart-related complications at the approved dose did not occur. The FDA

BOX 8.1   Gilenya side effects and monitoring

Bradyarrhythmia, atrioventricular block	First dose 6 hour monitoring, consider EKG
Infection	VZV antibody testing, if negative vaccination
Macular edema	Screening ophthalmologic exam, repeat 3 months after start
Respiratory effects	No specific monitoring recommended
Hepatic effects	Check CBC, LFTs before initiation, no specific serum monitoring after start
Fetal risk	Advise contraception

recommendations are that patients be monitored for 6 hours after the first dose. At our center, an EKG is obtained prior to drug initiation, pulse is measured every hour, and atropine is on hand. Fingolimod should be used judiciously in patients with known cardiac conditions. Patients not having fingolimod for 2 weeks need to be re-observed when the drug is reintroduced.

Macular edema was seen in 0.2% of patients at the approved dose in the TRANSFORMS trial, no cases were seen at this dose in FREEDOMS. Usually this is reversible with discontinuation of the drug, though 1 patient in each trial had a more permanent deficit. Because of concern for macular edema, the FDA has recommended that patients should undergo a screening ophthalmologic examination prior to drug initiation and at 3 months after starting fingolimod. Liver function tests should be drawn before treatment initiation. No specific monitoring was suggested for pulmonary function. Patients taking fingolimod did see a mild drop in forced expiratory volume (FEV1) at 1 month (2–3%), but no further reductions were observed. No changes in lung volumes or diffusion capacity were seen, and patients did not have an increased frequency of shortness of breath when compared with placebo. Routine monitoring of pulmonary function tests is not warranted but should be performed in cases where concerns arise. Discretion should be used in patients with pre-existing lung disease. Patients were advised to not be on fingolimod when trying to become pregnant, and should not breast-feed.

Mitoxantrone (Novantrone)

Mitoxantrone intercalates in DNA, reducing T cells, and serving as an immunomodulator and suppressant. It is the only medication approved by the FDA for the treatment of SPMS, though it also carries an indication for RRMS and progressive-relapsing MS. Two randomized-controlled trials suggest that mitoxantrone is efficacious in these settings. A trial by Edan et al. [43] randomized relapsing-remitting patients with recently enhancing lesions on MRI to mitoxantrone and methylprednisolone or methylprednisolone alone. An 86% reduction was seen in the proportion of patients with enhancing lesions in the mitoxantrone group when compared with placebo. A good effect was seen on relapse rate and EDSS as well, with relapse rate declining from a baseline 3.4 relapses/year to 0.7 relapse/year and EDSS improving rather than worsening with time. It is worth noting that clinician evaluators were not blind to treatment. The European Mitoxantrone in MS (MIMS) [44] study led to drug approval in the USA. It is considered as class II evidence due to incomplete blinding. Patients were admitted to the trial with either relapsing-remitting or secondary progressive disease. Again an effect on relapse rate was seen with an annualized relapse rate of 0.35 vs 1.02 (p = 0.001) in the mitoxantrone vs placebo groups at 2 years, as well as an improvement in EDSS. A post-hoc analysis found that patients with nonrelapsing secondary progressive MS responded to mitoxantrone as well as the secondary progressive patients with relapses, with favorable effects on EDSS progression and relapse rate seen in both groups. Mitoxantrone has many potential toxicities, but the two of primary concern are the development of acute leukemias and cardiac failure. Recent estimates are that acute leukemias occur in 0.8% of mitoxantrone-treated patients, cardiac systolic dysfunction in 12%, and heart failure in 0.8% [45]. At our center we use cyclophosphamide in preference to mitoxantrone because it has a more favorable side effect profile.

Off label MS medications

Immunosuppressives

Cyclophosphamide (Cytoxan)

Cyclophosphamide (Cytoxan) is a synthetic compound related to nitrogen mustards that becomes an alkylating agent after being metabolized in the liver. It interferes with the growth of cells, resulting in a variety of effects on the immune system. Many trials with cyclophosphamide have been conducted, with some showing a treatment response [46–49], others not [50, 51]. Over time it has become clear that certain characteristics suggest whether or not a patient will respond to cyclophosphamide (see Box 8.2). Because trials show that the effect of a cyclophosphamide induction lasts an average of 18 months, with some patient experiencing return of clinical activity at 6 months, we now favor a booster protocol [49]. Reader-blinded studies also show a favorable effect of cyclophosphamide on MRI measures [52–55]. A small open label trial of high-dose [50 mg/kg/d for 4 days) intravenous cyclophosphamide in patients with active disease showed a reduction in EDSS and T2 lesions [56]. Some open label trials of patients undergoing immunoablation with Cytoxan, with subsequent autologous stem cell transplantation, have reported impressive

---

BOX 8.2   Factor associated with a response to cyclophosphamide [122–133]

- Rapidly progressive course
- Gadolinium-enhancing lesions on MRI
- Relapses in the year prior to therapy
- Less than 2 years in the progressive phase
- Younger age
- Lower initial disability score

efficacy [57], though concerns about possible neurotoxicity from these aggressive treatments urge caution in over-application [58]. Open label reports of cyclophosphamide's efficacy in an active pediatric MS population also exist [59].

Our experience has been that monthly pulses of Cytoxan are generally well tolerated. At our center it is given in conjunction with IV methylprednisolone, anti-emetics, and aggressive (3L) intravenous fluid hydration on the day of treatment and the day after. As there is some evidence to suggest that methylprednisolone may augment cyclophosphamide's effects and cause less renal toxicity [60], it is our practice to co-administer steroids and cyclophosphamide. Alopecia is common with induction therapy, though less so with monthly pulses. Cyclophosphamide can cause infertility, with premature menopause more likely to occur in patients over the age of 25 or receiving >300 mg/kg cumulative dose [61]. Malignancies have been reported in patients receiving cyclophosphamide in the oncology and rheumatology literature, and the risk is thought to increase after a cumulative dose of 100 grams [62]. As bladder cancers have been reported quite frequently with cyclophosphamide treatment, we now perform annual urine cytologies at our institution. Opportunistic infections have been reported, including progressive multifocal leukoencephalopathy [63, 64]. Despite these concerns, a single follow-up study of MS patients undergoing pulse cyclophosphamide treatment found that it was well tolerated, with amenorrhea (33.3%), hypogammaglobulinemia (5.4%), and hemorrhagic cystitis (4.5%) being the most commonly reported side effects. Malignancies were diagnosed in 4 (3.6%) subjects, 30 of whom were previously treated with azathioprine (AZA). Interestingly, 81.8% of the patients judged the treatment regimen to be very, or relatively, acceptable and tolerable [65].

Mycophenolate mofetil (Cellcept)

Mycophenolate mofetil is a potent immunosuppressant that selectively inhibits inosine 5'-monophosphate dehydrogenase type II, the enzyme responsible for the de novo synthesis of the purine nucleotide guanine within activated T and B lymphocytes and macrophages. It has been used successfully to prevent organ rejection and has shown efficacy in treating other autoimmune diseases. Though no placebo-controlled trials have been completed in MS, open label reports are available. A trial of mycophenolate in 7 progressive patients [66] found that mycophenolate was well tolerated and either offered improvement or halted progression in 5 patients. MRI was available for only 2 patients, but was improved. One patient had a reduced dose because of frequent nonserious infections. Nausea was common. A retrospective review of patients on mycophenolate monotherapy, or in combination with INF-β or glatiramer acetate found again that mycophenolate was well tolerated, with 70% of patients continuing therapy [67]. Diarrhea was common, as was nausea. A case of cytomegalovirus diarrhea occurred, though no other serious infections were reported. Seven patients had disease progression, and clinical impression was that the others remained stable on therapy, though no formal evaluations were performed. An open label study in 30 active relapsing-remitting patients treated with a combination of INF-β-1a (Avonex) and mycophenolate reported a reduction in relapse rate (2 to 0.57), an average improvement in EDSS (2.9 to 2.6), and an absence of gadolinium lesions on MRI follow-up [68]. Six patients reported diarrhea, with one discontinuation. Eight patients reported transient abdominal pains, and 5 had transient nausea. During the 6-month study, relapses occurred more commonly in the first 2 months, suggesting some latency to drug effect.

At our center we tend to employ mycophenolate in MS patients progressing despite treatment with IFN or glatiramer. We have also had successful results in patients with neuromyelitis optica, an experience supported by a retrospective review [69]. We use the same dosages that were used in the open label studies: 250 mg twice daily for week 1, then 500 mg twice daily for week 2; 750 mg twice daily for week 3, then 1 gram twice daily thereafter. Laboratory studies – performed at baseline then at months 1, 2, 3, 6, and 12 – consist of liver function testing, a complete blood count, and basic metabolic panel. Though in the trials mycophenolate was well tolerated, immunosuppressive complications are known to occur and include progressive multifocal leukoencephalopathy [70]. Confirmed cases have been seen in solid organ transplant patients and patient with lupus, all of which were on concomitant immunosuppression.

Methotrexate

Methotrexate is a general immunosuppressant that acts primarily by inhibition of dihydrofolate reductase (Neuhaus 2007 [74]). Few randomized trials of methotrexate in MS have been conducted. Goodkin et al. [71] randomized 31 progressive patients to 7.5 mg of methotrexate and 29 to placebo for 36 months. In the treatment arm 23% of patients were PPMS, in the placebo arm 38% PPMS, with the remainder in each arm being SPMS patients. Neither sustained EDSS progression nor time to first relapse differed between the groups. MRI metrics were reported separately later [72] but also were unimpressive with no change in new T2 or gadolinium-enhancing lesions demonstrated between groups. Though it is fair to say that these results are unimpressive, some caveats should be offered. The first is that the trial did show a favorable effect of methotrexate on its primary outcome measure, a combination of EDSS, ambulation index, box and block test, and 9-hole PEG test. This effect was driven primarily by the 9-hole PEG test, with some support from the box and block test. A second caveat is that the T2 lesion area was significantly reduced compared to placebo when accounting for study week and baseline T2 lesion area. In this trial methotrexate was generally well tolerated with side effects reported no more frequently than in the placebo arm.

A recent study randomized patients with breakthrough disease while on Avonex, to combination treatment with either methotrexate 20 mg weekly, intravenous methylprednisolone 1 g bimonthly, or both [73]. Though again methotrexate was well tolerated, no significant benefit was observed in patients receiving Avonex combined with methotrexate when compared with those receiving Avonex alone on a number of metrics, including new or enlarged T2 lesions, gadolinium-enhancing lesions, MSFC, or brain parenchymal fraction. Because methotrexate's efficacy is questionable on the basis of currently available information, it is rarely used in our clinic.

Azathioprine (Immuran)

Azathioprine (Immuran) is a purine analogue that is metabolized to 6-mercaptopurine and thioinosine acid, which compete with DNA nucleotides, causing immunosuppression [74]. It has found use in autoimmune disorders such as myasthenia gravis and post-transplant organ rejection prevention. The largest trial of azathioprine (AZA) in MS [75] randomized 354 patients to either azathioprine 2.5 mg/kg daily or placebo and followed them for 3 years. Little change in EDSS (AZA 0.62 vs placebo 0.80) or relapse rate (AZA 2.2 vs placebo 2.5) was observed between the two groups, though ambulation index (AZA 0.84 vs placebo 1.25, CI 0.03–0.80) was significantly improved. About a third of patients were classified as having progressive disease, but a subgroup analysis revealed that neither disease course responded particularly to azathioprine. A meta-analysis looking at 698 patients included in placebo-controlled double-blind randomized trials of azathioprine in MS was recently conducted [76]. The authors concluded that the relapse rate declined at 2 years when compared with placebo (relative risk reduction 23%, 95% CI 12–33%). At 3 years there was a statistically significant reduction in risk of progression (RRR = 42%, 95% CI 7–64%). A study performed after this meta-analysis randomized 181 relapsing-remitting MS patients into one of three groups: Avonex or Avonex and 50 mg daily azathioprine, or Avonex and 50 mg oral daily azathioprine, and 10 mg oral prednisone every other day. Annualized relapse rate at 2 years [77] did not differ between groups. Cumulative probably of sustained disability progression also did not differ. Percent T2 lesion volume change favored the combination of azathioprine and Avonex, with a 14.5% increase vs 30.3% increase for Avonex alone, p < 0.05).

Generally mild side effects were seen, especially in the first year of azathioprine treatment. Leukopenia, macrocytic anemia, liver function abnormalities, pancytopenia, nausea, fever, and herpes zoster have been seen more commonly in MS than in placebo patients in trials. Some studies report increased hematologic malignancies with long-term azathioprine use [78] while others do not [79].

Other agents

Steroids

Steroids have historically been a mainstay of treatment for MS exacerbations. Many years ago it was demonstrated that daily low-dose oral steroid treatment was ineffective as maintenance therapy [80]. Two studies address the question of whether patients are better off in the long term for having received acute steroid treatment for a relapse. Miller et al. [81] found that at 1 month patients who had received 500 mg intravenous methylprednisolone for 5 days had lessened disability when compared with those who had not. Sellebjerg et al. [82] reported that at 8 weeks patients receiving 5 days of 500 mg of oral methylprednisolone with taper had improved EDSS compared to placebo. Recent work indicates that a steroid taper is probably not beneficial, except in particular circumstances [83]. It is not clear whether 3 or 5 days of IV methylprednisolone treatment is better, but it is likely that more than 5 days offers no additional benefit [84]. Oral dosage equivalents probably have the same clinical efficacy of a 1 g intravenous methylprednisolone course [85]. Prednisone 1250 mg has the same mean area under the concentration–time curve, suggesting equivalent absorption [86]. Because the peak concentration of methylprednisolone and prednisone differs, it remains our preference to give steroids intravenously, though for patients that have difficulty presenting for intravenous therapy, we do occasionally use oral prednisone in substitution. Patients may swallow the requisite 25 tablets of 50 mg, or crush and mix them in a fruit smoothie to make them more palatable. Though a few studies have also been performed with oral methylprednisolone, we use this less because in practice it tends to be more expensive for patients.

At our center pulsed steroids are often used for inflammatory breakthrough disease in combination with an injectable agent. A trial in an RRMS population giving patients 5 days of 1 g of methylprednisolone with oral taper every 4 months for 3 years, then every 6 months for 2 years, showed a reduction in brain T1-hypointensities and an improvement in brain parenchymal fraction and probability of sustained EDSS worsening (a 32% reduction) when compared with placebo [87]. No effect was seen on T2 lesion volume and annualized relapse rate. Recently completed trials looking at the combination of injectable agents with steroids are also of interest.

The Avonex combination trial employed a factorial design and was underpowered but showed a 30% reduction in relapse rate (p = 0.12) in patients receiving Avonex and 3 days of 1 g methylprednisolone bimonthly when compared to patients received Avonex alone [73]. The Nordic trial of oral methylprednisolone as add-on therapy to INF-β-1a for treatment of relapsing-remitting multiple sclerosis (NORMIMS) [88] randomized patients to Rebif with or without 200 mg oral methylprednisolone for 5 consecutive days monthly. Patients receiving oral methylprednisolone showed a 62% reduction in annualized relapse rate (p < 0.001). No effect was seen on disability progression, changes in MSFC, or normalized brain parenchymal volume, though T2 lesion volume was also decreased in the methylprednisolone group. Similar results were seen in methylprednisolone in combination with IFN-B-1a (MECOMBIN) study [89], which randomized patients to Avonex with or without 500 mg oral methylprednisolone for 3 days monthly. Again no effect on disability progression was seen, but the annualized relapse rate was reduced (38% relative reduction, p = 0.002) along with other measures such as the multiple sclerosis functional composite (MSFC), 9-hole PEG testing, change in T1 and T2 lesion volume. Taken together these results support the use of adjunctive steroids in patients with breakthrough disease.

We also employ pulse methylprednisolone in our progressive patients. Though no large-scale trials have been performed in this population some anecdotal evidence exists that this might be helpful. Goodkin et al. [90] randomized 108 patients with secondary progressive MS to receive either bimonthly pulses of 500 mg (high-dose) or 10 mg (low-dose) methylprednisolone every 8 weeks for 2 years. This trial found that the time to onset of sustained treatment failure was longer in the low dose methylprednisolone-treated patients. A trial of 35 Italian patients with a "primarily chronic progressive form of multiple sclerosis" who received 1 g of IV methylprednisolone daily for 5 days showed improvement on EDSS at 90 days (p < 0.001) when compared with placebo [91]. An open label trial including 18 patients with chronic progressive MS who received 1 g of methylprednisolone daily for 6 days showed a measurable improvement in EDSS at 12 months [92].

Pulse steroids are generally well tolerated, though they tend to have a higher rate of trial discontinuation than placebo. Common pulse steroid effects include a metallic taste in the mouth, agitation, insomnia, and flushing. It is our practice to monitor bone density every other year. We dissuade patients with osteoporosis from steroid treatment, though a recent trial found no effect on bone density scans obtained 39 months after treatment when compared with placebo [89]. Avascular necrosis of the hip [93] is probably an underappreciated complication, but has not arisen frequently in our practice. Infections related to immunosuppression can occur but are uncommon. Weight gain and cataracts can occur and patients should be monitored for this. In practice we use pulse methylprednisolone for relapsing patients on a platform agent with either clinical or radiologic evidence of breakthrough disease or for primary or secondary progressive MS patients experiencing slow decline.

Plasmapheresis and IVIg

Plasmapheresis and IVIg are used to treat other autoimmune neurologic disease such as myasthenia gravis and Guillain–Barre but both have shown limited success in MS. We employ plasmapheresis in patients suffering a catastrophic relapse that is not steroid responsive. Work by Weinshenker et al. [94] suggests that this subgroup of patients can benefit from plasmapheresis after an acute relapse. Multiple randomized-controlled studies have failed to show an effect of plasma exchange in chronic progressive patients [47, 51, 95]. Based on recommendations from the American Academy of Neurology [21] we reserve plasmapheresis for patients with a disabling relapse who have failed steroid therapy.

IVIg has also been tested in MS. A meta-analysis combining a number of small, randomized trials concluded that IVIg reduces relapse rate in RRMS with a magnitude of effect similar to the first line injectable agents [96]. A recently published study including 127 RRMS patients found that the proportion of relapse-free patients did not differ between IVIg and placebo with no effect observed on MRI measures, leading the authors to conclude that IVIG was ineffective for this population [97]. A trial employing IVIg in secondary progressive MS was unable to show an effect [98]. Two trials examining IVIg's ability to promote recovery after an acute relapse were unable to demonstrate an effect. IVIg has not been tested in primary progressive MS. Based on a trial by Haas et al. [99] there may be a role for postpartum treatment in active MS patients, though definitive conclusions cannot be made because the study was open label.

TOP TIPS 8.2: Treatment for acute MS relapses

- Relapses causing disability should be treated with IV methylprednisolone for 3–5 days.
- Plasmapheresis may be considered for patients who have not improved after methylprednisolone treatment.
- In extreme circumstances a high-dose cyclophosphamide induction may be considered.
- In cases when a patient cannot present for intravenous treatment 1250 mg of prednisone may be considered in substitution.

Rituximab (Rituxan)

Rituximab depletes CD20 + B cells through a combination of cell-mediated and complement dependent cytotoxic effects and the promotion of apoptosis. Its effect in MS may be related to decreased B cell cytokine secretion resulting in reduced T cell activation [100]. In a phase II trial it showed a relapse rate reduction of 58% and a 91% decrease in gadolinium enhancement compared to placebo [101]. One gram was given once then repeated 2 weeks later. It is unclear when a follow-up dose should be given after this. Some argue that it makes sense to wait until CD19 (a surrogate of CD20) returns to the low normal range, others are proponents of dosing about every 9 months, arguing that disease activity can return before CD19 counts normalize. In phase II rituximab-treated patients tended to react poorly to the first infusion with nearly 80% having an infusion-related reaction. Chills, nausea, headache, and pruritis were the most common symptoms. After the first dose, however, infusion-related reactions were seen more commonly in the placebo group. The overall incidence of infection was the same between placebo and rituximab groups, with no opportunistic infections reported, although urinary tract and sinus infections were somewhat more common in the rituximab group. Currently because of patent considerations there are no plans to pursue phase III trials with this drug. Ocrelizumab is an anti-CD20 antibody virtually identical to rituximab in its receptor binding site but its molecular backbone is more humanized. A phase II trial is ongoing though a recent trial in rheumatoid arthritis was stopped because of infection risk, some reported as opportunistic and fatal. We generally reserve rituximab for patients who have failed conventional agents. It is worth noting that PML has been seen with rituximab, though only when used in conjunction with other immuno-suppressives [102]. An open label report suggests that rituximab may be helpful for neuromyelitis optica [103]. A post-hoc analysis of a primary progressive trial found that patients <51 years old or with gadolinium-enhancing lesions responded to rituximab [104]. In this patient population we use rituximab if monthly intravenous pulse methylprednisolone appears ineffective.

In development

A number of medications have either completed phase III trials or are in trial. Table 8.2 lists these medications with initial trial results, and known side effects. We regard laquinimod and BG00012 as potentially exciting new medications. In phase II trials these oral medications were effective, well tolerated, and safe [106, 107]. Preliminary results of both the laquinimod and BG00012 phase III placebo-controlled trials have been released, though not published [108, 109]. Laquinimod showed a relapse rate reduction of 23% compared to placebo, with a 36% reduction in disability progression. New MRI T2 lesions were reduced 30%, brain atrophy 33%. It is taken daily

Table 8.2 Multiple sclerosis drugs currently in phase II or III trial (published results)

Drug	Phase	Comparator	No. patients	Admission Criteria	Trial Length	Outcome
BG00012 [106]	II	Placebo	257	RRMS, EDSS <5, 1 relapse prior year	24 wks	↓ Gd + lesions 69% (p<0.0001) ↓ relapse rate 32% (NS)
Laquinimod [107]	II	Placebo	306	RRMS, EDSS 1–5, 1 relapse prior year, 1 gd + lesion on screening MRI	36 wks	↓ cum. gd + lesions 40.4%, p=0.0048
Teriflunomide [124]	II	Placebo	179	RRMS or SPMS EDSS <6, 2 relapses prior 3 years, 1 relapse prior year	36 wks	↓ median # combined unique lesions 60% (p < 0.03)
Alemtuzimab [112]	II	Rebif	334	RRMS, EDSS ≤3, disease duration<3 years	36 wks	↓ rate of sustained accumulation of disability HR 0.29 (p < 0.001) ↓ relapse rate 74% (p < 0.001)
Daclizumab [125]	II	IFN + DAC or IFN + placebo	230	RRMS, EDSS <5, relapse or gd + lesion prior 6 months on IFN	24	↓ new or enlarging gd + lesions 72% (p = 0.004)
Abatacept	II	Abatacept or placebo	132	RRMS, EDSS <5, relapse or gd + lesion in prior year	24 weeks + extension to 64 weeks	mean number of new gd + lesions from weeks 8 to 24

HR = hazard ratio, RRMS = relapsing-remitting MS, EDSS = expanded disability status scale, gd + = gadolinium, cum = cumulative, IFN = interferon, DAC = daclizumab.

and other than LFT abnormalities (6.9% vs 2.7% in placebo), no side effects were seen. BG00012 showed a reduction in annualized relapse rate of 53%, disability 38%, new or enlarging T2 lesions about 85%. Results have also recently been released for Laquinimod and BG00012 phase III trials run in parallel with an active comparator, though not yet published. Though not designed for direct comparison the reduction is relapse rates and gadolinium enhancement vs. placebo are in line with what was reported in the first phase III trial for each drug. In the phase II BG00012 trial GI upset and flushing were seen in 52% of patients at 1 month, but were diminished to 4% at 6 months. Phase III results are reportedly similar. A phase III placebo-controlled trial demonstrated teriflunomide's favorable effect on MS, with a relapse rate reduction of 30% compared to placebo, 67% reduction in MRI total lesion volume [110]. It is our impression that this medication will be used sparingly because it is likely to be teratogenic and classified as pregnancy class X. In the appropriate patient, however, initial indications are that it is otherwise well tolerated. A number of add-on studies are ongoing. Daclizumab is being developed as a monthly injectable for MS. At our center we reported that the IV formulation showed a good efficacy and tolerability [111], though this is no longer available. It is also being explored as a potential add-on drug. Alemtuzumab (Campath), a monoclonal antibody

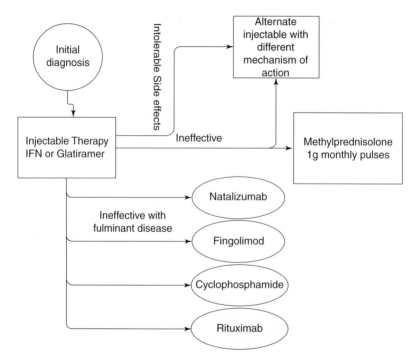

Figure 8.1 General schematic for treatment of relapsing-remitting multiple sclerosis.

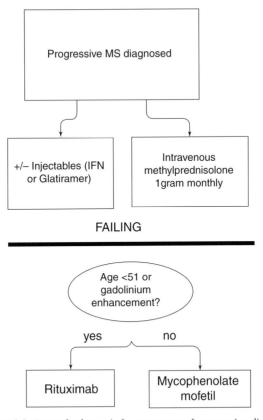

Figure 8.2 General schematic for treatment of progressive disease.

that target CD52 on lymphocytes and monocytes, performed impressively in phase II trials with a relapse rate reduction of 72% and a significant reduction in T2 lesion load when compared head-to-head against Rebif [112]. Though the phase II trial was not powered to look at disability an effect was still seen with an improvement in EDSS that compared favorably to the worsened EDSS seen with Rebif. In the trial there was a death related to a hemorrhagic complication from immune thrombocytopenia purpura, which is now an appreciated side effect of the drug. With proper monitoring this risk can be mitigated. Thyroid abnormalities were seen in 23% of treated patients. Mild to moderate respiratory tract infections were seen more commonly in the alemtuzumab group though no opportunistic infections were seen. At the time of this writing, results of two phase III trials with alemtuzumab have been released but not yet published. The first trial showed a 55% reduction in relapse rate vs. Rebif, but did not demonstrate an effect on sustained disability progression. The overall rate of disability progression in the trial was low for both alemtuzumab (8%) and Rebif (11%) treated patients. The second trial required patients to have a relapse while on therapy prior to enrollment. There was a 49% reduction in relapse rate vs. Rebif and 42% reduction in sustained disability progression, both significant results. Abatacept (CTLA4Ig, Orencia®) is a selective T cell co-stimulation modulator FDA approved for active rheumatoid arthritis (RA) in adults and active polyarticular juvenile idiopathic arthritis in pediatric patients. It has a favorable safety profile. A phase I trial of CTLA4Ig in MS was done at our center, showing that it was safe. It is currently in a phase II multicenter trial.

Conclusion

Great advances have been made in treatment of MS. Considering that the first MS medication was FDA approved less than two decades ago, our current armamentarium is impressive, and the breadth and depth of medications in development is encouraging. Currently we tend to start patients initially on an FDA-approved injectable. If new relapses or MRI activity occur we will either add a course of IV methylprednisolone monthly pulse therapy for 6 months or switch to a different medication. If the patient is experiencing some indications of failure but not significantly worsening we will tend to switch to an injectable with a different mechanism of action (i.e. IFN to Copaxone, or vice versa) (Figure 8.1]. If, on the other hand, the patient is significantly worse we favor beginning natalizumab, fingolimod, or cyclophosphamide. Though this is a general framework for beginning to think about where to employ medications, ultimately treatment decisions must be individualized. Unfortunately we have no bona fide treatments for progressive disease, but some literature supports trials of cellcept or rituximab and we have anecdotally at times had good results with these medicines (Figure 8.2). We look forward to the release of a number of exciting new options over the next few years, and expect that we will continue to make progress toward a cure.

References

1 Zhang J, Hutton G, Zang Y. A comparison of the mechanisms of action of interferon beta and glatiramer acetate in the treatment of multiple sclerosis. Clin Ther 2002 Dec; 24(12): 1998–2021.

2 Axtell RC, de Jong BA, Boniface K, van der Voort LF, Bhat R, De Sarno P, et al. T helper type 1 and 17 cells determine efficacy of interferon-beta in multiple sclerosis and experimental encephalomyelitis. Nat Med 2010 Apr; 16(4): 406–12.

3 Li DK, Paty DW. Magnetic resonance imaging results of the PRISMS trial: a randomized, double-blind, placebo-controlled study of interferon-beta 1a in relapsing-remitting multiple sclerosis. Prevention of Relapses and Disability by

Interferon-beta1a Subcutaneously in Multiple Sclerosis. Ann Neurol 1999 Aug; 46(2): 197–206.

4 O'Connor P, Filippi M, Arnason B, Comi G, Cook S, Goodin D, et al. 250 microg or 500 microg interferon beta-1b versus 20 mg glatiramer acetate in relapsing-remitting multiple sclerosis: a prospective, randomised, multicentre study. Lancet Neurol 2009 Oct; 8(10): 889–97.

5 Cadavid D, Wolansky LJ, Skurnick J, Lincoln J, Cheriyan J, Szczepanowski K, et al. Efficacy of treatment of MS with IFNbeta-1b or glatiramer acetate by monthly brain MRI in the BECOME study. Neurology 2009 Jun 9; 72(23): 1976–83.

6 Mikol DD, Barkhof F, Chang P, Coyle PK, Jeffery DR, Schwid SR, et al. Comparison of subcutaneous interferon beta-1a with glatiramer acetate in patients with relapsing multiple sclerosis (the REbif vs Glatiramer Acetate in Relapsing MS Disease REGARD] study): a multicentre, randomised, parallel, open-label trial. Lancet Neurol 2008 Oct; 7(10): 903–14.

7 Zivadinov R, Reder AT, Filippi M, Minagar A, Stuve O, Lassmann H, et al. Mechanisms of action of disease-modifying agents and brain volume changes in multiple sclerosis. Neurology 2008 Jul; 71(2): 136–44.

8 Rudick RA, Fisher E, Lee JC, Simon J, Jacobs L. Use of the brain parenchymal fraction to measure whole brain atrophy in relapsing-remitting MS. Multiple Sclerosis Collaborative Research Group. Neurology 1999 Nov; 53(8): 1698–704.

9 Khoury S, Bakshi R. Cerebral pseudoatrophy or real atrophy after therapy in multiple sclerosis. Ann Neurol 2010 Dec; 68(6): 778–9.

10 Pliskin NH, Hamer DP, Goldstein DS, Towle VL, Reder AT, Noronha A, et al. Improved delayed visual reproduction test performance in multiple sclerosis patients receiving interferon beta-1b. Neurology 1996 Dec; 47(6): 1463–8.

11 Fischer JS, Priore RL, Jacobs LD, Cookfair DL, Rudick RA, Herndon RM, et al. Neuropsychological effects of interferon beta-1a in relapsing multiple sclerosis. Multiple Sclerosis Collaborative Research Group. Ann Neurol 2000 Dec; 48(6): 885–92.

12 Barak Y, Achiron A. Effect of interferon-beta-1b on cognitive functions in multiple sclerosis. Eur Neurol 2002; 47(1): 11–14.

13 Metz LM, Patten SB, Archibald CJ, Bakker JI, Harris CJ, Patry DG, et al. The effect of immunomodulatory treatment on multiple sclerosis fatigue. J Neurol Neurosurg Psychiat 2004 Jul; 75(7): 1045–7.

14 Rojas JI, Romano M, Ciapponi A, Patrucco L, Cristiano E. Interferon Beta for primary progressive multiple sclerosis. Cochrane Database Syst Rev 2010 (1): CD006643.

15 Placebo-controlled multicentre randomised trial of interferon beta-1b in treatment of secondary progressive multiple sclerosis. European Study Group on interferon beta-1b in secondary progressive MS. Lancet 1998 Nov; 352(9139): 1491–7.

16 Panitch H, Miller A, Paty D, Weinshenker B. Interferon beta-1b in secondary progressive MS: results from a 3-year controlled study. Neurology 2004 Nov; 63(10): 1788–95.

17 Goodin DS, Frohman EM, Hurwitz B, O'Connor PW, Oger JJ, Reder AT, et al. Neutralizing antibodies to interferon beta: assessment of their clinical and radiographic impact: an evidence report: report of the Therapeutics and Technology Assessment Subcommittee of the American Academy of Neurology. Neurology 2007 Mar; 68(13): 977–84.

18 Tremlett HL, Yoshida EM, Oger J. Liver injury associated with the beta-interferons for MS: a comparison between the three products. Neurology 2004 Feb; 62(4): 628–31.

19 Panitch H, Goodin DS, Francis G, Chang P, Coyle PK, O'Connor P, et al. Randomized, comparative study of interferon beta-1a treatment regimens in MS: The EVIDENCE Trial. Neurology 2002 Nov; 59(10): 1496–506.

20 Durelli L, Verdun E, Barbero P, Bergui M, Versino E, Ghezzi A, et al. Every-other-day interferon beta-1b versus once-weekly interferon beta-1a for multiple sclerosis: results of a 2-year prospective randomised multicentre study (INCOMIN). Lancet 2002 Apr; 359(9316): 1453–60.

21 Goodin DS, Frohman EM, Garmany GP, Jr., Halper J, Likosky WH, Lublin FD, et al. Disease modifying therapies in multiple sclerosis: report of the Therapeutics and Technology Assessment Subcommittee of the American Academy of Neurology and the MS Council for Clinical Practice Guidelines. Neurology 2002 Jan; 58(2): 169–78.

22 Farina C, Weber MS, Meinl E, Wekerle H, Hohlfeld R. Glatiramer acetate in multiple sclerosis: update on potential mechanisms of action. Lancet Neurol 2005 Sep; 4(9): 567–75.

23 Johnson KP, Brooks BR, Cohen JA, Ford CC, Goldstein J, Lisak RP, et al. Copolymer 1 reduces relapse rate and improves disability in relapsing-remitting multiple sclerosis: results of a phase III multicenter, double-blind placebo-controlled trial. The Copolymer 1 Multiple Sclerosis Study Group. Neurology 1995 Jul; 45(7): 1268–76.

24 Ford C, Goodman AD, Johnson K, Kachuck N, Lindsey JW, Lisak R, et al. Continuous long-term immunomodulatory therapy in relapsing multiple sclerosis: results from the 15-year analysis of the US prospective open-label study of glatiramer acetate. Mult Scler 2010 Mar; 16(3): 342–50.

25 Rovaris M, Comi G, Rocca MA, Valsasina P, Ladkani D, Pieri E, et al. Long-term follow-up of patients treated with glatiramer acetate: a multicentre, multinational extension of the European/Canadian double-blind, placebo-controlled, MRI-monitored trial. Mult Scler 2007 May; 13(4): 502–8.

26 Weinstein A, Schwid SR, Schiffer RB, McDermott MP, Giang DW, Goodman AD. Neuropsychologic status in multiple sclerosis after treatment with glatiramer. Arch Neurol 1999 Mar; 56(3): 319–24.

27 Wolinsky JS, Narayana PA, O'Connor P, Coyle PK, Ford C, Johnson K, et al. Glatiramer acetate in primary progressive multiple sclerosis: results of a multinational, multicenter, double-blind, placebo-controlled trial. Ann Neurol 2007 Jan; 61(1): 14–24.

28 Bornstein MB, Miller A, Slagle S, Weitzman M, Drexler E, Keilson M, et al. A placebo-controlled, double-blind, randomized, two-center, pilot trial of Cop 1 in chronic progressive multiple sclerosis. Neurology 1991 Apr; 41(4): 533–9.

29 Caon CPJ, Tselis A, Ching W, Bao F, Latif Z, Zak I, Khan O.Twice weekly versus daily glatiramer acetate: results of a randomized, rater-blinded prospective clinical trial clinical and MRI study in relapsing-remitting MS. [Abstract presented at American Academy of Neurology.] In press 2010.

30 Cadavid D, Cheriyan J, Skurnick J, Lincoln JA, Wolansky LJ, Cook SD. New acute and chronic black holes in patients with multiple sclerosis randomised to interferon beta-1b or glatiramer acetate. J Neurol Neurosurg Psychiat 2009 Dec; 80(12): 1337–43.

31 Polman CH, O'Connor PW, Havrdova E, Hutchinson M, Kappos L, Miller DH, et al. A randomized, placebo-controlled trial of natalizumab for relapsing multiple sclerosis. N Engl J Med 2006 Mar; 354(9): 899–910.

32 Miller DH, Khan OA, Sheremata WA, Blumhardt LD, Rice GP, Libonati MA, et al. A controlled trial of natalizumab for relapsing multiple sclerosis. N Engl J Med 2003 Jan; 348(1): 15–23.

33 Mattioli F, Stampatori C, Capra R. The effect of natalizumab on cognitive function in patients with relapsing-remitting multiple sclerosis: preliminary results of a 1-year follow-up study. Neurol Sci 2010: Sep 25.

34 Miller DH, Soon D, Fernando KT, MacManus DG, Barker GJ, Yousry TA, et al. MRI outcomes in a placebo-controlled trial of natalizumab in relapsing MS. Neurology 2007 Apr; 68(17): 1390–401.

35 Kleinschmidt-DeMasters BK, Tyler KL. Progressive multifocal leukoencephalopathy complicating treatment with natalizumab and interferon beta-1a for multiple sclerosis. N Engl J Med 2005 Jul; 353(4): 369–74.

36 Langer-Gould A, Atlas SW, Green AJ, Bollen AW, Pelletier D. Progressive multifocal leukoencephalopathy in a patient treated with natalizumab. N Engl J Med 2005 Jul; 353(4): 375–81.

37 West TW, Cree BA. Natalizumab dosage suspension: are we helping or hurting? Ann Neurol 2010 Sep; 68(3): 395–9.

38 Miravalle A, Jensen R, Kinkel RP. Immune reconstitution inflammatory syndrome in patients with multiple sclerosis following cessation of natalizumab therapy. Arch Neurol 2011; 68(2): 186–91.

39 Killestein J, Vennegoor A, Strijbis EM, Seewann A, van Oosten BW, Uitdehaag BM, et al. Natalizumab drug holiday in multiple sclerosis: poorly tolerated. Ann Neurol 2010 Sep; 68(3): 392–5.

40 Gorelik L, Lerner M, Bixler S, Crossman M, Schlain B, Simon K, et al. Anti-JC virus antibodies: implications for PML risk stratification. Ann Neurol 2010 Sep; 68(3): 295–303.

41 Cohen JA, Barkhof F, Comi G, Hartung HP, Khatri BO, Montalban X, et al. Oral fingolimod or intramuscular interferon for relapsing multiple sclerosis. N Engl J Med 2010 Feb; 362(5): 402–15.

42 Kappos L, Radue EW, O'Connor P, Polman C, Hohlfeld R, Calabresi P, et al. A placebo-controlled trial of oral fingolimod in relapsing multiple sclerosis. N Engl J Med 2010 Feb; 362(5): 387–401.

43 Edan G, Miller D, Clanet M, Confavreux C, Lyon-Caen O, Lubetzki C, et al. Therapeutic effect of mitoxantrone combined with methylprednisolone in multiple sclerosis: a randomised multicentre study of active disease using MRI and clinical criteria. J Neurol Neurosurg Psychiat 1997 Feb; 62(2): 112–18.

44 Hartung HP, Gonsette R, Konig N, Kwiecinski H, Guseo A, Morrissey SP, et al. Mitoxantrone in progressive multiple sclerosis: a placebo-controlled, double-blind, randomised, multicentre trial. Lancet 2002 Dec; 360(9350): 2018–25.

45 Marriott JJ, Miyasaki JM, Gronseth G, O'Connor PW. Evidence Report: The efficacy and safety of mitoxantrone (Novantrone) in the treatment of multiple sclerosis: Report of the Therapeutics and Technology Assessment Subcommittee of the American Academy of Neurology. Neurology 2010 May; 74(18): 1463–70.

46 Zephir H, de Seze J, Duhamel A, Debouverie M, Hautecoeur P, Lebrun C, et al. Treatment of progressive forms of multiple sclerosis by cyclophosphamide: a cohort study of 490 patients. J Neurol Sci 2004 Mar; 218(1–2): 73–7.

47 Hauser SL, Dawson DM, Lehrich JR, Beal MF, Kevy SV, Propper RD, et al. Intensive immunosuppression in progressive multiple sclerosis. A randomized, three-arm study of high-dose intravenous cyclophosphamide, plasma exchange, and ACTH. N Engl J Med 1983 Jan; 308(4): 173–80.

48 Carter JL, Hafler DA, Dawson DM, Orav J, Weiner HL. Immunosuppression with high-dose i.v. cyclophosphamide and ACTH in progressive multiple sclerosis:

cumulative 6-year experience in 164 patients. Neurology 1988 Jul; 38 (7 Suppl 2): 9–14.

49 Weiner HL, Mackin GA, Orav EJ, Hafler DA, Dawson DM, LaPierre Y, et al. Intermittent cyclophosphamide pulse therapy in progressive multiple sclerosis: final report of the Northeast Cooperative Multiple Sclerosis Treatment Group. Neurology 1993 May; 43(5): 910–18.

50 Likosky WH, Fireman B, Elmore R, Eno G, Gale K, Goode GB, et al. Intense immunosuppression in chronic progressive multiple sclerosis: the Kaiser study. J Neurol Neurosurg Psychiat 1991 Dec; 54(12): 1055–60.

51 The Canadian cooperative trial of cyclophosphamide and plasma exchange in progressive multiple sclerosis. The Canadian Cooperative Multiple Sclerosis Study Group. Lancet 1991 Feb; 337(8739): 441–6.

52 Perini P, Gallo P. Cyclophosphamide is effective in stabilizing rapidly deteriorating secondary progressive multiple sclerosis. J Neurol 2003 Jul; 250(7): 834–8.

53 Gobbini MI, Smith ME, Richert ND, Frank JA, McFarland HF. Effect of open label pulse cyclophosphamide therapy on MRI measures of disease activity in five patients with refractory relapsing-remitting multiple sclerosis. J Neuroimmunol 1999 Sep; 99(1): 142–9.

54 Patti F, Reggio E, Palermo F, Fiorilla T, Politi G, Nicoletti A, et al. Stabilization of rapidly worsening multiple sclerosis for 36 months in patients treated with interferon beta plus cyclophosphamide followed by interferon beta. J Neurol 2004 Dec; 251(12): 1502–6.

55 Smith DR, Weinstock-Guttman B, Cohen JA, Wei X, Gutmann C, Bakshi R, et al. A randomized blinded trial of combination therapy with cyclophosphamide in patients-with active multiple sclerosis on interferon beta. Mult Scler 2005 Oct; 11(5): 573–82.

56 Krishnan C, Kaplin AI, Brodsky RA, Drachman DB, Jones RJ, Pham DL, et al. Reduction of disease activity and disability with high-dose cyclophosphamide in patients with aggressive multiple sclerosis. Arch Neurol 2008 Aug; 65(8): 1044–51.

57 Martino G, Franklin RJ, Van Evercooren AB, Kerr DA. Stem cell transplantation in multiple sclerosis: current status and future prospects. Nat Rev Neurol 2010 May; 6(5): 247–55.

58 Chen JT, Collins DL, Atkins HL, Freedman MS, Galal A, Arnold DL. Brain atrophy after immunoablation and stem cell transplantation in multiple sclerosis. Neurology 2006 Jun; 66(12): 1935–7.

59 Makhani N, Gorman MP, Branson HM, Stazzone L, Banwell BL, Chitnis T. Cyclophosphamide therapy in pediatric multiple sclerosis. Neurology 2009 Jun; 72(24): 2076–82.

60 Illei GG, Austin HA, Crane M, Collins L, Gourley MF, Yarboro CH, et al. Combination therapy with pulse cyclophosphamide plus pulse methylprednisolone improves long-term renal outcome without adding toxicity in patients with lupus nephritis. Ann Intern Med 2001 Aug; 135(4): 248–57.

61 Boumpas DT, Austin HA, 3rd, Vaughan EM, Yarboro CH, Klippel JH, Balow JE. Risk for sustained amenorrhea in patients with systemic lupus erythematosus receiving intermittent pulse cyclophosphamide therapy. Ann Intern Med 1993 Sep; 119(5): 366–9.

62 Talar-Williams C, Hijazi YM, Walther MM, Linehan WM, Hallahan CW, Lubensky I, et al. Cyclophosphamide-induced cystitis and bladder cancer in patients with Wegener granulomatosis. Ann Intern Med 1996 Mar; 124(5): 477–84.

63 Yokoyama H, Watanabe T, Maruyama D, Kim SW, Kobayashi Y, Tobinai K. Progressive multifocal leukoencephalopathy in a patient with B-cell lymphoma during rituximab-containing chemotherapy: case report and review of the literature. Int J Hematol 2008 Nov; 88(4): 443–7.

64 Morgenstern LB, Pardo CA. Progressive multifocal leukoencephalopathy complicating treatment for Wegener's granulomatosis. J Rheumatol 1995 Aug; 22(8): 1593–5.

65 Portaccio E, Zipoli V, Siracusa G, Piacentini S, Sorbi S, Amato MP. Safety and tolerability of cyclophosphamide 'pulses' in multiple sclerosis: a prospective study in a clinical cohort. Mult Scler 2003 Oct; 9(5): 446–50.

66 Ahrens N, Salama A, Haas J. Mycophenolate-mofetil in the treatment of refractory multiple sclerosis. J Neurol 2001 Aug; 248(8): 713–14.

67 Frohman EM, Brannon K, Racke MK, Hawker K. Mycophenolate mofetil in multiple sclerosis. Clin Neuropharmacol 2004 Mar–Apr; 27(2): 80–3.

68 Vermersch P, Waucquier N, Michelin E, Bourteel H, Stojkovic T, Ferriby D, et al. Combination of IFN beta-1a (Avonex) and mycophenolate mofetil (Cellcept) in multiple sclerosis. Eur J Neurol 2007 Jan; 14(1): 85–9.

69 Jacob A, Matiello M, Weinshenker BG, Wingerchuk DM, Lucchinetti C, Shuster E, et al. Treatment of neuromyelitis optica with mycophenolate mofetil: retrospective analysis of 24 patients. Arch Neurol 2009 Sep; 66(9): 1128–33.

70 http://www.fda.gov/downloads/Safety/MedWatch/SafetyInformation/SafetyAlertsforHumanMedicalProducts/ucm093666.pdf. [cited 2010 December 22].

71 Goodkin DE, Rudick RA, VanderBrug Medendorp S, Daughtry MM, Schwetz KM, Fischer J, et al. Low-dose (7.5 mg) oral methotrexate reduces the rate of progression in chronic progressive multiple sclerosis. Ann Neurol 1995 Jan; 37(1): 30–40.

72 Goodkin DE, Rudick RA, VanderBrug Medendorp S, Daughtry MM, Van Dyke C. Low-dose oral methotrexate in chronic progressive multiple sclerosis: analyses of serial MRIs. Neurology 1996 Nov; 47(5): 1153–7.

73 Cohen JA, Imrey PB, Calabresi PA, Edwards KR, Eickenhorst T, Felton WL, 3rd, et al. Results of the Avonex Combination Trial (ACT) in relapsing-remitting MS. Neurology 2009 Feb; 72(6): 535–41.

74 Neuhaus O, Kieseier BC, Hartung HP. Immunosuppressive agents in multiple sclerosis. Neurotherapeutics 2007 Oct; 4(4): 654–60.

75 Double-masked trial of azathioprine in multiple sclerosis. British and Dutch Multiple Sclerosis Azathioprine Trial Group. Lancet 1988 Jul; 2(8604): 179–83.

76 Casetta I, Iuliano G, Filippini G. Azathioprine for multiple sclerosis. Cochrane Database Syst Rev 2007 (4): CD003982.

77 Havrdova E, Zivadinov R, Krasensky J, Dwyer MG, Novakova I, Dolezal O, et al. Randomized study of interferon beta-1a, low-dose azathioprine, and low-dose corticosteroids in multiple sclerosis. Mult Scler 2009 Aug; 15(8): 965–76.

78 Lhermitte F, Marteau R, Roullet E. Not so benign long-term immunosuppression in multiple sclerosis? Lancet 1984 Feb; 1(8371): 276–7.

79 Amato MP, Pracucci G, Ponziani G, Siracusa G, Fratiglioni L, Amaducci L. Long-term safety of azathioprine therapy in multiple sclerosis. Neurology 1993 Apr; 43(4): 831–3.

80 Miller H, Newell DJ, Ridley A. Multiple sclerosis. Trials of maintenance treatment with prednisolone and soluble aspirin. Lancet 1961 Jan; 1(7169): 127–9.

81 Milligan NM, Newcombe R, Compston DA. A double-blind controlled trial of high dose methylprednisolone in patients with multiple sclerosis: 1. Clinical effects. J Neurol Neurosurg Psychiat 1987 May; 50(5): 511–16.

82 Sellebjerg F, Frederiksen JL, Nielsen PM, Olesen J. Double-blind, randomized, placebo-controlled study of oral, high-dose methylprednisolone in attacks of MS. Neurology 1998 Aug; 51(2): 529–34.

83 Perumal JS, Caon C, Hreha S, Zabad R, Tselis A, Lisak R, et al. Oral prednisone taper following intravenous steroids fails to improve disability or recovery from relapses in multiple sclerosis. Eur J Neurol 2008 Jul; 15(7): 677–80.

84 Filippini G, Brusaferri F, Sibley WA, Citterio A, Ciucci G, Midgard R, et al. Corticosteroids or ACTH for acute exacerbations in multiple sclerosis. Cochrane Database Syst Rev 2000 (4): CD001331.

85 Burton JM, O'Connor PW, Hohol M, Beyene J. Oral versus intravenous steroids for treatment of relapses in multiple sclerosis. Cochrane Database Syst Rev 2009 (3): CD006921.

86 Morrow SA, Stoian CA, Dmitrovic J, Chan SC, Metz LM. The bioavailability of IV methylprednisolone and oral prednisone in multiple sclerosis. Neurology 2004 Sep; 63(6): 1079–80.

87 Zivadinov R, Rudick RA, De Masi R, Nasuelli D, Ukmar M, Pozzi-Mucelli RS, et al. Effects of IV methylprednisolone on brain atrophy in relapsing-remitting MS. Neurology 2001 Oct; 57(7): 1239–47.

88 Sorensen PS, Mellgren SI, Svenningsson A, Elovaara I, Frederiksen JL, Beiske AG, et al. NORdic trial of oral Methylprednisolone as add-on therapy to Interferon beta-1a for treatment of relapsing-remitting Multiple Sclerosis (NORMIMS study): a randomised, placebo-controlled trial. Lancet Neurol 2009 Jun; 8(6): 519–29.

89 Ravnborg M, Sorensen PS, Andersson M, Celius EG, Jongen PJ, Elovaara I, et al. Methylprednisolone in combination with interferon beta-1a for relapsing-remitting multiple sclerosis (MECOMBIN study): a multicentre, double-blind, randomised, placebo-controlled, parallel-group trial. Lancet Neurol 2010 Jul; 9(7): 672–80.

90 Goodkin DE, Kinkel RP, Weinstock-Guttman B, VanderBrug-Medendorp S, Secic M, Gogol D, et al. A phase II study of i.v. methylprednisolone in secondary-progressive multiple sclerosis. Neurology 1998 Jul; 51(1): 239–45.

91 Cazzato G, Mesiano T, Antonello R, Monti F, Carraro N, Torre P, et al. Double-blind, placebo-controlled, randomized, crossover trial of high-dose methylprednisolone in patients with chronic progressive form of multiple sclerosis. Eur Neurol 1995; 35(4): 193–8.

92 Bergamaschi R, Versino M, Raiola E, Citterio A, Cosi V. High-dose methylprednisolone infusions in relapsing and in chronic progressive multiple sclerosis patients. One year follow-up. Acta Neurol (Napoli) 1993 Feb; 15(1): 33–43.

93 Ce P, Gedizlioglu M, Gelal F, Coban P, Ozbek G. Avascular necrosis of the bones: an overlooked complication of pulse steroid treatment of multiple sclerosis. Eur J Neurol 2006 Aug; 13(8): 857–61.

94 Weinshenker BG, O'Brien PC, Petterson TM, Noseworthy JH, Lucchinetti CF, Dodick DW, et al. A randomized trial of plasma exchange in acute central nervous system inflammatory demyelinating disease. Ann Neurol 1999 Dec; 46(6): 878–86.

95 Gordon PA, Carroll DJ, Etches WS, Jeffrey V, Marsh L, Morrice BL, et al. A double-blind controlled pilot study of plasma exchange versus sham apheresis in chronic progressive multiple sclerosis. Can J Neurol Sci 1985 Feb; 12(1): 39–44.

96 Sorensen PS, Fazekas F, Lee M. Intravenous immunoglobulin G for the treatment of relapsing-remitting multiple sclerosis: a meta-analysis. Eur J Neurol 2002 Nov; 9(6): 557–63.

97 Fazekas F, Lublin FD, Li D, Freedman MS, Hartung HP, Rieckmann P, et al. Intravenous immunoglobulin in relapsing-remitting multiple sclerosis: a dose-finding trial. Neurology 2008 Jul; 71(4): 265–71.

 98 Hommes OR, Sorensen PS, Fazekas F, Enriquez MM, Koelmel HW, Fernandez O, et al. Intravenous immunoglobulin in secondary progressive multiple sclerosis: randomised placebo-controlled trial. Lancet 2004 Sep–Oct; 364(9440): 1149–56.

 99 Haas J, Hommes OR. A dose comparison study of IVIG in postpartum relapsing-remitting multiple sclerosis. Mult Scler 2007 Aug; 13(7): 900–8.

100 Bar-Or A, Fawaz L, Fan B, Darlington PJ, Rieger A, Ghorayeb C, et al. Abnormal B-cell cytokine responses a trigger of T-cell-mediated disease in MS? Ann Neurol 2010 Apr; 67(4): 452–61.

101 Hauser SL, Waubant E, Arnold DL, Vollmer T, Antel J, Fox RJ, et al. B-cell depletion with rituximab in relapsing-remitting multiple sclerosis. N Engl J Med 2008 Feb 14; 358(7): 676–88.

102 Carson KR, Focosi D, Major EO, Petrini M, Richey EA, West DP, et al. Monoclonal antibody-associated progressive multifocal leucoencephalopathy in patients treated with rituximab, natalizumab, and efalizumab: a Review from the Research on Adverse Drug Events and Reports (RADAR) Project. Lancet Oncol 2009 Aug; 10(8): 816–24.

103 Jacob A, Weinshenker BG, Violich I, McLinskey N, Krupp L, Fox RJ, et al. Treatment of neuromyelitis optica with rituximab: retrospective analysis of 25 patients. Arch Neurol 2008 Nov; 65(11): 1443–8.

104 Hawker K, O'Connor P, Freedman MS, Calabresi PA, Antel J, Simon J, et al. Rituximab in patients with primary progressive multiple sclerosis: results of a randomized double-blind placebo-controlled multicenter trial. Ann Neurol 2009 Oct; 66(4): 460–71.

105 Giovannoni G, Comi G, Cook S, Rammohan K, Rieckmann P, Soelberg Sorensen P, et al. A placebo-controlled trial of oral cladribine for relapsing multiple sclerosis. N Engl J Med 2010 Feb; 362(5): 416–26.

106 Kappos L, Gold R, Miller DH, Macmanus DG, Havrdova E, Limmroth V, et al. Efficacy and safety of oral fumarate in patients with relapsing-remitting multiple sclerosis: a multicentre, randomised, double-blind, placebo-controlled phase IIb study. Lancet 2008 Oct; 372(9648): 1463–72.

107 Comi G, Pulizzi A, Rovaris M, Abramsky O, Arbizu T, Boiko A, et al. Effect of laquinimod on MRI-monitored disease activity in patients with relapsing-remitting multiple sclerosis: a multicentre, randomised, double-blind, placebo-controlled phase IIb study. Lancet 2008 Jun; 371(9630): 2085–92.

108 [cited 2011 April 23]; Available from: http://www.tevapharm.com/pr/2011/pr_1004.asp.

109 Available from:http://www.biogenidec.com/PRESS_RELEASE_DETAILS.aspx?ID = 5981&ReqId = 1548648.

110 P. O'Connor JW, C. Confavreux, G. Comi, L. Kappos, T. Olsson, H. Benzerdjeb, B. Wamil, L. Wang, A. Miller. Freedman for the Teriflunomide Multiple Sclerosis Trial Group. A placebo-controlled phase III trial (TEMSO) of oral teriflunomide in relapsing multiple sclerosis: clinical efficacy and safety outcomes. Mult Scler 2010; 16: S7–S39.

111 Ali EN, Healy BC, Stazzone LA, Brown BA, Weiner HL, Khoury SJ. Daclizumab in treatment of multiple sclerosis patients. Mult Scler 2009 Feb; 15(2): 272–4.

112 Coles AJ, Compston DA, Selmaj KW, Lake SL, Moran S, Margolin DH, et al. Alemtuzumab vs. interferon beta-1a in early multiple sclerosis. N Engl J Med 2008 Oct; 359(17): 1786–801.

113 Interferon beta-1b is effective in relapsing-remitting multiple sclerosis. I. Clinical results of a multicenter, randomized, double-blind, placebo-controlled trial. The IFNB Multiple Sclerosis Study Group. Neurology 1993 Apr; 43(4): 655–61.

114 Paty DW, Li DK. Interferon beta-1b is effective in relapsing-remitting multiple sclerosis. II. MRI analysis results of a multicenter, randomized, double-blind, placebo-controlled trial. UBC MS/MRI Study Group and the IFNB Multiple Sclerosis Study Group. Neurology 1993 Apr; 43(4): 662–7.

115 Interferon beta-1b in the treatment of multiple sclerosis: final outcome of the randomized controlled trial. The IFNB Multiple Sclerosis Study Group and The University of British Columbia MS/MRI Analysis Group. Neurology 1995 Jul; 45(7): 1277–85.

116 Jacobs LD, Cookfair DL, Rudick RA, Herndon RM, Richert JR, Salazar AM, et al. Intramuscular interferon beta-1a for disease progression in relapsing multiple sclerosis. The Multiple Sclerosis Collaborative Research Group (MSCRG). Ann Neurol 1996 Mar; 39(3): 285–94.

117 Simon JH, Jacobs LD, Campion M, Wende K, Simonian N, Cookfair DL, et al. Magnetic resonance studies of intramuscular interferon beta-1a for relapsing multiple sclerosis. The Multiple Sclerosis Collaborative Research Group. Ann Neurol 1998 Jan; 43(1): 79–87.

118 Rudick RA, Goodkin DE, Jacobs LD, Cookfair DL, Herndon RM, Richert JR, et al. Impact of interferon beta-1a on neurologic disability in relapsing multiple sclerosis. The Multiple Sclerosis Collaborative Research Group (MSCRG). Neurology 1997 Aug; 49(2): 358–63.

119 Randomised double-blind placebo-controlled study of interferon beta-1a in relapsing/remitting multiple sclerosis. PRISMS (Prevention of Relapses and Disability by Interferon beta-1a Subcutaneously in Multiple Sclerosis) Study Group. Lancet 1998 Nov; 352(9139): 1498–504.

120 Johnson KP, Brooks BR, Cohen JA, Ford CC, Goldstein J, Lisak RP, et al. Extended use of glatiramer acetate (Copaxone) is well tolerated and maintains its clinical effect on multiple sclerosis relapse rate and degree of disability. Copolymer 1 Multiple Sclerosis Study Group. Neurology 1998 Mar; 50(3): 701–8.

121 Comi G, Filippi M, Wolinsky JS. European/Canadian multicenter, double-blind, randomized, placebo-controlled study of the effects of glatiramer acetate on magnetic resonance imaging-measured disease activity and burden in patients with relapsing multiple sclerosis. European/Canadian Glatiramer Acetate Study Group. Ann Neurol 2001 Mar; 49(3): 290–7.

122 Hommers OR, Lamers KJ, Reekers P. Effect of intensive immunosuppression on the course of chronic progressive multiple sclerosis. J Neurol 1980; 223(3): 177–90.

123 Theys P, Gosseye-Lissoir F, Ketelaer P, Carton H. Short-term intensive cyclophosphamide treatment in multiple sclerosis. A retrospective controlled study. J Neurol 1981; 225(2): 119–33.

124 O'Connor PW, Li D, Freedman MS, Bar-Or A, Rice GP, Confavreux C, et al. A Phase II study of the safety and efficacy of teriflunomide in multiple sclerosis with relapses. Neurology 2006 Mar; 66(6): 894–900.

125 Wynn D, Kaufman M, Montalban X, Vollmer T, Simon J, Elkins J, et al. Daclizumab in active relapsing multiple sclerosis (CHOICE study): a phase 2, randomised, double-blind, placebo-controlled, add-on trial with interferon beta. Lancet Neurol 2010 Apr; 9(4): 381–90.

CHAPTER 9

Symptom Management

Lynn Stazzone[1] *and Brandon Brown*[2]

[1]Partners Multiple Sclerosis Center, Brigham and Women's Hospital, and Department of Neurology, Harvard Medical School, Boston, MA, USA

[2]Novartis Pharmaceuticals, West Roxbury, MA, USA

Introduction

Advances in the treatment of multiple sclerosis have made this field both exciting and challenging. Present and emerging medications appear to alter the progression of the disease, but certainly do not represent a "cure." Over time, the disease can affect a multitude of different body systems, which results in a wide variety of symptoms.

It is important to offer the patient ways in which to manage the wide variety of symptoms that can occur. This allows the patient some control in a disease that is otherwise unpredictable. This in turn can lead to improved quality of life.

Primary symptoms in MS are the direct result of demyelination within the brain and spinal cord as well as axonal loss. These include fatigue, bladder, bowel, and sexual dysfunction, weakness, pain, tremor, spasticity, numbness, cognitive issues, and depression. Secondary symptoms result from complications of primary symptoms. These may include, but are not limited to, urinary tract infections, skin breakdown, contractures, muscle atrophy, and osteoporosis. Tertiary symptoms occur when primary and secondary symptoms are not treated and result in difficulties for patients in other aspects of their lives. These include psychological, social, and vocational problems, leading to relationship difficulties, loss of employment, role reversals, and financial concerns.

There are a wide variety of interventions that can be used to treat symptoms of MS. By alleviating primary symptoms, secondary and tertiary symptoms may be reduced or prevented. It is important to point out to patients that although disease-modifying therapies may change the course of the disease, symptoms may still persist. As a consequence, it is not only imperative to treat the underlying disease, but is just as important to manage

Multiple Sclerosis: Diagnosis and Therapy, First Edition. Edited by Howard L. Weiner and James M. Stankiewicz.   © 2012 John Wiley & Sons, Ltd.
Published 2012 by John Wiley and Sons, Ltd.

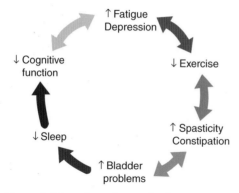

Figure 9.1 Interdependent cycle of MS symptoms

the symptoms as well. It's also important to note that symptoms rarely occur independently from one another. This interdependent cycle of MS symptoms presents a challenge to the patient as well as the healthcare providers caring for them. Commonly occurring symptoms will be discussed in this chapter, excluding depression and cognitive issues which are addressed in separate chapters in the book (Figure 9.1).

Fatigue

Fatigue in MS is a frequently experienced symptom, occurring in up to 90% of MS patients. It can significantly impact patients' quality of life [1–4]. Fatigue varies in severity and is not correlated to level of disability. Fatigue typically occurs midday with patients often getting "a second wind" late in the evening perhaps as a result of lower core body temperature. Fatigue is subjective, difficult to measure, and often misunderstood by employers, family and friends. Therefore, it is important for healthcare providers to address fatigue as a legitimate symptom of MS.

Though the pathophysiology remains unclear, many theories exist including alterations in GABAergic activity, voltage-gated Na^+ channel dysfunction, and imbalances in cortical activation and inhibition, among others [5]. Several pharmacological agents as well as nonpharmacological strategies are available for treating MS-related fatigue. Initial strategies should include identification and treatment of possible secondary causes of fatigue, such as sleep apnea, depression, anemia, infection, hypothyroidism, and side effects from other symptom management drugs or disease-modifying agents. This is followed by a multidisciplinary approach, including nonpharmacological and subsequent pharmacological interventions when necessary.

The nonpharmacological approach to treating MS-related fatigue may include energy conservation programs aimed at simplifying and pacing activities, resting and adjusting priorities, organizing workspace, using assistive technologies to conserve energy, and other strategies. Studies have shown that participating in such programs can improve symptoms as measured by the Fatigue Impact Scale and may improve health-related quality of life [6, 7] Conversely, the implementation of exercise programs for MS patients aimed to improve overall fitness, well-being, and fatigue has been examined extensively. Though results are often inconsistent, likely due to small sample sizes and differences in study design, evidence suggests that aerobic exercise, including cycling, aquatic and strength training may be helpful [8–10].

TOP TIPS 9.1

- MS-induced fatigue is extremely common, occurring in over 90% of patients.
- Fatigue is often debilitating at times and significantly impacts quality of life.
- Many management options exist, including nonpharmacologic coping strategies and medication when appropriate.

The use of cooling garments may also be effective for improving fatigue in MS patients. Most MS patients suffering from fatigue report that this particular symptom worsens significantly in the setting of elevated temperatures. Studies have shown that the intermittent use of cooling garments can reduce fatigue and this effect is sustained for several hours after removing the garment [11, 12]. Cooling systems generally consist of a vest or a vest-head garment connected to a box containing a cooling unit and pump system, which circulates the coolant fluid through tubes within the vest and cap. The garment is generally worn for 45 to 60 minutes, several times per day, maintaining a temperature around 50 °F.

Several medications for treating MS-related fatigue have been examined. Amantadine, an antiviral and anti-Parkinsonian medication is widely used to treat MS-related fatigue and has been shown to significantly improve fatigue in clinical trials [13–16]. Dosing of amantadine is 100 mg twice to three times daily. In patients with pre-existing renal disease, dose reduction to 100 mg once daily should be considered. Adverse events may include nausea, dizziness, insomnia, and nervousness and caution should be used in patients with a history of seizures, as amantadine may lower the seizure threshold. Modafinil is a medication indicated to improve wakefulness in adult patients with excessive sleepiness associated with narcolepsy, obstructive sleep apnea/hypopnea syndrome, and shift work sleep disorder. It is a central nervous system stimulant with an imprecisely defined mechanism of action. Its structure bares a distant similarity to dextroamphetamine, but lacks the sympathomimetic effects. Evidence suggests that when dosed appropriately, modafinil can help with MS related fatigue [17, 18]. Doses should start at 100 mg once daily, increasing to 100 mg twice daily if necessary. Second doses should be given no later than 2 pm to avoid insomnia. In individualized cases, doses may be increased slowly to a maximum daily dose of 400 mg; however, some data have shown that doses greater than 200 mg daily are no more effective than placebo [19]. One possible explanation for this is that higher doses may actually cause more insomnia, leading to increased fatigue so patients on higher doses should be monitored closely for insomnia, especially if fatigue persists. Nonetheless, doses should be titrated to individual response. Armodafinil, the R-enantiomer of modafinil, is also an option. With a longer half-life, armodafinil should be dosed once daily, starting at 150 mg and increasing to 250 mg once daily if necessary. Adverse events from modafinil and armodafinil occurring most commonly are insomnia, nausea, light-headedness, headache, lack of concentration, anorexia, depression, dry mouth, shaking, palpitations, and nervousness [18, 20]. Modafinil and armodafinil may reduce the effectiveness of birth control so careful assessment of sexual activity must be taken. Rare cases of serious or life-threatening rash, including Stevens–Johnson syndrome (SJS), toxic epidermal necrolysis (TEN), and drug rash with eosinophilia and systemic symptoms (DRESS) have been reported with modafinil, therefore therapy should be discontinued immediately if symptoms arise and medical attention should be sought.

Levocarnitine is an amino acid supplement important for cellular energy metabolism that is indicated for replacement therapy in patients with primary levocarnitine deficiency. Levocarnitine has proven to be effective for treating MS related fatigue at doses of 1 gram twice daily [21]. Higher doses, up to 6 grams daily in divided doses have also been used with good effect [22]. Levocarnitine is generally well tolerated, with insomnia and nervousness occasionally occurring. 4-Aminopyridine or 4-ap, a selective potassium channel blocker, may be effective in treating fatigue [23]. Dosing should start low with slow titration, as higher plasma concentrations have been associated with seizures. Other reported side effects include confusion, headache, and light-headedness.

Other medications that have been used to treat MS-related fatigue include CNS stimulants like methylphenidate or amphetamines, in their short- or long-acting formulations. The use of these products is largely based on the historic use of pemoline, a CNS stimulant that was removed from the market due to cases of hepatic failure. Clinical trials using pemoline to treat MS-related fatigue showed trends toward effectiveness, but tolerance for adverse events, specifically anorexia and irritability, was poor [24]. Anecdotally, amphetamine-containing products are beneficial but abuse potential is of concern and selected patients may not be candidates. Another strategy to treat fatigue would be the use of selective serotonin reuptake inhibitors. Agents such as fluoxetine or sertraline can be used even in the absence of depressive symptoms.

Spasticity

Spasticity is a common symptom occurring in up to 60% of MS patients, defined as an increase in muscle tone secondary to hyperexcitability of the stretch reflex resulting in a velocity dependent increase in tonic stretch reflexes [25]. Spasticity can effect mobility, cause painful muscle spasms, hinder transfers, cause contractures, as well as disturb sleep. It may worsen with concurrent problems such as infection, bladder and bowel retention, fatigue, or with interferon use, therefore these issues should always be addressed first. The nonpharmacological and pharmacological interventions are often used simultaneously. Pharmacological intervention is based on the clinical picture. For example, patients who are ambulatory with lower extremity weakness, rely on muscle tone to remain upright. By alleviating spasticity completely an inability to walk may result.

Physiotherapy plays a role in balancing muscle activity of antagonists and agonists. A thoroughly tailored stretching program can be beneficial. This can be done using both passive and active stretching. Exercising in a cool pool has shown to have effects on postural reflexes [26].

Baclofen is the most widely used antispastic agent. It is a gamma-amino butyric acid B agonist at the spinal and supraspinal levels. It suppresses both monosynaptic and polysynaptic transmissions, reducing spasticity, improving function, and increasing comfort [27]. Dose should be titrated to patient response and tolerability up to 160 mg total daily dose. Side effects include fatigue, nausea, dizziness, weakness, headache, and ataxia. Withdrawing from baclofen should be done slowly to prevent a rebound of spasms and to prevent seizures or hallucinations. Rare liver toxicities have been noted, but monitoring of enzymes is not routine.

TOP TIPS 9.2

- Spasticity in MS can be painful and often limits mobility, hinders sleep and may lead to permanent muscle contractures.
- Oral medications, such as baclofen and tizanidine may be combined to limit side effects and maximize efficacy.
- When oral medications fail, the placement of an intrathecal baclofen pump may be effective while minimizing systemic adverse events.

Tizanidine, an alpha-2-adrenergic agonist, is an imidazoline derivative thought to effect conduction in the descending noradrenergic pathways of the spinal cord. It may produce less weakness compared to baclofen but it is generally more sedating [28]. Dosing generally starts at 4 mg, titrating up to 36 mg daily in 3 divided doses. Tizanidine may cause hypotension, drowsiness, and dry mouth. Since baclofen and tizanidine have different mechanisms of action, the combination of the two may work well together for individual patients.

Benzodiazepines amplify the inhibitory action of GABA-A receptors, reducing the gain of stretch and flexor reflexes. These drugs are not first line and need to be used with discretion, secondary to the potential for serious side effects including dependency, weight gain, somnolence, and hallucinations [29].

Gabapentin is an antiepileptic drug which acts by stimulating GABA-B receptors. It was found to be effective in a double-blind, placebo-controlled, crossover study. Patients were dosed at 400 mg three times daily [30]. Gabapentin is well tolerated, but must be started at lower doses as drowsiness tends to be common.

When orally administered medications fail to be effective, intrathecal baclofen is a viable option. A test dose is generally given first and, if found to be effective, a programmable pump is implanted subcutaneously in the abdomen. A connected catheter is inserted into the thoracolumbar region and dispenses baclofen directly into the cerebrospinal fluid. The dose is adjusted to response and can be given at different rates and times as needed. Clinical efficacy has been demonstrated by different studies [31].

The local injection of botulinum toxin is an option for smaller muscle groups. Botulinum toxin works by blocking the release of acetylcholine leading to presynaptic inhibition of cholinergic transmission [32]. This costly procedure produces a local paralysis to the injected muscle, which lasts approximately 3 months. Side effects include injection site bruising and increased muscle weakness beyond the desired effect.

There has been evidence to support the use of cannabis in reducing spasticity and pain. Lakhan and Rowland reviewed studies using combined delta-9-tetrahydrocannabinol (THC) and cannabidiol (CBD) extracts, and found them to provide symptom relief as well as reduced intoxication and other side effects [33]. Although cannabis is an illegal substance, patients have reported subjective improvement and use it as they do many other unproven homeopathic remedies.

Ataxia and tremor

Ataxia and tremor are the least susceptible symptoms to drug interventions compared to other MS symptoms. Benzodiazepines, beta blockers, carbamazepine, gabapentin, ondansetron, isoniazid, and cannabis have been studied with minimal subjective response. Stereotactic neurosurgical procedures have demonstrated a positive response by creating a lesion in the ventrolateral nucleus of the thalamus. There is the inherent risk in using an invasive procedure.

Bladder dysfunction

About 80% of patients with MS will experience some level of bladder dysfunction during their course of disease. There is strong evidence to support that lower urinary tract dysfunction results from the disconnection between the brainstem and the sacral portion of the spinal cord [34]. Symptoms may include urinary urgency, frequency, hesitancy, incontinence, nocturia, and urinary tract infections. A careful history is important to determine the cause of symptoms and potential management strategies. Other neurological symptoms may occur in the presence of a urinary tract infection therefore obtaining a urinalysis, culture and sensitivities is part of a thorough assessment [35]. Studies have shown that patients have described urinary incontinence as one of the worst symptoms affecting quality of life [36]. There is also an increased cost associated with caretaker intervention and treatments provided for containment.

There are three types of bladder dysfunction. A small spastic or "failure to store" bladder results from demyelination of the spinal cord pathways between the brain and voiding reflex center. Voiding is a reflex activity that is no longer under voluntary control. "Failure to empty," or a flaccid bladder, occurs when demyelination presents in the area of the spinal voiding reflex center, and signals from, or to, the brain or bladder cannot be transmitted. A third type of dysfunction is a dyssynergic bladder. This problem is related to the coordination between bladder wall contraction and sphincter relaxation and not to the size of the bladder. It is however seen in combination with either a spastic or flaccid bladder.

Planning management strategies involve assessment of voiding history. Post micturation residual urine should also be measured. This can be done by a straight catheterization technique after a patient voids or by ultrasound post-voiding. A residual volume between 100 to 150 mL generally represents a normal or spastic bladder. A larger residual volume indicates a flaccid bladder. Urodynamic studies are usually reserved for patients with refractory symptoms who do not respond to initial interventions.

TOP TIPS 9.3

- Bladder dysfunction in MS may present as urinary urgency, frequency, hesitancy, incontinence, nocturia and urinary tract infections.
- Management must be tailored to the individual based on the symptoms being displayed.
- Self catheterization is a technique for both the flaccid bladder as well as patients with detrusor sphincter dyssynergy.

Functional difficulties can be a major cause of urinary dysfunction. If the patient cannot ambulate to the bathroom in a timely fashion, incontinence is a common result. The time required for a patient to ambulate to the bathroom from when he or first experiences the sensation to void, may be longer than the time needed. Scheduled voiding can eliminate this issue, as well as working with physical or occupational therapists to determine whether assistive devices are needed.

Bladder hyperactivity can be treated with physiotherapy to train pelvic floor muscles [37] or bladder-training protocols aimed at increasing bladder capacity through behavioral modification [38]. Micturation and urge incontinence can be effectively treated with anticholinergic agents [39]. Some of these agents include oxybutynin, tolterodine tartrate, hyoscyamine, flavoxate hydrochloride, and imipramine. Dosing depends on responsiveness as well as side effects, which include dry mouth, thirst, constipation, and confusion. Fluid management programs, in addition to eliminating caffeine-containing products, can be used in conjunction with the above agents for a better outcome.

Kegel exercises were developed by Dr Arnold Kegel in the 1940s to improve pelvic tone after childbirth and may be effective as an initial management strategy for incontinence [40]. Some patients can learn this technique by imagining holding back flatus. A patient should start by holding for 5 seconds, for 3 to 5 repetitions, increasing to 10 repetitions for 10 seconds. Baclofen can relax pelvic muscles which can help with external sphincter release, but can also increase incontinence if the muscle becomes too relaxed.

Hormone levels should be assessed in women as reduced estrogen levels may contribute to frequency and leakage. It is thought that estrogen promotes blood flow to the tissues of the vagina, decreasing swelling, which results in improved passive closure of the urethra.

Management strategies for impaired voiding with a flaccid bladder usually rely on alternative techniques for emptying rather than medications. The crude technique of applying a nonforceful, even pressure from the umbilicus toward the pubis can be utilized after a patient voids. This should not be used in the dyssynergic bladder because urine may back up into the kidneys. Supra-pubic vibration may help the detrusor to contract and improve bladder emptying when a patient has incomplete emptying and detrusor overactivity [41]. Self catheterization is a technique for both the flaccid bladder as well as patients with detrusor sphincter dyssynergy. When self catheterization is not possible, permanent catheterization is recommended. Suprapubic catheters are recommended over indwelling catheters and carry a lower risk of infection as well as progressive urethral damage [42]. Occasionally an ileal conduit procedure is done to surgically augment urinary diversion. This management strategy allows the patient or caregiver to easily change the bag avoiding incontinence and preventing decubiti. There is some evidence that alpha blockers, such as phenoxybenzamine, clonidine, or terazosin may reduce post-void residual volume by improving coordination and increased bladder control in the dyssynergic patient [43].

There is now evidence that injections of botulinum toxin into the detrusor muscle are effective in restoring continence. The need for self-catheterization may result and effects can last up to 9 months [44, 45]. Desmopressin has shown to decrease frequency during the day as well as nocturia. It slows the production of urine by the kidneys at doses of 100 to 400 mg daily, administered orally or intranasally. Sodium levels should be monitored as hyponatremia may result [46]. Desmopressin may also cause hypotension, dizziness, dry mouth, nausea, and ejaculatory failure.

Bowel dysfunction

Bowel dysfunction can be characterized as constipation, involuntary defecation, or diarrhea. It is a common symptom in MS but is probably under-reported due to the nature of the problem. It can exacerbate limb spasticity and bladder dysfunction. Demyelination in the brain and/or spinal cord may interfere with nerve transmission with attenuation of voluntary motor function and impaired anorectal sensation and reflexes. Generalized systemic factors need to be taken into consideration including altered diet, impaired mobility, and adverse drug effects.

The basic intention of any management program is to establish a scheduled defecation pattern by utilizing any manipulations of diet and lifestyle before utilizing laxatives, suppositories, or constipating agents [47]. Premorbid patterns and individual variations are important to consider in any bowel program. For constipation, an adequate diet of fiber and fluids combined with timed evacuation and stool softeners is beneficial. Minimizing the use of constipating medications such as anticholinergics, diuretics, and muscle relaxants needs to be balanced when treating other symptoms of MS. Oral and rectal stimulants can be used occasionally, but harsh laxatives should be limited.

Diarrhea can be the result of the overuse of laxatives. Poor muscle control and loose stool results in incontinence, so caffeine intake as well as artificial sweeteners and sorbitol should be limited. A warm drink and a small meal in the morning as well as abdominal massage may elicit the gastrocolic response, which may accelerate gut transit. Bulk-forming laxatives may also be useful. There have been reports that biofeedback may improve constipation and incontinence in those patients with a limited degree of disability [48]. If a management program fails, the need for a colostomy or ileostomy should be assessed. It can eliminate time spent on bowel care, promote independence, and improve quality of life [49, 50].

Sexual dysfunction

Sexuality is an integral part of who we are as humans. It is a complex part of life and is difficult to define because its expression is unique to each individual. It affects basic feelings of self-esteem, provides pleasure and relaxation, and is an important aspect of relationships. Sharing a sex life creates a special bond between partners. In a chronic disease like multiple sclerosis the process of sexual functioning can be altered physiologically, psychologically, and interpersonally. In a study comparing patients with MS, patients with other chronic diseases and normal controls, sexual dysfunction was found in 73, 39, and 13%, respectively [51].

A model of sexual dysfunction examining primary, secondary, and tertiary concepts helps to categorize sexual symptoms and provide manageable strategies for optimal outcomes [52, 53]. Primary sexual dysfunction comes from MS-related neurologic damage that directly affects the sexual response. In women, the main complaints are lack of sexual interest or desire, anorgasmia or hyporgasmia, altered genital sensation (including pain, burning, numbness, or hypersensitivity) and decreased vaginal lubrication. In men, the main complaints are erectile dysfunction or impotence, altered genital sensation, premature, slowed or retrograde ejaculation (orgasmic dysfunction), decreased force or frequency of ejaculation and decreased libido [51, 54–60]. Spinal cord lesions can dampen the transmission of nerve signals between the brain, spinal cord and the genitals. Psychogenic erections may be affected by upper motor neuron lesions in the brainstem or above the lumbar section of the spinal cord. Lower motor lesions in the sacral section of the cord may alter vasocongestion, causing weak or absent reflexive erections, reduced clitoral swelling, and a lack of vaginal lubrication [61]. Nerve impulses that facilitate vasocongestion between the brain and spinal cord may be altered by sensory changes in the genitalia. Lesions in the brain can affect the mechanisms in the brain that process sexual stimuli and libido [62, 63]. When looking at total brain lesions on MRI, Barack and colleagues found a correlation between anorgasmia and depression, total brain lesions as well as brainstem and pyramidal abnormalities [64].

Secondary sexual dysfunction occurs when physical changes caused by MS indirectly affect the sexual response. In both sexes these include fatigue, spasticity, bladder and bowel problems, weakness, pain and incoordination, which may also be a result of pharmacological nterventions [52,53].

Tertiary sexual dysfunction refers to the cultural, social and psychological issues that affect sexual functioning [52,53]. MS symptoms may alter body image and how one views herself or himself as attractive or sexy. Depression, anger, guilt, and anxiety can negatively affect sexual functioning as well as the quality of an intimate relationship. Social engagements may change as a result of loss of mobility or fatigue, changing how couples relate to each other. Roles within a family may change when an individual no longer works and is not seen as financially contributing. The need to help to care for an individual with MS may negatively impact the relationship when the partner becomes the caregiver as opposed to an intimate partner.

It is incumbent upon any healthcare provider to address sexual dysfunction as thoroughly and thoughtfully as any other symptom. Regardless of our own comfort level or lack of time, healthcare providers must offer assistance and options to patients with sexual dysfunction or refer them to someone who will. Management of sexual dysfunction should follow the conceptual model of addressing primary, secondary, and tertiary problems.

Erectile dysfunction can be treated with phosphodiesterase type 5 inhibitors like sildenafil, which increases cGMP concentrations and promotes tumescence. Penile injections into the base of the penis, such as papaverine can cause an erection but may lead to scarring and priapism. Muse, a prostaglandin E1 can be administered as a suppository into the urethra for the same effect without scarring. Surgical alternatives include inflatable and non-inflatable implanted devices. Risk of malfunction and infection are possible. Vacuum suction devices induce blood flow into the penis then a band is placed around the base preventing blood from flowing back out. Vaginal lubrication is often decreased in women and impacts satisfaction. The use of water-soluble lubricants such as K-Y Jelly or Replens can help. Sildenafil has been demonstrated to improve lubrication in women as well [65]. Altered genital sensation or hypersensitivity can be treated with anticonvulsants, topical anesthetics, changing positions or the use of a bag of frozen peas over the genitals. Discovering new and different pleasure zones can be done by a process of mapping and sensate focus. Decreased libido and difficulty with orgasm are contingent upon various nervous system pathways. Secondary and tertiary symptoms can negatively impact sexual interest and the ability to achieve orgasm. Becoming less goal-oriented and more exploratory can enhance intimacy and pleasure.

Minimizing secondary sexual symptoms as stated before, such as fatigue, spasticity, bowel and bladder problems, weakness, pain, and incoordination, through patient education and management is important to coordinate management with sexual dysfunction. For example, taking a nap before sexual activity or changing to a less strenuous sexual position may diminish fatigue. Changing positions may also decrease spasticity and enhance arousal. Eliminating bowel or bladder concerns will alleviate fear or embarrassment. A careful review of medications can eliminate sexual dysfunction such as with some antidepressants. Open communication is essential to tertiary sexual dysfunction. Patients may be experiencing anxiety, depression, and low self-esteem, which can interfere with positive sexual outcomes. Depression is treatable and counseling in a multitude of forms can diminish negative outcomes. Management of sexual dysfunction is multifactorial with interventions including pharmacologic, educational, medical and counseling. Communication between provider and patient is essential to solving problems or providing acceptable alternatives.

Pain

Pain is complex and difficult to define, occurring in up to 86% of MS patients [66–73]. The International Association for the Study of Pain defines pain as an individualistic, learned, and social response to an unpleasant sensory and emotional experience associated with actual or potential tissue damage [74]. Pain is associated with depression, anxiety, and fatigue and may heavily impact an individual's quality of life [66, 69, 73, 75–78]. In MS, pain can present at onset of disease and may occur over the course of a patient's life. It can be the result of central nervous system damage, as well as the sequelae of disability associated with disuse of muscles, tissues and joints [79]. Pain can be classified into acute with paroxysmal onset or chronic with insidious onset. Trigeminal neuralgia and painful optic neuritis represent acute pain, whereas musculoskeletal or painful spasticity represent chronic pain. Although these classifications are somewhat arbitrary it helps in developing a treatment plan.

Trigeminal neuralgia

Trigeminal neuralgia is a discrete pain syndrome affecting one or more branches of the trigeminal nerve, usually in the V2 or V3 distribution. In a young person it is highly suggestive of underlying demyelinating disease [80]. It is described as severe, intense, lancinating, sharp, shock-like pain that then eases to a burn, ache, or sense of numbness. These attacks are generally spontaneous but may be triggered by chewing, brushing teeth, touching, or facial movements. Trigeminal neuralgia may be associated with demyelination at the trigeminal route entry zone of the pons [81]. Interrupting the pain pathway through the use of anticonvulsant agents, which are known to stabilize cell membranes and decrease the hyperexcitability of sensory neurons via sodium and calcium channel regulation, are generally used as a first-line treatment [82, 83]. Carbamazepine at low doses with slow titration up to 200 mg four times daily is considered the gold standard [84]. Increased fatigue, ataxia, and decreased balance are associated side effects. Other agents such as phenytoin, gabapentin, lamotrigine, baclofen, clonazepam, and tramadol have demonstrated varying degrees of responsiveness [82, 85–87]. When drug intervention is not effective, pain relief may be obtained by blocking pain pathways through nerve blocks, radiofrequency, gamma knife surgery, cyberknife, or acupuncture [88–90].

Optic neuritis

Pain with optic neuritis is common, described as knife-like and may be associated with pressure behind or above the eye, often becoming worse upon movement of the eye [91]. This is due to inflammation and demyelination occurring around the pain sensitive meninges of the optic nerve. Treatment with high-dose corticosteroids generally resolves pain associated with optic neuritis.

Headache

Headache is a frequent problem in MS, occurring in up to 58% of patients [92]. The incidence is higher than in the general population and is characterized as migrainous, cluster or tension type. The pathophysiology is speculative but lesions in the midbrain have been associated with migraine headaches [93]. There is some evidence that migraine may present as the first MS symptom or as part of an exacerbation [94, 95]. When headache is associated with a relapse, high-dose steroids may be effective. Tricyclic antidepressants, acting by inhibiting the reuptake of serotonin and norepinephrine, have analgesic properties and are the mainstay treatment for headaches [94]. Duloxetine and venlafaxine act as neuromodulators of headache pain and have demonstrated effectiveness in neurogenic pain [96, 97]. Increasing serotonin and norepinephrine concentrations may be effective therapy in MS patients experiencing migraine headaches, as migraines may be related to changes in serotonin function and MS patients may have low serotonin levels [95].

TOP TIPS 9.4

- Pain is often an under-recognized symptom of MS and occurs in up to 86% of MS patients.
- Trigeminal neuralgia is more common in MS patients than the general population and is extremely painful, often requiring carbamazepine as first line therapy.
- Lhermitte's sign, a common pain syndrome in MS, is an electric shock sensation, spreading from the neck down the spinal column when a patient flexes their chin to their chest.

Painful tonic spasms, unlike spasticity from simple flexor spasms, can be a paroxysmal symptom not related to spasticity. The site of origin is the spinal cord, but spasms of the face suggest brainstem involvement [98]. Carbamazepine and gabapentin are effective forms of treatment [99]. Alternatives include phenytoin, topiramate, valproic acid, lamotrigine, or mexiletine [99–104].

Lhermitte's sign

Lhermitte's sign results from damage to the posterior columns of the spinal cord [105]. It manifests as a paresthesia or electric shock sensation that spreads from the neck down the spinal column possibly radiating to the extremities. Patients experience a range of feelings from a vibrating or buzzing sensation to painful, sharp, rapidly shooting sensations when bending the neck forward. Carbamazepine is often used first to treat this type of paroxysmal pain as less potent medications are typically ineffective.

Chronic pain syndromes

Chronic pain syndromes tend to be more difficult to treat and carbamazepine is less effective. The most common type of chronic pain is dysesthetic pain, which is characterized as pins and needles, prickling, burning, tingling, or band-like. It appears more often in patients with less disability and can affect the legs, feet, arms, trunk, and perineum [73,79]. It is generally worse at night and is exacerbated by temperature changes. This type of pain is associated with the feeling of cold or warmth throughout the extremities unrelated to temperature [106]. Tricyclics are considered first-line treatments, but have anticholinergic side effects which often limit their use. The combination of antidepressants with anticonvulsants may allow for effective pain control while minimizing side effects [107, 108].

Indirect pain in MS can be musculoskeletal resulting from spasticity, weakness, immobility and stress on muscles, bones, and joints. Careful assessment is required for any preventive or corrective condition. Prevention of musculoskeletal pain is essential and may include physical therapy, weight control, exercise, osteoporosis prevention, and supportive equipment, which all decrease stress on muscles, joints, and bones. Acetaminophen and nonsteroidal anti-inflammatory agents are appropriate first-line pharmacological treatments using the lowest effective dose [109].

The use of opioids is controversial and referral to a pain management program is highly recommended for retractable pain [110]. Studies have shown cannabis to have a greater effect on pain than placebo, but no greater than existing treatments [111]. Some states have legalized its use for medical purposes but the question of safety remains.

Gait

Gait disturbances in MS have important functional and emotional consequences for patients and family members alike, often leading to falls and subsequent trauma. Gait disturbances can result from a number of different neurologic manifestations including weakness, spasticity, ataxia, visual disturbances, sensory loss, and fatigue among others [112]. First-line therapy for gait disturbances should be aimed at correcting the underlying condition with appropriate pharmaceutical intervention and with the use of appropriate mobility aids.

In situations where the underlying condition cannot be treated adequately, dalfampridine (Ampyra) may provide some benefit. Dalfampridine, formerly fampridine, and also known as 4-aminopyridine or 4-ap (as previously discussed in the fatigue section) is a selective potassium channel blocker. In animal studies, by blocking potassium channels in the CNS, dalfampridine has been shown to increase conduction of action potentials in demyelinated axons [113]. In human clinical trials dalfampridine has been shown to improve walking speeds in patients with multiple sclerosis. Thirty-five percent of patients taking dalfampridine experienced a 25.2% increase in their 25-foot walking speed compared to only 8% of patients taking placebo who experienced only a 4.7% increase in speed [114]. Dosing of dalfampridine is one 10 mg sustained release tablet taken every 12 hours. Since higher peak concentrations have been associated with seizures, tablets should never be split or crushed and the dosing interval should never be more frequent than every 12 hours. Moderate or severe renal dysfunction is a contraindication as plasma concentrations may become elevated and other commonly experienced adverse events include urinary tract infection, insomnia, dizziness, headache, nausea, asthenia, back pain, balance disorder, multiple sclerosis relapse, paresthesia, nasopharyngitis, constipation, dyspepsia, and pharyngolaryngeal pain [113].

A comprehensive physical and functional assessment must focus on determining which manifestations are involved. Appropriate management strategies must focus on optimizing function as the goal.

Alternative medicine

There are seven FDA-approved medications to modify disease course and one medication, dalfampridine, to manage symptoms resulting from the disease. All other medications to treat MS as well as its symptoms are "off-label." As a result of limited controlled clinical trials, many people explore complementary and alternative medicine (CAM) to treat their symptoms and control their MS. Studies have shown that up to 70% of MS patients use CAM [115].

Commonly used CAM therapies include diet, omega-3 fatty acids and antioxidants [115–123]. Other therapies include massage, acupuncture, spirituality and chiropractic medicine. CAM users report empowerment and relief from physical and psychological symptoms [115, 117, 118, 120, 124]. Most MS patients perceive conventional and CAM therapies as both being beneficial and use them in conjunction [115, 116, 118, 121, 123].

Omega-3 fatty acids are available in many forms such as flaxseed oil, soy, and fish oils. They are thought to have immunomodulatory and anti-inflammatory effects. One study showed a trend in improvement in omega-3 fatty acid treated patients compared to placebo when measuring disease severity [125].

Ginseng studies have demonstrated both positive and negative outcomes related to MS fatigue. Excessive intake is associated with nervousness, irritability, insomnia, and diarrhea [126]. Ginkgo biloba has been studied for its effects on enhancing cognitive performance. There have been both positive and negative outcomes in clinical trials, although ginkgo biloba appears to be safe [127–131].

Epidemiology studies have demonstrated that low serum vitamin D levels and low intake may increase the risk of MS [132, 133]. This fat-soluble pro-hormone is also important in regulating calcium and phosphorus levels in the blood. A small study found that people with high vitamin D levels had an improved anti-inflammatory profile [134].

The role of dietary habits was initially explored by Dr Roy Swank starting in the late 1950s. The "swank diet" advocated a diet low in saturated fats together with supplementation with cod liver oil, a source of omega-3 fatty acids. Observational studies published by Swank between 1953 and 2003 implied that patients who followed the diet had reduced MS activity and disability progression compared to those who did not [135–138]. Unfortunately diet has not been subjected to well-controlled clinical trials, but the swank diet appears to be safe and cost contained.

Acupuncture and other Chinese medicine using herbs, massage, and stress reduction have been utilized by MS patients. Acupuncture has demonstrated in small studies to reduce pain, spasticity, bladder and bowel problems, tingling, incoordination, weakness, and sleep disorders [139]. Complications of acupuncture include fatigue and possible infection at the insertion site. Tai Chi, massage, and yoga are thought to decrease stress, increase balance, and promote the release of endorphins. All are low risk and well tolerated.

Rehabilitation

In 1991 the Disability Committee of the Royal College of Physicians defined rehabilitation as "an active process of change by which a person who has

Table 9.1 Symptom prevalence estimates

Common symptoms		Less common symptoms	
Fatigue [143]	> 90%	Speech disorders [163]	44%
Bowel and bladder dysfunction [144, 145]	68–75%	Swallowing disorders [163]	33%
Sexual dysfunction [51, 57, 64, 146–149]	40–74%	Seizures [164]	3.2%
Spasticity [25]	60–80%	Dizziness and vertigo [165, 166]	20%
Pain [150–157]	86%	Tremor [167]	37–58%
Depression [158]	50%	Pseudobulbar affect [168]	10%
Cognitive dysfunction [159–162]	34–70%		

become disabled acquires and uses the knowledge and skills necessary for optimal physical, psychological and social functioning." A multidisciplinary rehab approach in dealing with the dynamic changes that MS patients face will help to promote wellness and quality of life. Whether a patient is in the middle of an acute relapse or dealing with chronic symptoms, the healthcare provider should periodically reevaluate the need for rehabilitative services. During the lifetime of the disease, most patients will require the knowledge and skills of nursing, occupational and physical therapy, psychiatry, psychology, sexual counseling, wound care, urology, speech therapy, social services, and nutrition.

Trial designs, such as controlled studies, make evidence-based research difficult when assessing the effectiveness of rehabilitation [140]. The best evidence comes from studies with patients who have progressive disease. There is, however, newer evidence to support benefit from rehabilitation in patients with relapsing-remitting disease with incomplete recovery [141, 142]. New or chronic symptoms or clinical features perceived as progression in MS patients usually can benefit from a multidisciplinary approach in managing care (Table 9.1).

Conclusion

Recent changes advancing the treatment of MS have made this field both challenging and dynamic. Advances in disease modification affecting the course of the disease have been hopeful but monitoring for potential side effects can be challenging. At the same time managing the multitude of negative symptoms that may occur throughout an individual's disease adds additional complexity. In a chronic disease like MS, the healthcare provider builds a trusting relationship with the patient and family and helps them to understand the complex problems that MS may bring into their lives. By focusing on primary symptoms the healthcare provider may dampen the effects of secondary and tertiary symptoms. Since the disease is chronic and dynamic, secondary and tertiary symptoms will more than likely arise. Through careful assessment, symptomatic management, with a rehabilitative focus can be an effective intervention to promote quality of life.

References

1 Fisk JD, Pontefract A, Ritvo PG, Archibald CJ, Murray TJ (1994) The impact of fatigue on patients with multiple sclerosis. Can J Neurol Sci 21: 9–14.

2 Freal JE, Kraft GH, Coryell JK (1984) Symptomatic fatigue in multiple sclerosis. Arch Phys Med Rehabil 65: 135–8.

3 Kos D, Kerckhofs E, Nagels G, D'Hooghe MB, Ilsbroukx S (2008) Origin of fatigue in multiple sclerosis: review of the literature. Neurorehabil Neural Repair 22: 91–100.

4 Krupp LB, Alvarez LA, LaRocca NG, Scheinberg LC (1988) Fatigue in multiple sclerosis. Arch Neurol 45: 435–7.

5 Vucic S, Burke D, Kiernan MC (2010) Fatigue in multiple sclerosis: Mechanisms and management. Clin Neurophysiol 121: 809–17.

6 Mathiowetz VG, Finlayson ML, Matuska KM, Chen HY, Luo P (2005) Randomized controlled trial of an energy conservation course for persons with multiple sclerosis. Mult Scler 11: 592–601.

7 Finlayson M (2005) Pilot study of an energy conservation education program delivered by telephone conference call to people with multiple sclerosis. Neurorehabilitation 20: 267–77.

8 Mostert S, Kesselring J (2002) Effects of a short-term exercise training program on aerobic fitness, fatigue, health perception and activity level of subjects with multiple sclerosis. Mult Scler 8: 161–8.

9 Surakka J, Romberg A, Ruutiainen J, et al. (2004) Effects of aerobic and strength exercise on motor fatigue in men and women with multiple sclerosis: a randomized controlled trial. Clin Rehabil 18: 737–46.

10 Fragoso YD, Santana DLB, Pinto RC (2008) The positive effects of a physical activity program for multiple sclerosis patients with fatigue. Neurorehabilitation 23: 153–7.

11 Beenakker EAC, Oparina TI, Harting A, Teelken A, Arutjunyan AV, De Keyser J (2001) Cooling gament treatment in MS: Clinical improvement and decrease in leukocyte NO production. Neurology 57: 892–4.

12 NASA/MS Cooling Study Group (2003) A randomized controlled study of the acute and chronic effects of cooling therapy for MS. Neurology 60: 1955–60.

13 Cohen RA, Fisher M (1989) Amantadine treatment of fatigue associated with multiple sclerosis. Arch Neurol 46: 676–80.

14 Krupp LB, Coyle PK, Doscher C, et al. (1995) Fatigue therapy in multiple sclerosis: results of a double-blind, randomized, parallel trial of amantadine, pemoline, and placebo. Neurology 45: 1956–61.

15 Murray TJ (1985) Amantadine therapy for fatigue in multiple sclerosis. Can J Neurol Sci 12: 251–4.

16 The Canadian MS Research Group (1987) A randomized controlled trial of amantadine in fatigue associated with multiple sclerosis. Can J Neurol Sci 14: 273–8.

17 Langa R, Volkmer M, Heesen C, Liepert J (2009) Modafinil effects in multiple sclerosis patients with fatigue. J Neurol 256: 645–50.

18 Rammohan KW, Rosenberg JH, Lynn DJ, Blumenfeld AM, Pollack CP, Nagaraja HN (2002) Efficacy and safety of modafinil (Provigil) for the treatment of fatigue in multiple sclerosis: a two centre phase 2 study. J Neurol Neurosurg Psychiat 72: 179–83.

19 Stankoff B, Waubant E, Confavreux C, et al. (2005) Modafinil for fatigue in MS: A randomized placebo-controlled double-blind study. Neurology 64: 1139–43.

20 Littleton ET, Hobart JC, Palace J (2009) Modafinil for multiple sclerosis fatigue: Does it work? Clin Neurol Neurosurg 112(1): 29–31.

21 Tomassini V, Pozzilli C, Onesti E, et al. (2004) Comparison of the effects of acetyl L-carnitine and amantadine for the treatment of fatigue in multiple sclerosis: results of a pilot, randomized, double-blind, crossover trial. J Neurol Sci 218: 103–8.

22 Lebrun C, Alchaar H, Candito M, Bourg V, Chatel M (2006) Levocarnitine administration in multiple sclerosis patients with immunosuppressive therapy-induced fatigue. Mult Scler 12: 321–4.

23 Rossini PM, Pasqualetti P, Pozzilli C, et al. (2001) Fatigue in progressive multiple sclerosis: results of a randomized, double-blind, placebo-controlled, crossover trial of oral 4–aminopyridine. Mult Scler 7: 354–8.

24 Weinshenker BG, Penman M, Bass B, et al. (1992) A double-blind, randomized, crossover trial of pemoline in fatigue associated with multiple sclerosis. Neurology 42: 1468–71.

25 Lance JW. (1980) Symposium synopsis. In Feldman RG, Yound RR, Koclla WP (eds) Spasticity: Disordered Motor Control. Year Book Medical Publishers, Chicago, pp. 485–94.

26 Dietz V, Horstmann GA, Trippel M, Golhoter A (1989) Human postural reflexes and gravity. An underwater simulation. Neurosci Lett 106: 350–5.

27 Ha-Hab JR (1980) Review of European clinical trials with baclofen. In Feldman RG, Young RR, Koella WP (eds) Spasticity: Disordered Motor Control. Year Book Medical Publishers, Chicago, pp. 71–85.

28 Bes A, Eyssette M, Pierrot-Deseilligny E, Rohmer F, Warter JM (1988) A multi-centre, double-blind trial of tizanidine, a new antispastic agent, in spasticity associated with hemiplegia. Curr Med Res Opin 10(10): 709–18.

29 Glenn MB, Whyte J (1990) The practical management of spasticity in children and adults. JB Lippincott, Philidelphia.

30 Formica A, Verger K, Sol JM, Morralla C (2005) Gabapentin for spasticity: a randomized, double-blind, placebo-controlled trial. Med Clin (Barc) 124(3): 81–5.

31 Coffey JR, Cahill D, Steers W, et al. (1993) Intrathecal baclofen for intractable spasticity of spinal origin: results of a long-term multicenter study. J Neurosurg 78(2): 226–32.

32 Davis D, Jabbari B (1993) Significant improvement of stiff-person syndrome after paraspinal injection of botulinum toxin A. Mov Disord 8(3): 371–3.

33 Lakhan SE, Rowland M (2009) Whole plant cannabis extracts in the treatment of spasticity in multiple sclerosis: a systematic review. BMC Neurol 9: 59.

34 Fowler CJ, Panicker JN, Drake M, et al. (2009) A UK consensus on the management of the bladder in multiple sclerosis. J Neurol Neurosurg Psychiat 80: 470–7.

35 Buljevac D, Flach HZ, Hop WC, et al. (2002) Prospective study on the relationship between infections and multiple sclerosis exacerbations. Brain 125 (Pt 5): 952–60.

36 Hemmett L, Holmes J, Barnes M, Russell N (2004) What drives quality of life in multiple sclerosis? QJM 97(10): 671–6.

37 Glenn J (2003) Restorative Nursing Bladder Training program: recommending a strategy. Rehabil Nurs 28(1): 15–22.

38 Fantl J Newmann D, Colling J, et al. (1996) Urinary incontinence in adults: Acute and chronic management. Second Update. In: Research Agency of Health Care Policy and Research. Clinician's Handbook of Preventive Services: 2nd edn. Clinical Practice Guideline. Elsevier, Rockville, MD.

39 Abrams P, Freeman R, Anderstrom C, Mattiasson A (1998) Tolterodine, a new antimuscarinic agent: as effective but better tolerated than oxybutynin in patients with an overactive bladder. Br J Urol 81(6): 801–10.

40 Dierich M (2000) Bladder Dysfunction. In Burks J and Johnson K (eds) Multiple Sclerosis: Diagnosis, Medical Management and Rehabilitation: 1 edn. Demos Medical Publishing, New York, pp. 433–51.

41 Prasad RS, Smith SJ, Wright H (2003) Lower abdominal pressure versus external bladder stimulation to aid bladder emptying in multiple sclerosis: a randomized controlled study. Clin Rehabil 17(1): 42–7.

42 Branagan GW, Moran BJ (2002) Published evidence favors the use of suprapubic catheters in pelvic colorectal surgery. Dis Colon Rectum 45(8): 1104–8.

43 O'Riordan JI, Doherty C, Javed M, Brophy D, Hutchinson M, Quinlan D (1995) Do alpha-blockers have a role in lower urinary tract dysfunction in multiple sclerosis? J Urol 153(4): 1114–16.

44 Schurch B, Stohrer M, Kramer G, Schmid DM, Gaul G, Hauri D (2000) Botulinum-A toxin for treating detrusor hyperreflexia in spinal cord injured patients: a new alternative to anticholinergic drugs? Preliminary results. J Urol 164 (3 Pt 1): 692–7.

45 Leippold T, Reitz A, Schurch B (2003) Botulinum toxin as a new therapy option for voiding disorders: current state of the art. Eur Urol 44(2): 165–74.

46 Bosma R, Wynia K, Havlikova E, De Keyser J, Middel B (2005) Efficacy of desmopressin in patients with multiple sclerosis suffering from bladder dysfunction: a meta-analysis. Acta Neurol Scand 112(1): 1–5.

47 Anonymous (1998) Clinical practice guidelines. Neurogenic bowel management in adults with spinal cord injury. J Spinal Cord Med 21: 248–93.

48 Wiesel PH, Norton C, Roy AJ, Storrie JB, Bowers J, Kamm MA (2000) Gut focused behavioural treatment (biofeedback) for constipation and faecal incontinence in multiple sclerosis. J Neurol Neurosurg Psychiat 69(2): 240–3.

49 Rosito O, Nino-Murcia M, Wolfe VA, Kiratli BJ, Perkash I (2002) The effects of colostomy on the quality of life in patients with spinal cord injury: a retrospective analysis. J Spinal Cord Med 25(3): 174–83.

50 Safadi BY, Rosito O, Nino-Murcia M, Wolfe VA, Perkash I (2003) Which stoma works better for colonic dysmotility in the spinal cord injured patient? Am J Surg 186(5): 437–42.

51 Zorzon M, Zivadinov R, Bosco A, et al. (1999) Sexual dysfunction in multiple sclerosis: a case-control study. I. Frequency and comparison of groups. Mult Scler 5(6): 418–27.

52 Foley FW, Iverson J (1992) Sexuality and multiple sclerosis. In: Kalb RC, Scheinberg LC (eds) Multiple Sclerosis and the Family. Demos Publishing, New York.

53 Foley FW SA (1997) Sexualtiy, Multiple Sclerosis and Women. MS Management 4(1): 1–10.

54 Lilius HG, Valtonen EJ, Wikstrom J (1976) Sexual problems in patients suffering from multiple sclerosis. J Chronic Dis 29(10): 643–7.

55 Lilius HG, Valtonen EJ, Wikstrom J (1976) Sexual problems in patients suffering from multiple sclerosis. Scand J Soc Med 4(1): 41–4.

56 Ghezzi A, Malvestiti GM, Baldini S, Zaffaroni M, Zibetti A (1995) Erectile impotence in multiple sclerosis: a neurophysiological study. J Neurol 242(3): 123–6.

57 Mattson D, Petrie M, Srivastava DK, McDermott M (1995) Multiple sclerosis. Sexual dysfunction and its response to medications. Arch Neurol 52(9): 862–8.

58 McCabe MP ME, Deeks AA, et al. (1996) The impact of multiple sclerosis on sexuality and relationships. J Sex Res 33(3): 241–8.

59 Stenager E SE, Jensen K, et al. (1984) Multiple Sclerosis:Sexual dysfunction. J Sex Ed Ther 16(4): 242–69.

60 Valleroy ML, Kraft GH (1984) Sexual dysfunction in multiple sclerosis. Arch Phys Med Rehabil 65(3): 125–8.

61 Dewis ME, Thornton NG (1989) Sexual dysfunction in multiple sclerosis. J Neurosci Nurs 21(3): 175–9.

62 DeLisa JA, Miller RM, Mikulic MA, Hammond MC (1985) Multiple sclerosis: Part II. Common functional problems and rehabilitation. Am Fam Physic 32(5): 127–32.

63 Lundberg PO (1978) Sexual dysfunction in patients with multiple sclerosis. Sex Dis 1(3): 218–22.

64 Barak Y, Achiron A, Elizur A, Gabbay U, Noy S, Sarova-Pinhas I (1996) Sexual dysfunction in relapsing-remitting multiple sclerosis: magnetic resonance imaging, clinical, and psychological correlates. J Psychiat Neurosci 21(4): 255–8.

65 Bronner G, Elran E, Golomb J, Korczyn AD (2010) Female sexuality in multiple sclerosis: the multidimensional nature of the problem and the intervention. Acta Neurol Scand 121(5): 289–301.

66 Ehde DM, Gibbons LE, Chwastiak L, Bombardier CH, Sullivan MD, Kraft GH (2003) Chronic pain in a large community sample of persons with multiple sclerosis. Mult Scler 9(6): 605–11.

67 Stenager E, Knudsen L, Jensen K (1995) Acute and chronic pain syndromes in multiple sclerosis. A 5–year follow-up study. Ital J Neurol Sci 16(9): 629–32.

68 Stenager E, Knudsen L, Jensen K (1991) Acute and chronic pain syndromes in multiple sclerosis. Acta Neurol Scand 84(3): 197–200.

69 Osterberg A, Boivie J, Thuomas KA (2005) Central pain in multiple sclerosis–prevalence and clinical characteristics. Eur J Pain 9(5): 531–42.

70 Beiske AG, Pedersen ED, Czujko B, Myhr KM (2004) Pain and sensory complaints in multiple sclerosis. Eur J Neurol 11(7): 479–82.

71 Ehde DM, Osborne TL, Hanley MA, Jensen MP, Kraft GH (2006) The scope and nature of pain in persons with multiple sclerosis. Mult Scler 12(5): 629–38.

72 Hadjimichael O, Kerns RD, Rizzo MA, Cutter G, Vollmer T (2007) Persistent pain and uncomfortable sensations in persons with multiple sclerosis. Pain 127 (1-2): 35–41.

73 Solaro C, Brichetto G, Amato MP, et al. (2004) The prevalence of pain in multiple sclerosis: a multicenter cross-sectional study. Neurology 63(5): 919–921.

74 Merskey H, Bogduk N and the International Association for the Study of Pain, Task Force on Taxonomy (1994) Classification of Chronic Pain, Second Edition. IASP Press, Seattle.

75 Svendsen KB, Jensen TS, Overvad K, Hansen HJ, Koch-Henriksen N, Bach FW (2003) Pain in patients with multiple sclerosis: a population-based study. Arch Neurol 60(8): 1089–1094.

76 Ehde DM, Osborne TL, Jensen MP (2005) Chronic pain in persons with multiple sclerosis. Phys Med Rehabil Clin N Am 16(2): 503–512.

77 Kalia LV, O'Connor PW (2005) Severity of chronic pain and its relationship to quality of life in multiple sclerosis. Mult Scler 11(3): 322–327.

78 Portenoy RK, Yang K, Thorton D (1988) Chronic intractable pain: an atypical presentation of multiple sclerosis. J Neurol 235(4): 226–228.

79 Moulin DE, Foley KM, Ebers GC (1988) Pain syndromes in multiple sclerosis. Neurology 38(12): 1830–1834.

80 De Simone R, Marano E, Brescia Morra V, et al. (2005) A clinical comparison of trigeminal neuralgic pain in patients with and without underlying multiple sclerosis. Neurol Sci 26 (Suppl 2): s150–s151.

81 Olafson RA, Rushton JG, Sayre GP (1966) Trigeminal neuralgia in a patient with multiple sclerosis. An autopsy report. J Neurosurg 24(4): 755–759.

82 Albert ML (1969) Treatment of pain in multiple sclerosis – preliminary report. N Engl J Med 280(25): 1395.

83 Jensen TS (2002) Anticonvulsants in neuropathic pain: rationale and clinical evidence. Eur J Pain 6 (Suppl A): 61–8.

84 Hooge JP, Redekop WK (1995) Trigeminal neuralgia in multiple sclerosis. Neurology 45(7): 1294–6.

85 Bowsher D (1993) Pain syndromes and their treatment. Curr Opin Neurol Neurosurg 6(2): 257–63.

86 Andersson PB, Goodkin DE (1996) Current pharmacologic treatment of multiple sclerosis symptoms. West J Med 165(5): 313–17.

87 Lunardi G, Leandri M, Albano C, et al. (1997) Clinical effectiveness of lamotrigine and plasma levels in essential and symptomatic trigeminal neuralgia. Neurology 48(6): 1714–17.

88 Kaufmann AM (2006) Surgical treatment of trigeminal neuralgia. [cited 2010 Oct 28]; Available from: http://www.umanitoba.ca/cranial_nerves/surgical_management.pdf

89 Kondziolka D, Lunsford LD (2005) Percutaneous retrogasserian glycerol rhizotomy for trigeminal neuralgia: technique and expectations. Neurosurg Focus 18(5): E7.

90 Lim M, Villavicencio AT, Burneikiene S, et al. (2005) CyberKnife radiosurgery for idiopathic trigeminal neuralgia. Neurosurg Focus 18(5): E9.

91 Mathews WB (1985) Clinical aspects (symptoms and signs). In Mathews WB (ed.), McAlpine's Multiple Sclerosis. Churchill Livingstone, New York.

92 D'Amico D, La Mantia L, Rigamonti A, et al. (2004) Prevalence of primary headaches in people with multiple sclerosis. Cephalalgia 24(11): 980–4.

93 Gee JR, Chang J, Dublin AB, Vijayan N (2005) The association of brainstem lesions with migraine-like headache: an imaging study of multiple sclerosis. Headache 45(6): 670–7.

94 Rolak LA, Brown S (1990) Headaches and multiple sclerosis: a clinical study and review of the literature. J Neurol 237(5): 300–2.

95 Sandyk R, Awerbuch GI (1994) The co-occurrence of multiple sclerosis and migraine headache: the serotoninergic link. Int J Neurosci 76(3-4): 249–57.

96 Raskin J, Pritchett YL, Wang F, et al. (2005) A double-blind, randomized multicenter trial comparing duloxetine with placebo in the management of diabetic peripheral neuropathic pain. Pain Med 6(5): 346–56.

97 Sumpton JE, Moulin DE (2001) Treatment of neuropathic pain with venlafaxine. Ann Pharmacother 35(5): 557–559.

98 Ostermann PO, Westerberg CE (1975) Paroxysmal attacks in multiple sclerosis. Brain 98(2): 189–202.

99 Shibasaki H, Kuroiwa Y (1974) Painful tonic seizure in multiple sclerosis. Arch Neurol 30(1): 47–51.

100 Cianchetti C, Zuddas A, Randazzo AP, Perra L, Marrosu MG (1999) Lamotrigine adjunctive therapy in painful phenomena in MS: preliminary observations. Neurology 53(2): 433.

101 D'Aleo G, Sessa E, Di Bella P, Rifici C, Restivo DA, Bramanti P (2001) Topiramate modulation of R3 nociceptive reflex in multiple sclerosis patients suffering paroxysmal symptoms. J Neurol 248(11): 996–9.

102 Libenson MH, Stafstrom CE, Rosman NP (1994) Tonic "seizures" in a patient with brainstem demyelination: MRI study of brain and spinal cord. Pediat Neurol 11(3): 258–62.

103 Kuroiwa Y, Shibasaki H (1968) Painful tonic seizure in multiple sclerosis treatment with diphenylhydantoin and carbamazepine. Folia Psychiat Neurol Jpn 22(2): 107–19.

104 Sakurai M, Kanazawa I (1999) Positive symptoms in multiple sclerosis: their treatment with sodium channel blockers, lidocaine and mexiletine. J Neurol Sci 162(2): 162–8.

105 Lhermitte J, Bollack J, Nicholas M (1929) Les douleurs a type de decharge electrique consecutives a la flexion cephalique dans la sclerose en plaques: Un cas de forme sensitive de la sclerose multiple. Revue Neurol 31: 56–62.

106 Belgrade MJ (1999) Following the clues to neuropathic pain. Distribution and other leads reveal the cause and the treatment approach. Postgrad Med 106(6): 127–32, 135–40.

107 Sindrup S, Jensen TS (2003) Antidepressants in the treatment of neuropathic pain. In Hansson PT, Fields HL, Hill RG, Marchettini P (eds) Neuropathic Pain: Pathophysiology and Treatment. IASP Press, Seattle.

108 Gilron I, Max MB (2005) Combination pharmacotherapy for neuropathic pain: current evidence and future directions. Expert Rev Neurother 5(6): 823–30.

109 Department of Health and Human Services (2005) COX-2 selective and non-selective non-steroidal anti-inflammatory drugs. 2005 [cited 2010 Oct 29]; Available from: www.fda.gov

110 Rawbotham. M (2003) Efficacy of Opioids in Neuropathic Pain. IASP Press, Seattle.

111 Zajicek J, Fox P, Sanders H, et al. (2003) Cannabinoids for treatment of spasticity and other symptoms related to multiple sclerosis (CAMS study): multicentre randomised placebo-controlled trial. Lancet 362(9395): 1517–26.

112 Cattaneo D, De Nuzzo C, Fascia T, et al. (2002) Risks of falls in subjects with multiple sclerosis. Arch Phys Med Rehabil 83(6): 864–7.

113 Ampyra Package Insert (2010) Acorda Therapeutics Inc. Hawthorne, NY 10532, USA.

114 Goodman AD, Brown TR, Krupp LB, et al. (2009) Sustained-release oral fampridine in multiple sclerosis: a randomized, double-blind, controlled trial. Lancet 373: 732–8.

115 Berkman C, Pignotti M, Cavallo P, Holland N (1999) Use of ajternative treatments by people with multiple sclerosis. Neurorehabil Neural Repair 13: 243–54.

116 Leong EM, Semple SJ, Angley M, Siebert W, Petkov J, McKinnon RA (2009) Complementary and alternative medicines and dietary interventions in multiple sclerosis: what is being used in South Australia and why? Complement Ther Med. 17: 216–23.

117 Marrie RA, Hadjimichael O, Vollmer T (2003) Predictors of alternative medicine use by multiple sclerosis patients. Mult Scler 9: 461–6.

118 Nayak S, Matheis RJ, Schoenberger NE, Shiflett SC (2003) Use of unconventional therapies by individuals with multiple sclerosis. Clin Rehabil 17: 181–91.

119 Page SA, Verhoef MJ, Stebbins RA, Metz LM, Levy JC (2003) The use of complementary and alternative therapies by people with multiple sclerosis. Chronic Dis Can 24: 75–9.

120 Schwartz CE, Laitin E, Brotman S, LaRocca N (1999) Utilization of unconventional treatments by persons with MS: is it alternative or complementary? Neurology 52: 626–9.

121 Schwarz S, Knorr C, Geiger H, Flachenecker P (2008) Complementary and alternative medicine for multiple sclerosis. Mult Scler 14: 1113–19.

122 Stuifbergen AK, Harrison TC (2003) Complementary and alternative therapy use in persons with multiple sclerosis. Rehabil Nurs 28: 141–7.

123 Yadav V, Shinto L, Morris C, Senders A, Baldauf-Wagner S, Bourdette D (2006) Use and self-reported benefit of complementary and alternative medicine (CAM) among multiple sclerosis patients. Int J MS Care 8: 5–10.

124 Shinto L, Yadav V, Morris C, Lapidus JA, Senders A, Bourdette D (2006) Demographic and health-related factors associated with complementary and alternative medicine (CAM) use in multiple sclerosis. Mult Scler 12: 94–100.

125 Bates D, Cartlidge NE, French JM, et al. (1989) A double-blind controlled trial of long chain n-3 polyunsaturated fatty acids in the treatment of multiple sclerosis. J Neurol Neurosurg Psychiat 52(1): 18–22.

126 Siegel RK (1979) Ginseng abuse syndrome. Problems with the panacea. J Am Med Assoc 241(15): 1614–15.

127 Rao SM, Leo GJ, Bernardin L, Unverzagt F (1991) Cognitive dysfunction in multiple sclerosis. I. Frequency, patterns, and prediction. Neurology 41(5): 685–91.

128 Amato MP, Ponziani G, Siracusa G, Sorbi S (2001) Cognitive dysfunction in early-onset multiple sclerosis: a reappraisal after 10 years. Arch Neurol 58(10): 1602–6.

129 Napryeyenko O, Sonnik G, Tartakovsky I (2009) Efficacy and tolerability of Ginkgo biloba extract EGb 761 by type of dementia: analyses of a randomised controlled trial. J Neurol Sci 283(1–2): 224–9.

130 Mazza M, Capuano A, Bria P, Mazza S (2006) Ginkgo biloba and donepezil: a comparison in the treatment of Alzheimer's dementia in a randomized placebo-controlled double-blind study. Eur J Neurol 13(9): 981–5.

131 Le Bars PL, Katz MM, Berman N, Itil TM, Freedman AM, Schatzberg AF (1997) A placebo-controlled, double-blind, randomized trial of an extract of Ginkgo biloba for dementia. North American EGb Study Group. J Am Med Assoc 278(16): 1327–32.

132 Munger KL, Levin LI, Hollis BW, Howard NS, Ascherio A (2006) Serum 25-hydroxyvitamin D levels and risk of multiple sclerosis. J Am Med Assoc 296(23): 2832–8.

133 Munger KL, Zhang SM, O'Reilly E, et al. (2004) Vitamin D intake and incidence of multiple sclerosis. Neurology 62(1): 60–5.

134 Smolders J, Thewissen M, Peelen E, et al. (2009) Vitamin D status is positively correlated with regulatory T cell function in patients with multiple sclerosis. PLoS One 4(8): e6635.

135 Swank RL (1953) Treatment of multiple sclerosis with low-fat diet. AMA Arch Neurol Psychiat 69(1): 91–103.

136 Swank RLM (1970) Multiple sclerosis: twenty years on low fat diet. Arch Neurol 23(5): 460–74.

137 Swank RL, Dugan BB (1990) Effect of low saturated fat diet in early and late cases of multiple sclerosis. Lancet 336(8706): 37–9.

138 Swank RL, Goodwin J (2003) Review of MS patient survival on a Swank low saturated fat diet. Nutrition 19(2): 161–2.

139 NIH Consensus Development Panel on Acupuncture (1998) Acupuncture. J Am Med Assoc 280(17): 1518–24.

140 Kesselring J (2004) Neurorehabilitation in multiple sclerosis – what is the evidence-base? J Neurol 251 (Suppl 4): IV25–9.

141 Craig J, Young CA, Ennis M, Baker G, Boggild M (2003) A randomised controlled trial comparing rehabilitation against standard therapy in multiple sclerosis patients receiving intravenous steroid treatment. J Neurol Neurosurg Psychiat 74(9): 1225–30.

142 Liu C, Playford ED, Thompson AJ (2003) Does neurorehabilitation have a role in relapsing-remitting multiple sclerosis? J Neurol 250(10): 1214–18.

143 Branas P, Jordan RE, Fry-Smith A, Burls A, Hyde CJ (2000) Treatments for fatigue in multiple sclerosis: a rapid and systematic review. Health Technol Assess 4: 27.

144 Chia YW, Fowler CJ, Kamm MA, et al. (1995) Prevalence of bowel dysfunction in patients with multiple sclerosis and bladder dysfunction. J Neurol 242(2): 105–8.

145 Marrie RA, Cutter G, Tyry T, et al. (2007) Disparities in the management of multiple sclerosis-related ladder symptoms. Neurology 68: 1971–8.

146 Hulter BM, Lundberg PO (1995) Sexual function in women with advanced multiple sclerosis. J Neurol Neurosurg Psychiat 59: 83–6.

147 Minderhoud JM, Leemhuis JG, Kremer J, Laban E, Smits PM (1984) Sexual disturbances arising from multiple sclerosis. Acta Neurol Scand 70: 299–306.

148 Szasz G, Paty D, Lawton-Speert S, Eisen K (1984) A Sexual Functioning Scale in multiple sclerosis. Acta Neurol Scand Suppl 101: 37–43.

149 Demirkiran M, Sarica Y, Uguz S, Yerdelen D, Aslan K (2006) Multiple sclerosis patients with and without sexual dysfunction: are there any differences? Mult Scler 12: 209–14.

150 Ehde DM, Gibbons LE, Chwastiak L, Bombardier CH, Sullivan MD, Kraft GH (2003) Chronic pain in a large community sample of persons with multiple sclerosis. Mult Scler 9(6): 605–11.

151 Stenager E, Knudsen L, Jensen K (1995) Acute and chronic pain syndromes in multiple sclerosis. A 5-year follow-up study. J Neurol Sci 16(9): 629–32.

152 Stenager E, Knudsen L, Jensen K (1991) Acute and chronic pain syndromes in multiple sclerosis. Acta Neurol Scand 84(3): 197–200.

153 Osterberg A, Boivie J, Thuomas KA (2005) Central pain in multiple sclerosis– prevalence and clinical characteristics. Eur J Pain 9(5): 531–42.

154 Beiske AG, Pedersen ED, Czujko B, Myhr KM (2004) Pain and sensory complaints in multiple sclerosis. Eur J Neurol 11(7): 479–82.

155 Ehde DM, Osborne TL, Hanley MA, Jensen MP, Kraft GH (2006) The scope and nature of pain in persons with multiple sclerosis. Mult Scler 12(5): 629–38.

156 Hadjimichael O, Kerns RD, Rizzo MA, Cutter G, Vollmer T (2007) Persistent pain and uncomfortable sensations in persons with multiple sclerosis. Pain 127(1-2): 35–41.

157 Solaro C, Brichetto G, Amato MP, et al. (2004) The prevalence of pain in multiple sclerosis: a multicenter cross-sectional study. Neurology 63(5): 919–21.

158 Minden SL, Schiffer RB (1990) Affective disorders in multiple sclerosis. Review and recommendations for clinical research. Arch Neurol 47: 98–103.

159 Heaton RK, Nelson LM, Thompson DS, et al. (1985) Neuropsychological findings in relapsing-remitting and chronic progressive multiple sclerosis. J Consult Clin Psychol 53, 101–10.

160 Maurelli M, Marchioni E, Cerretano R, et al. (1992) Neuropsychological assessment in MS: Clinical, neurophysiological and neuroradiological relationships. Acta Neurol Scand 86: 124–8.

161 McIntosh-Michaelis SA, Roberts MH, Wilkinson SM, et al. (1991) The prevalence of cognitive impairment in a community survey of multiple sclerosis. Br J Clin Psychol 30: 333–48.

162 Rao SM, Leo GJ, Bernardin L, et al. (1991) Cognitive dysfunction in multiple sclerosis I: Frequency, patterns, and predictions. Neurology 41: 685–91.

163 Hartelius L, Svensson P (1994) Speech and swallowing symptoms associated with Parkinson's disease and multiple sclerosis: a survey. Folia Phoniatrica et Logopedica 46(1): 9–17.

164 Kelley BJ, Rodriguez M (2009) Seizures in patients with multiple sclerosis. CNS Drugs 23(10): 805–15.

165 Turkington C, Hoopas KD (2005) The A to Z of Multiple Sclerosis. New York: Checkmark Books.

166 Schapiro RT (2007) Managing the Symptoms of Multiple Sclerosis, 5th edn. New York: Demos Publishing.

167 Alusi SH, Worthington J, Glickman S, Bain PG (2001) A study of tremor in multiple sclerosis. Brain 124(4): 720–30.

168 Surridge D (1969) An investigation into some psychiatric aspects of multiple sclerosis. Br J Psychiat 115(524): 749–64.

CHAPTER 10

Cognitive Dysfunction in Multiple Sclerosis

Bonnie I. Glanz and Maria K. Houtchens

Partners Multiple Sclerosis Center, Brigham and Women's Hospital, and Department of Neurology, Harvard Medical School, Boston, MA, USA

Prevalence of cognitive dysfunction in MS

Charcot described dementia as a feature of MS in 1877. He wrote that his patients had a "marked enfeeblement of the memory, conceptions are formed slowly and intellectual and emotional facilities are blunted in their totality" [1]. Similar observations of cognitive impairment were reported by others during the first half of the twentieth century [2, 3]. Despite these reports, most agreed that cognitive dysfunction was uncommon in MS. In 1970, Kurtzke [4], on the basis of clinical examination, estimated that fewer than 5% of MS patients were cognitively impaired.

Over the next two decades, researchers began applying more sensitive methods of neuropsychological testing to document cognitive changes. Peyser et al. [5] compared cognitive test performance and physicians' judgment of cognitive functioning in 55 patients with MS. Patients were administered the Halstead Category Test, a measure of abstract conceptualization, and the Comprehension, Similarities, and Vocabulary subtests of the Wechsler Adult Intelligence Scale (WAIS). Fifty-four percent of subjects were impaired on the Category Test. Verbal IQ was estimated to be in the average range. Of the 45 patients who were clinically judged by their neurologists to have intact cognition, 22 (48.9%) scored within the impaired range. In a study of 30 patients with definite or probable MS of less than 2 years' duration, Lyon-Caen et al. [6] observed mild to moderate cognitive impairment in 60% of patients. Deficits were primarily related to affected visual and/or verbal efficiency. None of the patients showed clinical signs of cognitive impairment.

In 1991, Rao et al. [7] pointed out that earlier studies may have overestimated the prevalence of cognitive impairment in MS because

Multiple Sclerosis: Diagnosis and Therapy, First Edition. Edited by Howard L. Weiner and James M. Stankiewicz. © 2012 John Wiley & Sons, Ltd.
Published 2012 by John Wiley and Sons, Ltd.

they relied on patients recruited from university-based medical centers. These patients were presumed to have greater physical disability and more active disease than the general MS population. Rao et al. [7] reasoned that these patients may also display a higher rate of cognitive impairment. In an attempt to establish the frequency of cognitive impairment in the general MS population, Rao et al. [7] recruited a community-based sample of MS patients from a membership listing of a local MS society. One hundred patients and 100 matched controls were enrolled. Subjects were administered a battery of 31 tests that included measures of verbal intelligence, immediate and remote verbal memory, immediate and remote visual spatial memory, abstract reasoning, attention/concentration, language, and visual spatial perception. Test scores that fell below the 5th percentile based on the performance of the healthy control group were considered failed tests. Subjects with four or more failed tests were classified as cognitively impaired. Forty-eight percent of MS patients and 5% of healthy controls met criteria for cognitive impairment. By subtracting the false positive rate (5%) from the true positive rate (48%), the frequency rate of cognitive impairment in the MS sample was estimated to be 43%.

In a second community-based study of cognitive impairment in MS, McIntosh-Michaelis et al. [8] recruited subjects from a population-based MS registry that included 411 individuals with MS. One hundred and 47 patients with MS and 34 patients with rheumatoid arthritis (RA) were interviewed at home and completed a battery of neuropsychological tests. Subjects who demonstrated impairment on more than three measures were defined as cognitively impaired. Forty-six percent of MS patients and 12% of RA patients met criteria for cognitive impairment. In addition, 34% of patients with MS demonstrated memory impairment and 33% of patients with MS demonstrated impairment on tests of frontal lobe function.

Pattern of cognitive dysfunction in MS

Cognitive function has been studied extensively in MS. Researchers have focused on overall intellectual functioning as well as specific cognitive domains including processing speed and working memory, new learning and memory, spatial processing, language, and executive function. These domains are discussed separately below.

Intelligence

Cross-sectional studies have used the Wechsler Scales [9–11] to estimate IQ in patients with MS. The results suggest that patients with MS have full scale

IQ scores in the average range (90 to 110) [12–15]. In addition, studies have used the Wechsler scales to compare IQ scores in MS patients and various control groups. Jambor [16], for example, compared the performances of patients with MS, psychiatric patients, disabled patients without CNS involvement, and healthy controls on the verbal subtests of the WAIS. There were no differences among groups. Goldstein and Shelly [13] reported similar IQ scores in patients with MS, psychiatric disease, and non-MS-related brain damage. Rao [17] pointed out that in these studies, the standard deviations for the MS groups were larger than for the control groups. This may explain why the MS groups overlap with both healthy and brain-damaged controls.

Several longitudinal studies have reported a decline in intellectual functioning in patients with MS. Canter [18] studied 23 males who completed the Army General Classification Test at the time of their induction into the military and subsequently developed MS. He re-tested subjects after an interval of approximately 4 years and observed a highly significant drop of 13.5 IQ points. Ivnik [14] examined 14 patients with MS and 14 neurological and neurosurgical controls matched for age and education. Subjects were administered the WAIS at baseline and 3 years. The MS group showed declines of 3 to 4 points on verbal, performance, and full-scale IQs. The control group showed slight improvement which may have been related to recovery of function in control subjects with a history of head trauma. Other studies have failed to find evidence of MS-related intellectual decline. Fink and Houser [19], for example, administered the verbal subtests of the WAIS to 44 patients with recent-onset MS. The test-retest interval was 1 year. A significant 4-point increase in verbal IQ was observed.

Discrepancies between verbal and performance IQs have also been reported in patients with MS. Numerous studies have observed performance IQs seven to 14 points lower than verbal IQs [12, 13, 15]. In a study of 57 patients with relapsing-remitting MS (RRMS) and 43 patients with chronic progressive MS (CPMS), Heaton et al. [15] reported that the VIQ/PIQ differences were 4.5 (110.7/106.2) for the RRMS group and 11.5 (109.8/98.3) for the CPMS group. The fact that the performance subtests rely on fine motor speed and coordination which may be reduced in MS may explain this observation.

In summary, cross-sectional studies suggest that IQ scores are intact in MS. The results of longitudinal studies of intellectual functioning in MS are inconsistent. Some studies report a slight deterioration in intellectual functioning over time while others report stable IQs. There are clear discrepancies between verbal and performance IQs in patients with MS. These discrepancies may be related to sensorimotor deficits in MS and could explain any observed deterioration in overall IQ functioning.

Attention and speed of information processing

Reduced attention and speed of information processing are commonly reported in patients with MS. Speed of information processing has been assessed using a variety of cognitive tasks including the Paced Auditory Serial Addition Test [20]. The subject hears a series of 61 randomly selected digits and is required to add sequential pairs so that each digit is added to the digit immediately preceding it. The task can be presented at different rates. Those rates have generally varied from 1.2 to 4 seconds. Numerous studies have reported impaired performance on the PASAT in patients with MS compared to healthy controls [7, 21, 22]. There is growing evidence, however, to suggest that performance strategies may need to be considered in evaluating PASAT scores [23]. A subject, for example, may ignore every third test item in order to cluster the remaining items into a manageable task. This subject may end up with a score in the average range, but will have managed to avoid the intended goal of performing several cognitive tasks simultaneously. The PASAT has been used as a core outcome measure in clinical trials evaluating the efficacy of new MS therapies and it is one of the three components of the MS Functional Composite (MSFC) [24].

Demaree et al. [25] used a PASAT-like protocol designed to measure speed of information processing by adjusting the presentation rate to control for accuracy of performance between patients with MS and healthy controls. Interstimulus intervals that resulted in a 50% success rate were determined for each subject. As a group, patients with MS had a significantly longer interstimulus interval. When subjects performed the task at their own threshold speed, there was no significant difference in the accuracy rates of patients with MS and healthy controls.

The Symbol Digit Modalities Test (SDMT) [26] has also been used to assess information processing speed in MS. The task requires subjects to verbally substitute numbers for symbols as part of a set code. Scores are the number of correct responses in 90 seconds. Performance on the SDMT has been shown to be impaired in MS. Benedict et al. [27] administered the SDMT to 291 patients with clinically definite MS and 56 healthy controls as part of the Minimal Assessment of Cognitive Function in MS (MACFIMS) battery. They reported that 51.9% of patients demonstrated impairment. In study of 92 patients with early MS, Glanz et al. [22] reported that 15% of patients performed in the impaired range.

Given the reported sensitivity of the SDMT to cognitive changes in MS, Parmenter et al. [28] have suggested that it be used as a screen for cognitive impairment. They administered the MACFIMS battery to 100 patients with MS and 50 healthy controls. Patients were considered cognitively impaired if they performed one and a half standard deviations below controls on two or more MACFIMS variables, excluding the SDMT. Fifty-five percent of patients demonstrated cognitive impairment. Bayesian statistics showed that a total score of 55 or lower on the SDMT accurately categorized 72% of patients. Parmenter et al. [28] argued that the SDMT could be used as an effective screen for cognitive dysfunction in MS and that it could be administered during regular neurology clinic appointments in less than 5 minutes.

To summarize, reduced speed of information processing has been shown to be a key cognitive deficit in MS. It has been assessed using a variety of measures including the PASAT and SDMT. Deficits in processing speed have been reported in as many as 50% of patients with MS including those in the early stages of disease. There is evidence to support the use of the SDMT as a quick screening instrument for cognitive dysfunction in MS.

Memory

Memory function has been widely studied in MS and numerous studies have examined the exact nature of MS-related memory dysfunction. Short-term memory, long-term memory, implicit memory, and remote memory function have all been investigated.

Short-term memory is responsible for the immediate recall of small amounts of verbal and spatial information and can be assessed using simple tests of digit or visual memory span. Early reports suggested that patients with MS had intact or mildly impaired short-term memory [6, 7, 15, 29, 30]. In a meta-analysis of short-term memory function in MS, Thornton and Raz [31] analyzed 22 studies and found evidence for small-to-medium (d = 0.35] MS-related deficits in short-term memory capacity. The authors concluded that earlier findings might reflect power limitations in studies with small sample sizes.

Long-term memory refers to memory for tasks that exceed the limits and capacity of short-term memory. These tasks include prose memory, visual spatial memory, paired associate memory, and list learning across both immediate and delayed learning trials. Impaired long-term memory has been reported in 30–60% of patients with MS [29, 32, 33]. Rao et al. [7] administered the Selective Reminding Test (SRT), Story Recall Test, and 7/ 24 Spatial Recall Test (7/24) as part of a 31–test battery to 100 patients with MS and 100 normal controls. The SRT is a verbal learning test. The subject is read a list of 12 words and asked to recall as many of the words as possible. On subsequent learning trials the subject is read only the words that were not recalled on the previous learning trial. Six trials are administered. The 7/24 is a test of visual spatial learning. Subjects are shown a checkerboard with randomly placed checkers. After a 10–second exposure, subjects are asked to reproduce the design on an empty board. There are three learning trials. Consistent long-term retrieval (CLTR) on the SRT, the number of words recalled consistently on all subsequent trials, and total recall on the 7/24 (TR) were the two most sensitive measures in the battery. Based on the performance of the control group, 31 of patients were impaired on the SRT CLTR and 31% were impaired on 7/24 (TR). Twenty-five percent of patients were impaired on a story recall test.

More recently, Benedict et al. [27] administered the California Verbal Learning Test, 2nd edition (CVLT-II) and the revised Brief Visuospatial Memory Test (BVMT-R) to 291 patients with MS and 56 healthy controls. The CVLT-II gives patients five trials to learn a 16–word list. The BVMT-R uses a matrix of six visual designs that are presented for 10 seconds during each of three trials. The CVLT-II and BVMT-R include immediate recall, delayed recall, and recognition trials. Patients with MS were significantly impaired on both immediate and delayed recall of the CVLT-II and BVMT-R. On all measures, patients with RRMS performed better than patients with secondary progressive disease.

Several researchers have identified greater impairment on tests of recall than recognition in patients with MS [17, 34–36]. This discrepancy has led researchers to suggest that the primary deficit in MS is deficient retrieval as opposed to impaired encoding [32, 34]. It is possible, however, that patients with MS initially acquired less information than controls. In this case, reduced delayed recall could be due to either poor learning or poor retrieval. In studies where researchers controlled for the amount of information initially learned, patients with MS required more trials to learn, but showed similar rates of retrieval [37, 38].

Implicit and remote memory have also been studied in MS. Implicit memory does not rely on conscious recall and includes priming and motor skills. Research studies have shown that patients with MS have intact semantic and lexical priming [39, 40]. They also perform normally on tests of procedural learning [40]. Remote memory function in patients with MS is unclear. Using a famous faces recognition task, Beatty et al. [39] reported memory deficits in a group of patients with secondary progressive MS (SPMS). Rao et al. [7], on the other hand, found no evidence of impaired remote memory on the President's Test which required patients to recall the past eight US presidents.

In summary, memory dysfunction is common in patents with MS. Short-term memory is intact or mildly impaired. Patients consistently show impairment on tests of verbal and nonverbal long-term memory. There is less impairment on tests of recognition than recall, which may indicate greater difficulty with retrieval than encoding. It is also possible that the long-term memory impairment observed in MS is a consequence of inadequate initial learning. Implicit memory appears to be intact. Remote memory has not been widely studied in patients with MS.

Concept formation and abstract reasoning

Concept formation and abstract reasoning have been examined in MS using a variety of tasks. The Wisconsin Card Sorting Test (WCST) [41] consists of four cards placed in front of the subject. The subject is given two decks containing 64 cards each and asked to match each of the cards in the decks to one of the four key cards and is given feedback each time whether he or she is right or wrong. The WCST has been shown to reliably differentiate patients with MS from healthy controls [7, 15, 42]. These findings have led researchers to conclude that patients with MS have difficulty identifying abstract concepts, shifting set, and responding to environmental feedback. Beatty and Monson [43] used the WCST and the California Card Sorting Test to discriminate between impaired concept formation and perseveration when an incorrect problem-solving strategy was used. They concluded that patients with MS demonstrate impaired concept formation rather than increased perseveration.

More recently, the Delis-Kaplan Executive Function System Sorting Test (D-KEFS) [44] has been used to study abstract reasoning in MS. Subjects are presented with six cards each depicting a single word. The cards vary in different ways that allow for conceptual sorting according to at least eight different principles such as card shape or color. Benedict et al. [27] administered the D-KEFS to 100 patients with MS and 50 healthy controls. The frequency of impairment in patients with MS was 16%.

In summary, patients with MS have shown impaired performance on measures of concept formation and abstract reasoning. They have difficulty identifying abstract concepts, shifting set, and responding to environmental feedback. There is no strong evidence of increased perseveration.

Language

Impaired language expression and reduced comprehension are rarely reported in MS [45]. Heaton et al. [15] administered a screening test for aphasic symptoms to RRMS, CPMS, and healthy control groups. They reported a significantly higher aphasia error score in patients with CPMS than RRMS. Patients with RRMS did not differ from healthy controls. The precise nature of the errors made was not reported.

There are numerous studies showing reduced verbal fluency in patients with CIS, RRMS and SPMS [7, 15, 27, 32, 46]. The Controlled Oral Word Association Test (COWAT) [47] is a commonly used measure of verbal fluency. Subjects are given 60 seconds to produce as many words as possible that begin with a given letter of the alphabet. Proper names, numbers, and multiple forms of a word are prohibited. Scores are the sum of all admissible words across the three trials. A single study comparing cognitive function in RRMS, SPMS, and primary progressive MS (PPMS) groups found that patients with RRMS performed significantly worse than patients with PPMS on the COWAT [48].

Naming ability has not been widely studied in MS. Rao et al. [7] found no differences between MS and healthy control groups on the Abbreviated Boston Naming Test. Jambor [16] administered a battery of naming, reading, spelling, and comprehension tests to patients with MS and disabled, non-neurologic, psychiatric, and healthy controls. As a group, patients with MS performed slightly worse than controls on naming and reading. There were no differences on tests of spelling or comprehension.

In summary, aphasia has rarely been reported in MS. Verbal fluency deficits are common and easy to assess using the COWAT. Naming appears to be intact or mildly impaired.

Visuospatial processing

Visuospatial processing has been shown to be impaired in patients with MS. Scores on the performance subtests of the WAIS including Block Design and Object Assembly have consistently been shown to be lower in patients with MS than healthy controls [12, 13, 15]. It is not clear, however, whether reduced functioning is the result of impaired visuospatial problem solving or primary sensorimotor deficits [17]. Poor conceptual reasoning and organizational skills may also contribute [45]. Rao et al. [7] found no significant difference between patients with MS and normal controls on the Hooper Visual Organization Test (HVOT), a fragmented figures test. Conflicting results have been reported on Judgment of Line Orientation with some studies showing impaired performance [7, 27, 49] and others showing no significant differences between groups [50, 51].

In a recent study, Vleugels et al. [33] administered a series of 31 tests of visuoperceptual ability to 49 patients with MS and 30 healthy volunteers. Applying a cut-off of four failed tasks, 32.6% of patients with MS and 6.6% of healthy controls were considered impaired. The four most sensitive measures were a color discrimination task, perception of the Muller–Lyer Illusion, and two object recognition tasks.

In summary, there is some evidence to suggest that visuospatial processing is impaired in patients with MS. In some studies, primary sensorimotor deficits may have contributed to the reported findings. It is also possible that the tasks used to measure visuospatial functions are measuring additional functions such as conceptual reasoning and organizational skills. Additional research is needed to clarify visuospatial functioning in MS.

TOP TIPS 10.1: Important features of cognitive dysfunction in MS

- Intellectual functioning (IQ) is generally intact.
- Reduced speed of information processing/working memory is a key cognitive deficit.

- Short-term memory is mildly impaired.
- Long-term verbal and visual spatial memory deficits are common.
- Implicit memory is spared.
- Executive functions such as concept formation and abstract reasoning are impaired.
- Aphasia is rare.
- Naming is intact or mildly impaired.
- Verbal fluency is reduced.
- Visuospatial processing is impaired.

Influence of disease course, disease duration, and disability

Cross-sectional studies suggest that cognitive dysfunction may occur early in the course of MS. Callanan et al. [52] administered a one and a half hour test battery to 48 patients with clinically isolated lesions (CIL) and 40 rheumatologic and neurologic controls. Mild deficits in cognitive functioning were observed. The most striking cognitive abnormalities were on tests of visual and auditory attention. In a study of 67 patients with new-onset neurologic symptoms and the diagnosis of probable MS, Achiron and Barak [46] reported cognitive impairment in 54% of patients. Glanz et al. [22] identified cognitive impairment in 49% of patients with a clinically isolated syndrome (CIS) or the diagnosis of MS within the last 3 years.

Early studies consistently showed greater cognitive dysfunction in patients with CPMS than with RRMS [15, 53]. These studies used an older disease classification system that combined patients with PPMS and SPMS into a single group. In a study that distinguished between PPMS and SPMS, Comi et al. [54] reported that 53% of patients with SPMS and 7% of patients with PPMS showed evidence of cognitive impairment. Foong et al. [55], on the other hand, could not distinguish between the performance of PPMS and SPMS patients on cognitive tasks. Both groups performed worse than healthy controls on most cognitive measures.

A more recent study [48] compared the pattern of cognitive function in RRMS ($n = 108$), SPMS ($n = 71$), PPMS ($n = 55$), and healthy controls ($n = 67$). Subjects were administered the Brief Repeatable Battery of Neuropsychological Tests in Multiple Sclerosis (BRB). Cognitive impairment was observed in all three MS groups. Deficits were most severe in SPMS, followed by PPMS, and then RRMS. The RRMS group differed from controls on three of five cognitive tasks. Using the MACFIMS test battery, Benedict et al. [27] reported that all nine cognitive variables significantly discriminated RRMS and SPMS patients at a probability of $p < 0.01$. In each case, RRMS patients performed better than SPMS patients.

Disease duration and disability level measured using the Expanded Disability Status Scale (EDSS) have generally been shown to be weak predictors of cognitive dysfunction in patients with MS. Rao et al. [56] administered a comprehensive cognitive test battery to 53 patients with MS and found no relationship between duration of illness and severity of cognitive dysfunction. In a study of 100 patients with MS, Rao et al. [7] reported that EDSS correlated significantly ($p < 0.05$] with cognitive test performance, but accounted for only 6% of the shared variance. There was no association between duration of disease and cognitive function.

In summary, cognitive impairment occurs in patients with CIS as well as patients with RRMS, SPMS, and PPMS. There is consistent evidence to suggest a higher prevalence and greater severity of cognitive dysfunction in patients with progressive rather than relapsing MS. Disease duration and disability do not appear to be significantly associated with cognitive dysfunction patients with MS.

Longitudinal changes

There are several longitudinal studies of cognitive functioning in MS. Researchers have reported both cognitive decline [21, 57, 58] and cognitive stability [59–61] in MS patients followed for periods ranging from 1 to 10 years. Amato et al. [62] compared 50 early-onset MS patients and 70 healthy controls at 4- and 10-year intervals. At baseline, MS patients demonstrated deficits on tests of attention/concentration, verbal memory, and abstract reasoning. At 4 years, deficits in verbal fluency and comprehension were also identified and at 10 years new deficits in spatial memory had emerged. Amato et al. [62] concluded that as the disease progresses, the profile of cognitive deficits expands. Jonsson et al. [61], on the other hand, reported improved performance on tests of attentional control, mental processing, and visual spatial memory over a 4-year period. There were no changes on measures of problem solving or naming. Cognitive deterioration was observed on measures of visual organization. The authors suggested that improved performance on cognitive measures was largely attributable to practice effects. The fact that performance improved on some, but not all, measures suggests that certain tests may be more sensitive to the effects of practice than others.

There are many explanations for the discrepant findings reported in the literature. First, studies differ in terms of the clinical characteristics of the patients enrolled. Second, studies rely on different neuropsychological test batteries and varied criteria for the identification of cognitive impairment. Third, there is great variation in the length of follow-up. Fourth, studies have several methodological limitations including small sample sizes, high drop-out rates, and large practice effects.

In summary, longitudinal changes in cognitive functioning have been described in MS. There are also reports of cognitive stability. Practice effects on cognitive testing may lead to an underestimate of cognitive deterioration in MS. The best approach to understanding practice effects in longitudinal research is to serially assess healthy volunteers.

Impact of depression and fatigue

Depression occurs in as many as half of all patients with MS at some point during the course of the disease [63–65]. Although the impact of depression on cognitive functioning is well known [66–68], most early studies failed to find any clear association between depression and cognitive impairment in MS [7, 69–71]. These studies have been criticized for relying on correlation analyses rather than the use of high- and low-depression groups and for using cognitive measures that are not sensitive to the cognitive effects of depression [72, 73].

Some recent studies have shown that information processing speed and working memory may be affected by depressive symptoms in MS. Arnett et al. [74] compared 19 depressed and 41 non-depressed patients with MS on a highly effortful working memory task (reading span) and a short-term memory task that did not tax working memory (word span). Subjects with depression were significantly impaired on the effortful task compared to subjects without depression. No group differences were observed on the passive task. Demaree et al. [72] administered a battery of cognitive tests to 23 patients with MS and 23 healthy controls. The Beck Depression Inventory was used to assess severity of depressive symptomatology, and patients with MS were divided into high-BDI and low-BDI groups. The high-BDI group performed significantly worse than the low-BDI and healthy control groups on the PASAT. The high-BDI group also required significantly more trials to learn a word list. There were no differences between high- and low-BDI groups on WAIS-R verbal subtests including Vocabulary, Similarities, and Digit Span. The authors concluded that depression may augment the severity of learning and processing speed deficits in patients with MS.

Fatigue is common in patients with MS with a reported prevalence of more than 50% [75–78]. The impact of fatigue on cognitive functioning in MS is unclear. Most studies support a positive correlation between subjective fatigue and cognitive dysfunction [79–81], although other studies fail to find a significant association [82–84]. The discrepant results are thought to be related to small sample sizes, limited cognitive test batteries, and the failure to control for depression.

In a large-scale study that used both cross-sectional ($n = 465$] and longitudinal ($n = 69$] designs, Morrow et al. [85] reported that patients with MS had significantly higher scores on the Fatigue Severity Scale (FSS) than a group of healthy controls ($n = 70$). No significant correlations were found between cognitive (MACFIMS) measures and FSS scores in either cross-sectional or longitudinal analyses. There was, however, a significant correlation between fatigue (FSS) and depression (BDI) scores.

In summary, early studies suggested that there was no clear relationship between depression and cognitive impairment in patients with MS. More recent studies indicate that depressive symptoms may impact performance on effortful working memory tasks. There is no strong evidence to suggest that fatigue is related to cognitive impairment in MS.

Treatment strategies for cognitive dysfunction

Treatment of cognitive impairment in MS is a challenging subject. Pharmacologic therapy focuses on treatment of underlying disease as well as symptomatic manifestations of declining mental function, such as difficulties with attention, memory and fatigue. Cognitive neuro-rehabilitation programs have been used to improve communication skills, memory impairment, and concentration [86]). Appropriate management of the comorbid psychiatric disease often improves cognitive performance.

Pharmacologic intervention

Pharmacological treatment of cognitive dysfunction in MS can be divided into two major categories: (a) disease-modifying therapies (DMTs) alter the course of the disease and thus may help with cognitive impairment, and (b) symptomatic therapies that may target specific cognitive symptoms.

The observation that some magnetic resonance imaging (MRI) disease measures, including lesion load and brain volume [87] correlate with cognitive impairment, suggests that DMTs reduce lesion development and may also prevent or delay cognitive decline. However, the potential cognitive benefits of DMTs in patients with MS have not been addressed as primary outcome measures in pivotal clinical trials which led to the approval of these drugs for MS treatment [88]. Some of the trials included cognitive metrics, but only as secondary outcomes [89, 90]. In general, trials that selected patients with impaired cognitive scores showed some treatment benefit on cognition [90, 91], while trials that included many patients with cognitive scores comparable to healthy controls failed to show improvement post-therapy [92].

The COGIMUS (COGnitive Impairment in MUltiple Sclerosis) study was performed specifically to evaluate the progression of cognitive decline in patients with early (EDSS < 4, no prior treatment history) relapsing-remitting MS (RRMS) receiving treatment with interferon beta-1a (IFN-β-1a), 22 or 44 mcg administered subcutaneously three times weekly. In this study, treatment with the higher interferon dose was predictive of lower cognitive impairment at 3 years of follow-up [89, 93]. It is important to note that the cognitive impairment was significantly lower at 3 years than at the baseline in both treatment groups, indicating improved cognitive function over the course of the study, whih is likely due to practice effects. An earlier trial of intramuscular IFN-β-1a showed a 47% reduction in cognitive decline on PASAT testing over 2 years of follow-up [90]. Therefore, treatment with interferons may have dose-dependent cognitive benefits in mildly disabled patients with RRMS. Positive effects of IFN-β-1a on cognitive function were also observed in patients with secondary progressive MS (SPMS) when Multiple Sclerosis Functional Composite (MSFC) showed longitudinal improvement, especially evident in upper extremity function and the PASAT [94].

Treating MS relapses with high-dose steroids may have reversible negative effects on cognition. Declarative memory and long-term memory function can be affected shortly after steroid administration, but both tend to recover fully within 2 months post-treatment [94, 95].

Many different medications were tried to address symptoms of cognitive impairment in MS patients. Through the years, these included amantadine, pemoline, 4–aminopyridine, fampridine, modafinil, L-amphetamine, and acetylcholine esterase inhibitors. The majority of these studies have been underpowered, small, and uncontrolled. Results from the studies have, therefore, been mixed [82].

There is some evidence that treatment with L-amphetamine is associated with improved learning and memory in cognitively impaired MS patients [96, 97]. Modafinil may improve fatigue, focused attention, and dexterity. It has a favorable safety profile and can be used for symptomatic management of MS patients with severe fatigue and decreased focus [98]. There is some evidence that cholinesterase inhibitors improve memory in MS patients, although the results have not been consistent across the small studies. One study assessed the effects of donepezil on SPMS patients who were residents in a nursing home, documenting improvement in several cognitive domains after 8 weeks of therapy [99]. A larger randomized controlled trial of donepezil examined 69 patients over 24 weeks and demonstrated improved verbal learning and memory compared to placebo on formal neuropsychological assessment, and some improvement in quality of life measures [100]. However, recently, published results from a multicenter randomized trial of 120 patients showed no evidence of efficacy of donepezil over placebo. SRT and participants' impression of memory improvements were used an primary outcome measures, and both failed to reach significance [101].

There are additional anecdotal reports of efficacy in small numbers of subjects. Interestingly, memantine failed to improve cognitive function in MS patients in a recent randomized, placebo-controlled trial [102].

Considering the domain of alternative medicine, a pilot study with 22 MS patients showed no side effects and modest benefit on some functional cognitive domains with the use of gingko biloba. Fatigue was one of the measures that demonstrated improvement with therapy in some patients [103].

Cognitive neurorehabilitation

Cognitive-behavioral therapy, family and individual counseling, strategies to improve day-to-day function, as well as necessary job modifications and accommodations can be of great help to MS patients suffering from cognitive decline. Various but heterogeneous studies report improvement of cognitive performance as a result of specific attention-training tasks or neuropsychological counseling [104, 105]. The results support the idea that a specific cognitive intervention is superior to a nonintervention [106]. Attention training in MS patients may result in improved deficit compensation patterns by recruiting additional brain regions as seen on fMRI study [107]. A fairly recent comprehensive review of psychological treatments for MS [108] concludes that cognitive therapy can help MS patients to adjust better to the disease and to better control their comorbid depression.

Psychiatric disease

Cross-sectional studies have shown some degree of affective disturbance in a significant number of patients with MS [109, 110]. Major depressive disorder (MDD) is the most common manifestation and is in part secondary to the burden of having to cope with a chronic, incurable disease. However, it is more prevalent in MS than in other chronic diseases, suggesting an organic component. The lifetime risk of major depression in patients with MS is up to 50%, compared with 12.9% in patients with chronic medical conditions in another study. Adequate treatment of depression in MS patients may improve cognitive function. Selective serotonin reuptake inhibitors with or without psychotherapy are effective [111] and will be discussed in more detail elsewhere in this book.

Some data indicate a comorbid association between bipolar illness and MS. The prevalence of bipolar disease in MS patients is double that of the general population. Suicide rates are higher in patients with MS and bipolar disease than in the general population or when compared to patients with other chronic illnesses [112]. Mood stabilizers and lithium carbonate can be used successfully to control bipolar affective disorder.

Euphoria, formerly considered to be common in MS, is actually infrequent and is usually associated with moderate or severe cognitive impairment and greater disease burden on MRI [113]. Patients may manifest a dysphoric state with swings from depression to elation.

Pseudobulbar affect refers to a condition where mood and affect are basically disconnected: patients laugh when they do not feel mirth, or they cry when they do not feel sad, or they may show a mix of laughing and crying without the matching internal mood states [114]. An estimated 10% of MS patients are affected with this syndrome and treatment may be attempted with SSRI, amitriptyline, or a combination of dextromethorphan/quinidine [115]. Neudexta is a new medication, recently approved for treatment of the pseudobulbar affect in patients with MS and Amyotrophic Lateral Sclerosis (ALS). It is a combination of dextromethorphan hydrobromide and quinidine sulfate. It is thought to help to regulate excitatory neurotransmission through presynaptic inhibition of glutamate release, and through postsynaptic glutamate response modulation via uncompetitive, low-affinity NMDA antagonist activity. In trials, it was effective to decrease the number of laughing and crying episodes over the 12 weeks of the study [116]. A pseudobulbar affect, if present and troublesome in MS patients, tends to be associated with worse cognitive performance on frontally mediated tasks, greater physical neurologic disability, and higher MRI lesion load [117].

In summary, when considering the treatment options for cognitive impairment in MS, it is important to utilize the platform disease-modifying MS therapies as well as symptomatic treatments that may enhance memory, improve attention, and decrease fatigue. A multimodal approach should include both medical and cognitive-behavioral modalities. Underlying psychiatric disease, if present, should also be appropriately treated.

TOP TIPS 10.2: Key aspects of treatment of cognitive dysfunction in MS

- There is no FDA approved therapy for cognitive dysfunction in MS.
- Maintaining patients on disease-modifying therapy may positively affect cognitive function in MS.
- Symptomatic treatments with wakefulness promoting and memory-enhancing agents may occasionally be helpful, although trial results have been conflicting.
- Brain atrophy, especially deep gray matter loss, correlates with severity of cognitive impairment in MS.
- Depression is a common psychiatric co-morbidity in MS and may also affect cognitive performance.
- Neurorehabilitation efforts may be helpful in improving functioning in cognitively impaired MS patients.

Imaging correlates of cognitive impairment in MS

Cognitive impairment in MS has been associated with a variety of MRI metrics of disease activity and progression. Early studies reported high correlations with the total T2 lesion burden and volume [34]. Lesions located in frontal and parietal lobes showed stronger correlations with tasks of processing speed, attention, and verbal memory [60]. Periventricularly located lesions are significantly related to decreased psychomotor speed, supporting the idea that periventricular lesions have a determinant impact on cognition in patients with MS. Global and regional atrophy plays a role in cognitive impairment. Third ventricular width as a measure of central atrophy has a substantial predictive value for cognitive dysfunction [118]. Thalamic atrophy appears to correlate particularly well with impairment on a variety of cognitive tests in MS patients [119]. Hippocampal atrophy and abnormalities in limbic circuitry functional connectivity are evident in MS patients even before cognitive impairment is detected on NP testing [120]. The contribution of cortical lesions [121, 122] and loss of cortical ribbon thickness [123] are important. Cognitively impaired patients have abnormalities in normal appearing white and gray matter as measured by magnetization transfer ratio (MTR) that are not seen in cognitively intact MS patients [124]. Diffusion tensor imaging shows the difference in the fractional anisotropy between the mildly impaired MS patients and control subjects in corpus callosum, cingulum, and superior and inferior longitudinal fasciculi. In addition, different diffusion measures correlate with PASAT scores for cognitive decline in parietal, frontal, as well as temporal white matter regions in MS patients [125].

In summary, when reviewing MRI correlates to cognitive impairment, it is important to remember that both conventional and nonconventional imaging metrics show various degrees of correlation with cognitive deficits. Large-scale clinical-imaging trials will need to further elucidate the most robust association between MRI disease and cognitive decline in MS patient population.

Conclusion

Overall, cognitive impairment is quite prevalent in MS, and may lead to significant patient disability. It is more common in patients with progressive rather than relapsing MS, but is seen across all disease states. Disease duration and physical disability are not strongly associated with cognitive impairment. Well-described cognitive deficits are present on tests of verbal memory, visuospatial memory, verbal fluency, concept formation, abstract reasoning, and spatial reasoning. Reduced attention and speed of information processing is a key cognitive deficit in MS with as many as half of patients performing below the expected range. Longitudinal studies have been inconsistent with some studies showing cognitive decline and others showing cognitive stability over periods ranging from 1 to –10 years. Depression may play a role in decreased performance on certain effortful working memory tasks. Fatigue, although common in MS, does not appear to directly impact cognition. Pharmacologic treatment of cognitive impairment focuses on treatment of the underlying disease of MS, as well as on treatment of symptoms, such as poor attention, fatigue, memory impairment, depression and anxiety. Cognitive-behavioral therapy, psychological counseling, assistance with job retraining, and disability matters may also be helpful. MRI correlates of cognitive dysfunction in MS are currently being investigated. Atrophy of deep gray matter structures, such as thalamus, correlates well with MS-related cognitive decline. More rigorous studies are needed to further elucidate the nature of cognitive impairment in MS patients, and to assess the best therapeutic modalities for this significant problem.

References

1 Feinstein A. The Clinical Neuropsychiatry of Multiple Sclerosis. Cambridge, UK: Cambridge University Press; 1999.
2 Ross DM. The mental symptoms in disseminated sclerosis. Rev Neurol Psychiat 1917; 13: 361–73.
3 Dercum FX. A case of multiple cerebrospinal sclerosis presenting unusual symptoms suggesting paresis. J Am Med Assoc 1912; 59: 1612–13.
4 Kurtzke JF. Neurologic impairment in multiple sclerosis and the Disability Status Score. Acta Neurol Scand 1970; 46: 493–512.
5 Peyser JM, Edwards K.R., Poser C.M., Filskov, S.B. Cognitive function in patients with multiple sclerosis. Arch Neurol 1980; 37: 437–40.
6 Lyon-Caen O, Jouvent R, Hauser S, Chaunu MP, Benoit N, Widlocher D, et al. Cognitive function in recent-onset demyelinating diseases. Arch Neurol 1986 Nov; 43(11): 1138–41.
7 Rao SM, Leo GJ, Bernardin L, Unverzagt F. Cognitive dysfunction in multiple sclerosis. I. Frequency, patterns, and prediction. Neurology 1991 May; 41(5): 685–91.
8 McIntosh-Michaelis SA, Roberts MH, Wilkinson SM, Diamond ID, McLellan DL, Martin JP, et al. The prevalence of cognitive impairment in a community survey of multiple sclerosis. Br J Clin Psychol 1991 Nov; 30 (Pt 4): 333–48.
9 Wechsler D. Wechsler Adult Intelligence Scale. New York: The Psychological Corporation; 1955.
10 Wechsler D. Wechsler Adult Intelligence Scale – Revised. New York: The Psychological Corporation; 1981.

11 Wechsler D. Wechsler Adult Intelligence Scale – III. New York: The Psychological Corporation; 1991.

12 Matthews CG, Cleeland CS, Hopper CL. Neuropsychological patterns in multiple sclerosis. Dis Nerv Syst 1970 Mar; 31(3): 161–70.

13 Goldstein G, Shelly CH. Neuropsychological diagnosis of multiple sclerosis in a neuropsychiatric setting. J Nerv Ment Dis 1974 Apr; 158(4): 280–90.

14 Ivnik RJ. Neuropsychological stability in multiple sclerosis. J Consult Clin Psychol 1978 Oct; 46(5): 913–23.

15 Heaton RK, Nelson LM, Thompson DS, Burks JS, Franklin GM. Neuropsychological findings in relapsing-remitting and chronic-progressive multiple sclerosis. J Consult Clin Psychol 1985 Feb; 53(1): 103–10.

16 Jambor KL. Cognitive functioning in multiple sclerosis. Br J Psychiat 1969 Jul; 115(524): 765–75.

17 Rao SM. Neuropsychology of multiple sclerosis: a critical review. J Clin Exp Neuropsychol 1986 Oct; 8(5): 503–42.

18 Canter AH. Direct and indirect measures of psychological deficit in multiple sclerosis. J Gen Psychol 1951; 44: 3–50.

19 Fink SL, Houser HB. An investigation of physical and intellectual changes in multiple sclerosis. Arch Phys Med Rehabil 1966 Feb; 47(2): 56–61.

20 Gronwall D, Wrightson P. Delayed recovery of intellectual function after minor head injury. Lancet 1974 Sep; 2(7881): 605–9.

21 Feinstein A, Kartsounis LD, Miller DH, Youl BD, Ron MA. Clinically isolated lesions of the type seen in multiple sclerosis: a cognitive, psychiatric, and MRI follow up study. J Neurol Neurosurg Psychiat 1992 Oct; 55(10): 869–76.

22 Glanz BI, Holland CM, Gauthier SA, Amunwa EL, Liptak Z, Houtchens MK, et al. Cognitive dysfunction in patients with clinically isolated syndromes or newly diagnosed multiple sclerosis. Mult Scler 2007 Sep; 13(8): 1004–10.

23 Fisk JD, Archibald CJ. Limitations of the Paced Auditory Serial Addition Test as a measure of working memory in patients with multiple sclerosis. J Int Neuropsychol Soc 2001 Mar; 7(3): 363–72.

24 Fischer JS, Rudick RA, Cutter GR, Reingold SC. The Multiple Sclerosis Functional Composite Measure (MSFC): an integrated approach to MS clinical outcome assessment. National MS Society Clinical Outcomes Assessment Task Force. Mult Scler 1999 Aug; 5(4): 244–50.

25 Demaree HA, DeLuca J, Gaudino EA, Diamond BJ. Speed of information processing as a key deficit in multiple sclerosis: implications for rehabilitation. J Neurol Neurosurg Psychiat 1999 Nov; 67(5): 661–3.

26 Smith A. Symbol Digit Modalities Test. Los Angeles: Western Psychological Services; 1991.

27 Benedict RH, Cookfair D, Gavett R, Gunther M, Munschauer F, Garg N, et al. Validity of the minimal assessment of cognitive function in multiple sclerosis (MACFIMS). J Int Neuropsychol Soc 2006 Jul; 12(4): 549–58.

28 Parmenter BA, Weinstock-Guttman B, Garg N, Munschauer F, Benedict RH. Screening for cognitive impairment in multiple sclerosis using the Symbol digit Modalities Test. Mult Scler 2007 Jan; 13(1): 52–7.

29 Rao SM, Hammeke TA, McQuillen MP, Khatri BO, Lloyd D. Memory disturbance in chronic progressive multiple sclerosis. Arch Neurol 1984 Jun; 41(6): 625–31.

30 Kujala P, Portin R, Ruutiainen J. Memory deficits and early cognitive deterioration in MS. Acta Neurol Scand 1996 May; 93(5): 329–35.

31 Thornton AE, Raz N. Memory impairment in multiple sclerosis: a quantitative review. Neuropsychology 1997 Jul; 11(3): 357–66.

32 Caine ED, Bamford KA, Schiffer RB, Shoulson I, Levy S. A controlled neuropsychological comparison of Huntington's disease and multiple sclerosis. Arch Neurol 1986 Mar; 43(3): 249–54.

33 Beatty WW, Goodkin DE, Monson N, Beatty PA, Hertsgaard D. Anterograde and retrograde amnesia in patients with chronic progressive multiple sclerosis. Arch Neurol 1988 Jun; 45(6): 611–19.

34 Rao SM, Leo GJ, St Aubin-Faubert P. On the nature of memory disturbance in multiple sclerosis. J Clin Exp Neuropsychol 1989 Oct; 11(5): 699–712.

35 Armstrong C, Onishi K, Robinson K, D'Esposito M, Thompson H, Rostami A, et al. Serial position and temporal cue effects in multiple sclerosis: two subtypes of defective memory mechanisms. Neuropsychologia 1996 Sep; 34(9): 853–62.

36 Beatty WW, Krull KR, Wilbanks SL, Blanco CR, Hames KA, Paul RH. Further validation of constructs from the selective reminding test. J Clin Exp Neuropsychol 1996 Feb; 18(1): 52–5.

37 DeLuca J, Gaudino EA, Diamond BJ, Christodoulou C, Engel RA. Acquisition and storage deficits in multiple sclerosis. J Clin Exp Neuropsychol 1998 Jun; 20(3): 376–90.

38 Demaree HA, Gaudino EA, DeLuca J, Ricker JH. Learning impairment is associated with recall ability in multiple sclerosis. J Clin Exp Neuropsychol 2000 Dec; 22(6): 865–73.

39 Beatty WW, Monson, N. Semantic priming in multiple sclerosis. Bull Psychonom Soc 1990; 28: 397–400.

40 Rao SM, Grafman, J., DiGiulio D., Mittenberg, W., Bernardin, L., Leo, J.G., Luchetta, T., Unverzagt, F. Memory dysfunction in multiple sclerosis: it's relation to working memory, semantic encoding, and implicit learning. Neuropsychology 1993; 7: 364–74.

41 Berg EA. A simple objective technique for measuring flexibility in thinking. J Gen Psychol 1948; 39: 15–22.

42 Beatty WW, Goodkin DE, Beatty PA, Monson N. Frontal lobe dysfunction and memory impairment in patients with chronic progressive multiple sclerosis. Brain Cogn 1989 Sep; 11(1): 73–86.

43 Beatty WW, Monson N. Problem solving by patients with multiple sclerosis: comparison of performance on the Wisconsin and California Card Sorting Tests. J Int Neuropsychol Soc 1996 Mar; 2(2): 134–40.

44 Delis DC, Kaplan, E., Kramer, J.H. Delis-Kaplan Executive Function System. San Antonio: The Psychological Corporation; 2001.

45 Fennell EB, Smith, M.C. Neuropsychological assessment. In: Rao SM, editor. Neurobehavioral aspects of multiple sclerosis. NewYork: Oxford University Press; 1990. pp. 63–81.

46 Achiron A, Barak Y. Cognitive impairment in probable multiple sclerosis. J Neurol Neurosurg Psychiat 2003 Apr; 74(4): 443–6.

47 Spreen O, Benton, A.L. Neurosensory Center Comprehensive Examination For Aphasia. Victoria: University of Victoria Neuropsychology Laboratory; 1969.

48 Huijbregts SC, Kalkers NF, de Sonneville LM, de Groot V, Reuling IE, Polman CH. Differences in cognitive impairment of relapsing remitting, secondary, and primary progressive MS. Neurology 2004 Jul; 63(2): 335–9.

49 Benedict RH, Weinstock-Guttman B, Fishman I, Sharma J, Tjoa CW, Bakshi R. Prediction of neuropsychological impairment in multiple sclerosis: comparison of

conventional magnetic resonance imaging measures of atrophy and lesion burden. Arch Neurol 2004 Feb; 61(2): 226–30.

50 Beatty WW, Paul RH, Wilbanks SL, Hames KA, Blanco CR, Goodkin DE. Identifying multiple sclerosis patients with mild or global cognitive impairment using the Screening Examination for Cognitive Impairment (SEFCI). Neurology 1995 Apr; 45(4): 718–23.

51 Beatty WW, Hames KA, Blanco CR, Paul RH, Wilbanks SL. Verbal abstraction deficits in multiple sclerosis. Neuropsychology 1995; 9: 198–205.

52 Callanan MM, Logsdail SJ, Ron MA, Warrington EK. Cognitive impairment in patients with clinically isolated lesions of the type seen in multiple sclerosis. A psychometric and MRI study. Brain 1989 Apr; 112 (Pt 2): 361–74.

53 Rao SM, Hammeke TA, Speech TJ. Wisconsin Card Sorting Test performance in relapsing-remitting and chronic-progressive multiple sclerosis. J Consult Clin Psychol 1987 Apr; 55(2): 263–5.

54 Comi G, Filippi M, Martinelli V, Campi A, Rodegher M, Alberoni M, et al. Brain MRI correlates of cognitive impairment in primary and secondary progressive multiple sclerosis. J Neurol Sci 1995 Oct; 132(2): 222–7.

55 Foong J, Rozewicz L, Chong WK, Thompson AJ, Miller DH, Ron MA. A comparison of neuropsychological deficits in primary and secondary progressive multiple sclerosis. J Neurol 2000 Feb; 247(2): 97–101.

56 Rao SM, Leo GJ, Haughton VM, St Aubin-Faubert P, Bernardin L. Correlation of magnetic resonance imaging with neuropsychological testing in multiple sclerosis. Neurology 1989 Feb; 39 (2 Pt 1): 161–6.

57 Amato MP, Ponziani G, Pracucci G, Bracco L, Siracusa G, Amaducci L. Cognitive impairment in early-onset multiple sclerosis. Pattern, predictors, and impact on everyday life in a 4–year follow-up. Arch Neurol 1995 Feb; 52(2): 168–72.

58 Zivadinov R, Sepcic J, Nasuelli D, De Masi R, Bragadin LM, Tommasi MA, et al. A longitudinal study of brain atrophy and cognitive disturbances in the early phase of relapsing-remitting multiple sclerosis. J Neurol Neurosurg Psychiat 2001 Jun; 70(6): 773–80.

59 Jennekens-Schinkel A, Laboyrie PM, Lanser JB, van der Velde EA. Cognition in patients with multiple sclerosis After four years. J Neurol Sci 1990 Nov; 99(2–3): 229–47.

60 Sperling RA, Guttmann CR, Hohol MJ, Warfield SK, Jakab M, Parente M, et al. Regional magnetic resonance imaging lesion burden and cognitive function in multiple sclerosis: a longitudinal study. Arch Neurol 2001 Jan; 58(1): 115–21.

61 Jonsson A, Andresen J, Storr L, Tscherning T, Soelberg Sorensen P, Ravnborg M. Cognitive impairment in newly diagnosed multiple sclerosis patients: a 4–year follow-up study. J Neurol Sci 2006 Jun; 245(1–2): 77–85.

62 Amato MP, Ponziani G, Siracusa G, Sorbi S. Cognitive dysfunction in early-onset multiple sclerosis: a reappraisal after 10 years. Arch Neurol 2001 Oct; 58(10): 1602–6.

63 Minden SL, Orav J, Reich P. Depression in multiple sclerosis. Gen Hosp Psychiat 1987 Nov; 9(6): 426–34.

64 Joffe RT, Lippert GP, Gray TA, Sawa G, Horvath Z. Mood disorder and multiple sclerosis. Arch Neurol 1987 Apr; 44(4): 376–8.

65 Sadovnick AD, Remick RA, Allen J, Swartz E, Yee IM, Eisen K, et al. Depression and multiple sclerosis. Neurology 1996 Mar; 46(3): 628–32.

66 Shenal BV, Harrison DW, Demaree HA. The neuropsychology of depression: a literature review and preliminary model. Neuropsychol Rev 2003 Mar; 13(1): 33–42.

67 Elliott D, Ricker KL, Lyons J. The control of sequential goal-directed movement: learning to use feedback or central planning? Motor Control 1998 Jan; 2(1): 61–80.

68 Hartlage S, Alloy LB, Vazquez C, Dykman B. Automatic and effortful processing in depression. Psychol Bull 1993 Mar; 113(2): 247–78.

69 DeLuca J, Barbieri-Berger S, Johnson SK. The nature of memory impairments in multiple sclerosis: acquisition versus retrieval. J Clin Exp Neuropsychol 1994 Apr; 16(2): 183–9.

70 Grafman J, Rao S, Bernardin L, Leo GJ. Automatic memory processes in patients with multiple sclerosis. Arch Neurol 1991 Oct; 48(10): 1072–5.

71 Minden SL, Moes EJ, Orav J, Kaplan E, Reich P. Memory impairment in multiple sclerosis. J Clin Exp Neuropsychol 1990 Aug; 12(4): 566–86.

72 Demaree HA, Gaudino E, DeLuca J. The relationship between depressive symptoms and cognitive dysfunction in multiple sclerosis. Cogn Neuropsychiat 2003 Aug; 8(3): 161–71.

73 Siegert RJ, Abernethy DA. Depression in multiple sclerosis: a review. J Neurol Neurosurg Psychiat 2005 Apr; 76(4): 469–75.

74 Arnett PA, Higginson CI, Voss WD, Bender WI, Wurst JM, Tippin JM. Depression in multiple sclerosis: relationship to working memory capacity. Neuropsychology 1999 Oct; 13(4): 546–56.

75 Krupp LB, Alvarez LA, LaRocca NG, Scheinberg LC. Fatigue in multiple sclerosis. Arch Neurol 1988 Apr; 45(4): 435–7.

76 Freal JE, Kraft GH, Coryell JK. Symptomatic fatigue in multiple sclerosis. Arch Phys Med Rehabil 1984 Mar; 65(3): 135–8.

77 Fisk JD, Pontefract A, Ritvo PG, Archibald CJ, Murray TJ. The impact of fatigue on patients with multiple sclerosis. Can J Neurol Sci 1994 Feb; 21(1): 9–14.

78 Putzki N, Katsarava Z, Vago S, Diener HC, Limmroth V. Prevalence and severity of multiple-sclerosis-associated fatigue in treated and untreated patients. Eur Neurol 2008; 59(3–4): 136–42.

79 Schwid SR, Tyler CM, Scheid EA, Weinstein A, Goodman AD, McDermott MP. Cognitive fatigue during a test requiring sustained attention: a pilot study. Mult Scler 2003 Oct; 9(5): 503–8.

80 Simioni S, Ruffieux C, Bruggimann L, Annoni JM, Schluep M. Cognition, mood and fatigue in patients in the early stage of multiple sclerosis. Swiss Med Wkly 2007 Sep; 137(35–36): 496–501.

81 Diamond BJ, Johnson SK, Kaufman M, Graves L. Relationships between information processing, depression, fatigue and cognition in multiple sclerosis. Arch Clin Neuropsychol 2008 Mar; 23(2): 189–99.

82 Geisler MW, Sliwinski M, Coyle PK, Masur DM, Doscher C, Krupp LB. The effects of amantadine and pemoline on cognitive functioning in multiple sclerosis. Arch Neurol 1996 Feb; 53(2): 185–8.

83 Parmenter BA, Denney DR, Lynch SG. The cognitive performance of patients with multiple sclerosis during periods of high and low fatigue. Mult Scler 2003 Mar; 9(2): 111–18.

84 Bailey A, Channon S, Beaumont JG. The relationship between subjective fatigue and cognitive fatigue in advanced multiple sclerosis. Mult Scler 2007 Jan; 13(1): 73–80.

85 Morrow SA, Weinstock-Guttman B, Munschauer FE, Hojnacki D, Benedict RH. Subjective fatigue is not associated with cognitive impairment in multiple sclerosis: cross-sectional and longitudinal analysis. Mult Scler 2009 Aug; 15(8): 998–1005.

86 Chiaravalloti ND, DeLuca J. Cognitive impairment in multiple sclerosis. Lancet Neurol 2008 Dec; 7(12): 1139–51.

87 Amato MP, Zipoli V, Portaccio E. Multiple sclerosis-related cognitive changes: a review of cross-sectional and longitudinal studies. J Neurol Sci 2006 Jun; 245(1–2): 41–6.

88 Montalban X, Rio J. Interferons and cognition. J Neurol Sci 2006; 245: 137–40.

89 Patti F, Amato MP, Bastianello S, Caniatti L, Di Monte E, Ferrazza P, et al. Effects of immunomodulatory treatment with subcutaneous interferon beta-1a on cognitive decline in mildly disabled patients with relapsing-remitting multiple sclerosis. Mult Scler 2010 Jan; 16(1): 68–77.

90 Fischer JS, Priore RL, Jacobs LD, Cookfair DL, Rudick RA, Herndon RM, et al. Neuropsychological effects of interferon beta-1a in relapsing multiple sclerosis. Multiple Sclerosis Collaborative Research Group. Ann Neurol 2000 Dec; 48(6): 885–92.

91 Pliskin NH, Hamer DP, Goldstein DS, Towle VL, Reder AT, Noronha A, et al. Improved delayed visual reproduction test performance in multiple sclerosis patients receiving interferon beta-1b. Neurology 1996 Dec; 47(6): 1463–8.

92 Weinstein A, Schwid SR, Schiffer RB, McDermott MP, Giang DW, Goodman AD. Neuropsychologic status in multiple sclerosis after treatment with glatiramer. Arch Neurol 1999 Mar; 56(3): 319–24.

93 Patti F, Amato MP, Trojano M, Bastianello S, Tola MR, Goretti B, et al. Cognitive impairment and its relation with disease measures in mildly disabled patients with relapsing-remitting multiple sclerosis: baseline results from the Cognitive Impairment in Multiple Sclerosis (COGIMUS) study. Mult Scler 2009 Jul; 15(7): 779–88.

94 Uttner I, Muller S, Zinser C. Reversible impaired memory induced by pulsed methylprednisolone in patients with MS. Neurology 2005; 64: 1971–3.

95 Brunner R. D. S, Hess K. Effects of corticosteroids on short-term and long-term memory. Neurology 2005; 64: 335–7.

96 Benedict RH, Munschauer F, Zarevics P, Erlanger D, Rowe V, Feaster T, et al. Effects of l-amphetamine sulfate on cognitive function in multiple sclerosis patients. J Neurol 2008 Jun; 255(6): 848–52.

97 Morrow SA, Kaushik A, Zarevics P. The effects of L-amphetamine sulfate on cognitive function in multiple sclerosis patients: results of a randomized controlled trial. J Neurol 2009; 256: 1095–102.

98 Lange R, Volkmer M, Heesen C, Liepert J. Modafinil effects in multiple sclerosis patients with fatigue. J Neurol 2009 Apr; 256(4): 645–50.

99 Greene YM, Tariot PN, Wishart H, Cox C, Holt CJ, Schwid S, et al. A 12-week, open trial of donepezil hydrochloride in patients with multiple sclerosis and associated cognitive impairments. J Clin Psychopharmacol 2000 Jun; 20(3): 350–6.

100 Krupp LB, Christodoulou C, Melville P, Scherl WF, MacAllister WS, Elkins LE. Donepezil improved memory in multiple sclerosis in a randomized clinical trial. Neurology 2004 Nov; 63(9): 1579–85.

101 Krupp LB, Christodoulou C, Melville P, Scherl WF, Pai LY, Muenz LR, et al. Multicenter randomized clinical trial of donepezil for memory impairment in multiple sclerosis. Neurology Apr; 76(17): 1500–7.

102 Lovera JF, Frohman E, Brown TR, Bandari D, Nguyen L, Yadav V, et al. Memantine for cognitive impairment in multiple sclerosis: a randomized placebo-controlled trial. Mult Scler 2010 Jun; 16(6): 715–23.

103 Johnson SK, Diamond BJ, Rausch S, Kaufman M, Shiflett SC, Graves L. The effect of Ginkgo biloba on functional measures in multiple sclerosis: a pilot randomized controlled trial. Explore (NY) 2006 Jan; 2(1): 19–24.

104 Benedict RH, Shapiro A, Priore R, Miller C, Munschauer F, Jacobs L. Neuropsychological counseling improves social behavior in cognitively-impaired multiple sclerosis patients. Mult Scler 2000 Dec; 6(6): 391–6.

105 Plohmann AM, Kappos L, Ammann W. Computer assisted retraining of attentional impairments in patients with multiple sclerosis. J Neurol Neurosurg Psychiat 1999; 64: 455–62.

106 Winkelmann A, Engel C, Apel A, Zettl UK. Cognitive impairment in multiple sclerosis. Neurology 2008; 255: 309–10.

107 Penner I, Kappos L, Opwis K, editors. Induced changes in brain activation using a computerized attention training in patients with Multiple Sclerosis (MS). Proceedings of KogWis05 The German Cognitive Science Conference; 2005; Schwabe, Basel.

108 Thomas PW, Thomas S, Hillier C, Galvin K, Baker R. Psychological interventions for multiple sclerosis. Cochrane Database Syst Rev 2006 (1): CD. 004431.

109 Minden SL, Schiffer RB. Affective disorders in multiple sclerosis. Review and recommendations for clinical research. Arch Neurol 1990 Jan; 47(1): 98–104.

110 Arnett PA. Longitudinal consistency of the relationship between depression symptoms and cognitive functioning in multiple sclerosis. CNS Spectr 2005 May; 10(5): 372–82.

111 Mohr DC, Boudewyn AC, Goodkin DE, Bostrom A, Epstein L. Comparative outcomes for individual cognitive-behavior therapy, supportive-expressive group psychotherapy, and sertraline for the treatment of depression in multiple sclerosis. J Consult Clin Psychol 2001 Dec; 69(6): 942–9.

112 Bronnum-Hansen H, Stenager E, Nylev Stenager E, Koch-Henriksen N. Suicide among Danes with multiple sclerosis. J Neurol Neurosurg Psychiat 2005 Oct; 76(10): 1457–9.

113 Benedict RH, Carone DA, Bakshi R. Correlating brain atrophy with cognitive dysfunction, mood disturbances, and personality disorder in multiple sclerosis. J Neuroimaging 2004 Jul; 14 (3 Suppl): 36S–45S.

114 Feinstein A. Neuropsychiatric syndromes associated with multiple sclerosis. J Neurol 2007 May; 254Suppl 2: II73–6.

115 Panitch HS, Thisted RA, Smith RA, Wynn DR, Wymer JP, Achiron A, et al. Randomized, controlled trial of dextromethorphan/quinidine for pseudobulbar affect in multiple sclerosis. Ann Neurol 2006 May; 59(5): 780–7.

116 Pioro EP, Brooks BR, Cummings J, Schiffer R, Thisted RA, Wynn D, et al. Dextromethorphan plus ultra low-dose quinidine reduces pseudobulbar affect. Ann Neurol 2010 Nov; 68(5): 693–702.

117 Feinstein A, O'Connor P, Gray T, Feinstein K. Pathological laughing and crying in multiple sclerosis: a preliminary report suggesting a role for the prefrontal cortex. Mult Scler 1999 Apr; 5(2): 69–73.

118 Tiemann L, Penner IK, Haupts M, Schlegel U, Calabrese P. Cognitive decline in multiple sclerosis: impact of topographic lesion distribution on differential cognitive deficit patterns. Mult Scler 2009 Oct; 15(10): 1164–74.

119 Houtchens MK, Benedict RH, Killiany R, Sharma J, Jaisani Z, Singh B, et al. Thalamic atrophy and cognition in multiple sclerosis. Neurology 2007 Sep; 69(12): 1213–23.

120 Roosendaal SD, Hulst HE, Vrenken H, Feenstra HE, Castelijns JA, Pouwels PJ, et al. Structural and functional hippocampal changes in multiple sclerosis patients with intact memory function. Radiology 2010 May; 255(2): 595–604.

121 Bakshi R, Ariyaratana S, Benedict RH, Jacobs L. Fluid-attenuated inversion recovery magnetic resonance imaging detects cortical and juxtacortical multiple sclerosis lesions. Arch Neurol 2001 May; 58(5): 742–8.

122 Calabrese M, Agosta F, Rinaldi F, Mattisi I, Grossi P, Favaretto A, et al. Cortical lesions and atrophy associated with cognitive impairment in relapsing-remitting multiple sclerosis. Arch Neurol 2009 Sep; 66(9): 1144–50.

123 Calabrese M, Mattisi I, Rinaldi F, Favaretto A, Atzori M, Bernardi V, et al. Magnetic resonance evidence of cerebellar cortical pathology in multiple sclerosis. J Neurol Neurosurg Psychiat 2010 Apr; 81(4): 401–4.

124 Amato MP, Portaccio E, Stromillo ML, Goretti B, Zipoli V, Siracusa G, et al. Cognitive assessment and quantitative magnetic resonance metrics can help to identify benign multiple sclerosis. Neurology 2008 Aug; 71(9): 632–8.

125 Hecke WV, Nagels G, Leemans A, Vandervliet E, Sijbers J, Parizel PM. Correlation of cognitive dysfunction and diffusion tensor MRI measures in patients with mild and moderate multiple sclerosis. J Magn Reson Imaging 2010 Jun; 31(6): 1492–8.

CHAPTER 11

Depression and Other Psychosocial Issues in Multiple Sclerosis

David J. Rintell

Partners Multiple Sclerosis Center, Brigham and Women's Hospital, Boston, MA, USA

Introduction

There are many aspects of life with MS which present a significant challenge to the patient and his/her family. The threat of life-altering disability, the variability of the illness, the lack of predictability, and the specific limitations that are present daily can be experienced as obstacles to performing the roles and functions of family, work, etc. Despite these challenges, most people living with MS are able to adapt to this new life circumstance and function well, although often differently than their premorbid mode of functioning.

The challenges of chronic, potentially disabling illness can contribute to psychological problems which, on their own, can contribute to disability. In addition, the biological aspects of the illness can be contributors to psychological problems. There is a body of literature describing psychopathology in MS, which will be reviewed in this chapter. Unfortunately, the factors that contribute to successful adaptation have not been the subject of many studies, despite the fact that patients and their families often seek help with the adaptational process from MS professionals. Much more information is needed about how to help patients through a successful transition from health to living well with chronic illness. A number of psychosocial interventions have been attempted, some to treat depression and other psychological problems, and others to enhance the adaptational process, and these too will be reviewed on these pages.

Multiple Sclerosis: Diagnosis and Therapy, First Edition. Edited by Howard L. Weiner and James M. Stankiewicz. © 2012 John Wiley & Sons, Ltd.
Published 2012 by John Wiley and Sons, Ltd.

Psychological problems experienced by MS patients

Depression

MS patients have a high rate of depression compared to the general population as well as patients with other neurological and chronic illnesses. Depression in MS is prevalent, highly disabling, and likely related to organic as well as reactive etiology. As depression carries a high morbidity and can be life threatening, its assessment and treatment are highly important in treating patients with MS.

Prevalence

Estimates of the prevalence of depression among people with MS vary according to the mechanism of measurement, the population studied, and whether the estimate is based on cross-sectional or longitudinal measurement. Despite the methodological variability of the studies, the incidence of depression in this population is very high and warrants attention. Screening for, and diagnosing depression in MS patients is complicated by the fact that some symptoms indicative of depression are also common symptoms of MS. For example, among the DSM IV criteria for major depression are fatigue, insomnia, and difficulty concentrating and thinking, which are all common MS symptoms [1]. A number of instruments have been used to screen for depression in this population. Most commonly the Center for Epidemiologic Studies Depression Scale (CES-D) [2] and the Beck Depression Inventory (BDI) [3] have been utilized. Some researchers prefer the CES-D due to concern that the items relating to somatic symptoms on the BDI may overlap with the symptoms of MS; however the BDI has been determined to be reliable and valid for this population [4]. Nevertheless, there is no universal standard cutoff score utilized in these studies, and the diagnostic definitions of depression can vary [5]. For example, Chwastiak et al. [6] found a 41.8% rate of patients in the clinical range on the CES-D [2] (Scale Score ≥16) in a community sample derived from membership in an MS organization, but a lower rate when a higher cutoff – signifying moderate to severe depression – was used (Scale Score ≥21). Recent point-prevalence rates of depression include 31.4% [7], 25.7% [8], and 57.4% [9]. Cetin and colleagues found a 51% rate of current depression in a recent large survey using the CES-D cutoff score of ≥16 [10].

Lifetime prevalence of major depression (by age 59) has been found to be over 50% [5] in a representative clinical population, which excluded patients with an EDSS of ≥6.5 and used a structured psychiatric interview based on the DSM-IV [11], but actual prevalence is likely to be higher. Some studies find that more advanced illness has been shown to be a risk factor for depression in MS [6]. (See Box 11.1.)

> **BOX 11.1   Diagnostic criteria for major depressive disorder**
>
> A. A prominent and persistent disturbance in mood predominates in the clinical picture and is characterized by either (or both) of the following:
>
>   **1** Depressed mood or markedly diminished interest or pleasure in all, or almost all, activities.
>
>   **2** Elevated, expansive, or irritable mood.
>
> B. There is evidence from the history, physical examination, or laboratory findings that the disturbance is the direct physiological consequence of a general medical condition.
>
> C. The disturbance is not better accounted for by another mental disorder.
>
> D. The disturbance does not occur exclusively during the course of a delirium.
>
> E. The symptoms cause clinically significant distress or impairment in social, occupational, or other important areas of functioning.
>
> *Source*: American Psychiatric Association [105].

Depression can be found very early in MS. In fact, it has been reported that 30% of patients with clinically isolated syndrome (CIS) were found to experience depression [12]. We have found that in patients with a first demyelinating event or new diagnosis, 32% of patients were experiencing depression [13].

Depression which does not meet the criteria for major depressive disorder (MDD) can still impose functional limitations and disability on the patient. One wonders what the measured incidence of depression in MS patients would be if the criteria for mood disorder due to a general medical condition [14] (see Box 11.2) were utilized. This diagnosis requires a depressed mood or diminished interest or pleasure which causes distress and impairment. Such results might also occur using a clinical rather than a MDD score on the CES-D to indicate depression. In Minden's 1987 sample [15], where one-third of the MS patients met the criteria for major depression, 64% were reported to have low mood. Minden points out that depression in their sample was more in the mild to moderate range, often referred to as dysthymia, and characterized by anger, irritability, worry, and discouragement. Further, subsyndromal symptoms of depression can be associated with a great deal of distress and can be debilitating, but are responsive to therapy [16].

The incidence of depression in MS greatly exceeds that of the general population [17] and most medical populations [18], and has also been found to exceed the incidence of depression in other chronic medical illnesses in a large population-based study [19]. Depression is common in chronic illness [20]. Higher rates of depression in MS as compared with other neurological disorder were found in a 1993 meta-analysis [21]. Depression is found in such disorders as hypertension, diabetes mellitus, coronary artery

---

BOX 11.2 Diagnostic criteria for mood disorder due to a general medical condition

A. Five (or more) of the following:
    Must include at least of (1) depressed mood or (2) diminished interest or pleasure.
    1 Depressed mood most of the day.

    2 Markedly diminished interest or pleasure in all, or almost all, activities.

    3 Significant weight loss when not dieting or weight gain $> +/- 5\%$ every month.

    4 Insomnia or hypersomnia nearly every day.

    5 Psychomotor agitation or retardation every day.

    6 Fatigue or less or energy nearly every day.

    7 Feelings of worthlessness or excessive or inappropriate guilt nearly every day.

    8 Diminished ability to think or concentrate, or indecisiveness, nearly every day.

    9 Recurrent thoughts of death (not just fear of dying), recurrent suicidal ideation.

B. Symptoms do not meet criteria for a mixed episode.

C. Symptoms cause clinically significant distress or impairment in social, occupational, or other important areas of functioning.

D. Symptoms are not due to physiological effects of a substance of a medical condition.

E. Symptoms are not better accounted for by bereavement (loss of a loved one), symptoms persist for more than 2 months or are characterized by marked functional impairment, morbid preoccupation with worthlessness, suicidal ideation, psychotic symptoms, or psychomotor retardation.

Source: American Psychiatric Association [106].

---

disease, congestive heart failure, stroke, chronic obstructive pulmonary disease, and end-stage renal disease, but at rates lower than those found in MS patients [22]. However, a recent study found comparable rates of depression between MS patients and those with ulcerative colitis [23] and, by self-report, with GI disease and other syndromes [24]. Treatment of mental health issues in MS will be discussed later in this chapter; however, it is important to point out here that depression in MS often goes unrecognized and untreated. In one study, for example, 25% of patients with depression were unaware that they were depressed, and received no treatment [25]. In a second study, over 16% of patients had CES-D scores ≥ 21 without awareness or treatment for a measured serious depression [26].

Questions related to the increased incidence of depression in MS compared to other disorders also relate to questions on the etiology of depression in MS, whether it is reactive to the existence or possibility of decreasing physical and cognitive abilities, or whether the depression has an organic cause. Psychosocial causes, such as the uncertainty of living with chronic illness, decreased social support, and decreased physical functioning, have been cited [27]. Evidence for an organic cause is strengthened by the observation that patients who have lesions limited to their spinal cord have a lower rate of depression than those who have lesions in the brain [28]. There is growing strength of MRI evidence of physical changes in the brain which are linked to depression in MS. This evidence has been linked to lesions and T1 black holes in the frontal and parietal lobes [29].

The severity of depression has also been linked to MRI changes in the brain. Increased frequency of T1–weighted lesions in the frontal, parietal and temporal lobes, and atrophy were seen in patients with more severe depression. Bakshi [29] found a relationship between depression and white matter lesions and atrophy on the MRI, but this relationship was independent of neurological disability. A growing literature has demonstrated a relationship between depression and hyperintense and hypointense lesion volume and atrophy [30]. Feinstein et al. [31] reported that patients with major depression had a greater T2-weighted lesion volume and more extensive T1–weighted lesion volume in the left medial inferior prefrontal cortex and less gray matter volume and more CSF volume in the left anterior temporal region, concluding that lesion burden and atrophy are involved in depression in MS, but stressed that psychosocial causes should also be explored.

Depression in CIS patients also seems, at least in part, to be related to MRI changes. Di Legge et al. found that the severity of depressive symptoms in CIS was correlated with the number and size of lesions in the right temporal region [12].

There is growing evidence that depressed patients who do not have MS also have structural changes in their brains [32]. This finding can be seen as supporting the organic basis of depression in MS, or complicating the picture due to lack of certainty that the changes seen on MRI in depressed MS patients are due to MS or due to the depression itself.

Depression and interferon-beta

Concerns about increased rates of depression among MS patients taking interferon-beta came about as a result of reports of a suicide and suicide attempts among patients in the initial trial of this medication in MS [33] as well as reports of depression linked to interferon use in other illnesses [34]. Although increased levels of depression were not reported in a number of successive studies, a trial of interferon-beta for a first demyelinating event did show significantly higher rates of depression among the treated patients [35]. Wallin et al. [16] point out that thyroid dysfunction, which has also been linked to the use of interferon-beta, may play a role in this inconsistent finding of depression in MS. In any case, clinicians would be wise to monitor not only their patients on interferons, but all MS patients for depression, and treat and/or refer them when appropriate.

Correlates of depression: disability

Measures of physical impairment such as the EDSS and their relationship to depression yield mixed results. For example, Chwastiak [6] described such a relationship in a population-based study; however, Bakshi [36] found no association between physical disability and depression.

There is some evidence, however, that depressive episodes or an increase of severity of depression may follow MS exacerbations [15].

While the relationship between overall disability and depression in MS is unclear, specific components of disability do have a variable impact on depression in MS. Williams and colleagues found that falls and bowel dysfunction were linked to increased levels of depression in their population [37].

Correlates of depression: fatigue

Fatigue – perhaps the most common and one of the most disabling aspects of multiple sclerosis – has been found to be present in up to 88% of MS patients [38], and fatigue in MS has been found to be highly correlated with depression. Patients with fatigue were more likely to be depressed than patients without fatigue, and fatigue levels were linked to the severity of depression. Since fatigue was also found in the absence of depression, there are clearly other additional causes of fatigue in MS [39].

It is often difficult to distinguish psychomotor retardation (a vegetative sign of depression) from fatigue in multiple sclerosis. It has been proposed that items that measure vegetative symptoms of depression should be eliminated from scales used to measure depression in MS patients [40].

Poor sleep and lack of sleep are likely to contribute to fatigue. Since sleep disturbance is common in MS, and as sleep disturbance commonly occurs in depression, the complex relationship between depression, fatigue, and sleep in MS deserves further study. Bamer et al. [41] found that depression was highly associated with sleep problems among MS patients, and explains much of the variance (33%) of sleep problems in a large mailed health outcomes study.

Correlates of depression: quality of life and social support

Depression has been found to be a major contributing factor to a reduced quality of life (QoL) in people with MS. Even after adjusting for disability and fatigue levels, depression's association with QoL is highly significant [42]. In fact, D'Alisa and colleagues have shown that much of the variance of the the the Short Form [36] Health Survey (SF36), the main component of the quality of life measures most commonly used in MS, the Multiple Sclerosis Quality of Life Inventory (MSQLI) [43], and the Multiple Sclerosis Quality of Life-54 Instrument (MSQOL 54) [44], can be accounted for by depression [45]. These findings are supported by those of Benedict et al. [46], using the MSQOL-54. Significant correlations between depression and all QoL subscales were recently found in a study of patients with early MS [47].

Reduced levels of social support have been found to be linked to depression in people with MS [48], and increased levels of social support were found to be associated with reduced depression in MS [49]. Tapping into deficits in social support, unmarried status was linked to depression in a large study of veterans with MS [37]. A further discussion of the role of social support is given below.

Correlates of depression: cognition

Depressed MS patients had lower scores in processing speed and sustained attention [50]. Arnett and colleagues demonstrated that depressed MS patients performed lower capacity-demanding attentional tasks than non-depressed MS patients, including the Paced Auditory Serial Addition Test (PASAT) [51] and the Symbol Digit Modalities Test (SDMT) [52].

Verbal fluency has also been shown to be related to depression scores with higher levels of depression associated with lower verbal fluency scores [47]. Impairment in cognitive functioning has been shown to be predictive of depression in a longitudinal study [53], although the impact can be mediated by coping style.

"Pseudodementia" [54] has been described in MS [55]. Due to lowered attention, concentration, and processing speed as symptoms of depression, patients can appear to have a cognitive dysfunction which improves after treatment of depression.

Correlates of depression: adherence

Depression is related to poor adherence to disease-modifying medication, and treatment of depression has been shown to increase adherence [56].

Treatment of depression

Depression is largely a very treatable disorder. Unfortunately, since many patients with MS do not receive treatment for depression, untreated depression is likely to persist [16].

Depression can occur early in MS. Di Legge and colleagues [12] found that 30% of CIS patients experienced depression, but none of these patients had received any treatment for their depression. The benefits of treating patients with MS who have depression go beyond the patient, to the medical care system itself. Patients with depression and anxiety tend to be high users of medical care, increasing the frequency of contact with medical professionals [57].

The Goldman Consensus Statement on Depression in MS [58] notes that both psychopharmacological and psychotherapeutic treatment for depression are effective in MS, and established the "gold standard" of treatment, consisting of a combination of psychotherapy and pharmacological intervention.

It is now common practice for neurologists and other providers to prescribe modern antidepressant medication such as selective serotonin reuptake inhibitors (SSRIs) to people with MS [10]. It is surprising, however, that there is little research studying the efficacy of such treatment in MS. Schiffer and Wineman [59] conducted a small double-blind study utilizing the tricyclic antidepressant desiprimine together with psychotherapy, comparing the intervention group with controls who received psychotherapy and a placebo, and found significant improvements in the medication group on clinical assessment and the Hamilton Rating Scale [60], but not on the BDI. Ehde and colleagues [61] describe the use of paroxetine with MS patients, but did not find that the use of the medication improved depressive symptoms significantly above placebo. It has been reported that in a clinic population, most (65%) of patients with a major depressive disorder did not receive antidepressant treatment, and most received less than optimal doses for the treatment of depression [62].

There are few studies of the efficacy of psychotherapy in MS. One of the difficulties in this area is that, as an intervention, psychotherapy is highly variable depending on the theoretical framework and training of the provider, frequency and length of meetings, and inclusion of others (family members, group interventions). Nevertheless, it has been shown that various types of psychotherapy constitute effective treatment for depression in MS [63]. There are, however, models of psychosocial treatment that operate from a standard manual. One such model is cognitive behavioral therapy (CBT). Mohr recently published a detailed guide to conducting CBT with MS patients [64]. CBT has been shown to be effective as a treatment for depression in MS, and the intervention can be conducted over the telephone [65].

In addition to psychotherapy and medication, specific behavioral patterns have been shown to be effective in reducing depression in MS and other populations. Dalgas and colleagues [66] demonstrated that exercise is linked to reduced depression in MS. Helping others has also been found to reduce depression. Arnstein et al. [67], for example, found that volunteering was linked to reduced depression in patients with chronic pain.

Anxiety in MS

Clinical levels of anxiety are present in many patients with MS, yet study of this problem has been limited. While the point prevalence rate of anxiety may be lower, the lifetime prevalence of anxiety disorders approaches the prevalence of depression. Lifetime prevalence of anxiety in MS has been shown to be 35.7% [68]. Korostil and Feinstein identify female gender, lifetime experience of major depression, suicidal thoughts, alcohol abuse, high social stress, and low social support as correlates of lifetime anxiety [68]. The link between anxiety and suicidal thinking should be underlined, as it is likely that anxiety contributes to suicide. Anxiety and depression have been shown to be often comorbid conditions [69]. Bieske identified lower EDSS and younger age as correlates of clinical anxiety in MS [70]. Poder et al. found that over 30% of the MS patients they studied experienced social anxiety [71].

It is important to note that anxiety problems occur not only in the patient but in family members. Janssens [72] found that 34% of newly diagnosed MS patients scored in the clinical range of an anxiety measure, as well as 40% of their partners. This finding contributes to the idea that anxiety in MS is reactive rather than organic. Supporting this assumption is the lack of MRI findings linking anxiety in MS [68, 73].

It is possible that the uncertainty about the future that a diagnosis brings contributes to high anxiety levels, and this has been reported by patients [74]. Anxiety has also been found to contribute to poor treatment adherence in MS [75].

Unfortunately, since anxiety problems are rarely recognized in MS treatment settings, they are also rarely treated. For example, only about 10% of patients with clinical anxiety received treatment in Beiske's sample [70]. Of note, none of the patients experiencing clinical anxiety in the Korostil and Feinstein [68] study received a diagnosis of anxiety disorder. Cognitive behavioral therapy in group and individual formats has been shown to be effective in the treatment of anxiety in MS [76]. Selective serotonin reuptake inhibitors are effective in the general public [77]. Benzodiazapines have been used to treat anxiety in MS, but they tend to increase fatigue and can impair cognition. Benzodiazapines have also been shown to be addictive. [78]

Bipolar disorder

Bipolar disorder is twice as prevalent in people who have MS than in the general population [79]. Bipolar disorder is characterized by periods of elevated, expansive mood, with inflated self-esteem, reduced need for sleep, pressured or excessive speech, and excessive pursuit of pleasurable activities. Manic periods often alternate with periods of major depression. Suicide is a significant risk for patients with bipolar disorder: 10–15% of patients with bipolar disorder are lost through completed suicide [14]. If a patient has a history of mania or hypomania, she or he should be referred to a psychiatrist for treatment [70]. Selective serotonin uptake inhibitors as well as corticosteroids can sometimes induce mania in these patients.

Pathological laughing and crying

Pathological laughing and crying (PLC), also referred to as the pseudobulbar affect, has been reported in the MS literature for some time. The clinical definition and prevalence, however, were established by Feinstein et al. in 1997 [80]. PLC is characterized by incidents of crying, laughing, or both, which are involuntary and do not match the patient's perception of his or her mood state. The prevalence is reported to be close to 10% of people with MS. Prevalence was not found to be correlated with age or gender, but was found to be related to increased disability and the course of progressive disease. MRI indicators of PLC were identified by Ghaffar and colleagues [81].

There is increased interest in PLC since the approval by the FDA of a medication that has been shown to be effective in its treatment [82]. In the past, low-dose antidepressants were found to be effective for this disorder [83].

Risk of suicide

Depression is a major risk factor for suicidal ideation and suicide. Suicide is a major public health problem in the USA, taking about 30,000 lives per year, and constituting the fourth leading cause of death for ages 25–44 [84], a prime age group for the diagnosis of MS. Chronic illness is thought to be a motivating factor in 25% of suicides, and chronic pain has also been linked to suicide [44]. MS patients have an increased rate of suicide compared to the general and matched populations. Sadovnik et al. [85] found that suicide accounted for 15% of all deaths in an MS clinic population. Feinstein [86], who studied 140 patients in an MS clinic, found that 28.6% had experienced suicidal intent and that 9 of the 140 had actually attempted suicide. While there was no increased risk of suicide for age, sex, duration of disease, or cognitive impairment, the presence and severity of depression, alcohol abuse, and social isolation had an 85% predictive accuracy for suicidal intent in the MS patients studied. Additional risk factors shown include being male, onset of MS prior to age 30 [87], current age between 40 and 49, previous suicidal tendencies, worsening of illness, presence of a mental disorder, and a moderate level of disability [88]. Other factors include diagnosis at an earlier age, primary or secondary progressive disease, being unmarried, lower social support, no longer driving, and increased disability including mobility, bowel, and bladder problems [89]. Clinicians should also be aware of characteristics of completed suicides in the general population: male, Caucasian, older, widowed, socially isolated [90], firearm availability [91], and alcohol use. In fact, alcohol is a factor in 50% of suicides, and 18% of alcoholics die from suicide [92].

Screening for mental health problems

Given the prevalence of mental health problems in MS, it seems clear that screening for these disorders should occur when MS patients come for medical care. Unfortunately, outside of screening for research studies, such screening does not routinely occur. Thus, identification and treatment of mental health problems is well behind the prevalence of such problems. In a survey of patients in four university-affiliated MS Centers [93], 60% of the patients were found to have mental health problems, while only 46% of the patients received any form of treatment. Increased screening is indicated in these circumstances.

Given the risk of suicide in the MS patient population, medical care providers, if they are not already screening their patients for depression, should begin to do so. The CES-D [2] and the BDI [3] are commonly used instruments. A form of the BDI which eliminates the items that overlap with MS symptoms has been referred to as the BDI-18 and can be used with confidence [94]. A two-item screen for depression has also been identified by Mohr, and found to be as valid as the BDI [94] (see Box 11.3). Screening for anxiety and other mental disorders should also be considered.

BOX 11.3   Two-item screen for depression

1 Effective screening for depression in MS patients can be quickly accomplished by asking two questions.

2 A referral to the National MS Society can help patients and family increase their social support network, which may lead to improvements in quality of life.

Source: Mohr et al. [107].

Treatment of mental health problems

Among MS patients who received treatment for mental health problems, in a large, multi-site study, treatment was sought for depression and anxiety, but the largest group sought help to cope with MS and family issues (see Figure 11.1). It is important to note that half of the patients who received treatment for mental health problems were provided treatment by neurologists (see Figure 11.2).

Successful adaptation to multiple sclerosis

Given the documentation of mental health and other problems experienced by people with MS, the reader could develop an understanding that few if any people affected with the illness can achieve lives free of psychopathology. However, half of patients never experience a major depressive episode, and many are free of mental health problems despite their illness [95]. In fact, contact with patients easily reveals that many patients are able to manage the multiple demands of their illness and live happy, productive lives. A careful observer also notes that successful adaptation to MS does not

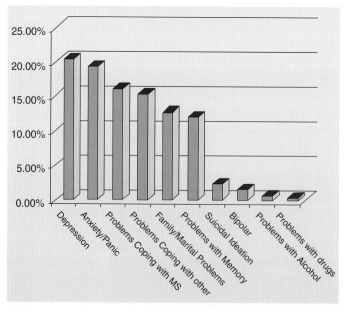

Figure 11.1 Reasons for seeking treatment. (Reproduced from Rintell et al. [108] with permission from ACTRIMS.)

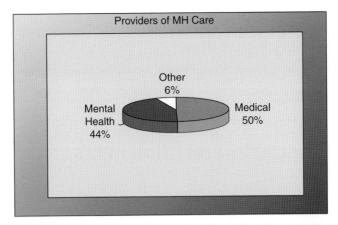

Figure 11.2 Who provided treatment. (Reproduced from Rintell et al. [108] with permission from ACTRIMS.)

seem to be dependent on the level of physical impairment – an observation made by Bandura [96]. One wishes for a literature with a breadth such as that which documents psychopathology, but unfortunately we know little about what helps people with MS and their families to achieve positive, productive, and happy lives [97]. Such research is needed to provide models for psychosocial adjustment and adaptation to life with MS.

The research documenting psychopathology in MS does provide support for a model which seeks to identify protective and strength-promoting factors in adaptation to MS. Principal among these factors is social support. As stated above, social support has been linked to lower levels of depression [49] and anxiety in MS [68]. Social support has also been found to predict marital satisfaction in MS [98]. The social support literature provides additional evidence of the potential value of social networks in successful adaptation to MS, and social support has been linked to reduced morbidity and mortality in illness and disability [99]. In addition, social support has been found to reduce cognitive decline in an elderly population [100]. It would appear that helping patients maintain and augment their social support networks would assist them in the process of positive adaptation [101]. One way to help patients to increase their sources of social support is a referral to the National MS Society, which offers educational and social support to patients and families whose lives have been affected by MS.

There is growing interest in benefit finding in MS. Benefit finding refers to the ability to identify positive growth in the midst of adversity. Post-traumatic growth is another term that is understood to refer to the same concept [102]. MS patients have been shown to identify a number of areas of benefit finding. One-third of the patients in a study by Pakenham [103] reported that they had experienced personal growth as a result of their MS. They also reported benefits accrued in interpersonal relationships, appreciation of life, health gains, and alteration of life priorities and goals.

While it has not been shown that intervening to increase social support or benefit finding in patients with MS can improve patient outcomes, those of us who care for people with MS and their families should increase our awareness of these factors. Additionally, we should begin to design trials of interventions aimed at increasing social support, benefit finding, and other variables found to be related to positive patient and family adaptation.

Psychosocial intervention in MS

Psychosocial intervention studies published prior to January 2006 were reviewed by Malcomson et al. [104]. Thirty-three studies fulfilled the criteria for methodological quality. Studies included wellness groups, psychotherapy, exercise, relaxation, stress management, music therapy, and CBT. The reader is referred to this review.

Conclusion

Psychological problems secondary to MS increase disability. In particular, the high rate of depression, anxiety, and suicidality are well established in this population. It is essential that patients are screened for these conditions during medical appointments. Effective treatments are available, and functioning can be improved. Since neurologists provide much of the mental healthcare for MS patients, it is recommended that they are prepared for this role, and have good referral sources for those patients in need of additional care. Less is known about the factors that contribute to successful adaptation, despite the fact that patients and their families often seek help with the adaptational process from MS professionals. More study is needed about how to help patients through a successful transition from health to living well with chronic illness.

References

1 Patten SB. Diagnosing Depression in MS in the Face of Overlapping Symptoms. Int MS J 2010; 17(1): 3–5.
2 Radloff L. The CES-D Scale: A Self Report Depression Scale for Research in the General. Appl Psychol Measur 1977; 1(3): 385–401.
3 Beck A, Steer R, Brown G. Manual for the Beck Depression Inventory-II. San Antonio, TX: Psychological Corporation 1996, pp. 1–82.
4 Moran P, Mohr D. The validity of Beck Depression Inventory and Hamilton Rating Scale for Depression items in the assessment of depression among patients with multiple sclerosis. J Behav Med 2005; 28(1): 35–41.

5 Sadovnick A, Remick R, Allen J, Swartz E, Yee I, Eisen K, et al. Depression and multiple sclerosis. Neurology 1996; 46(3): 628–32.

6 Chwastiak L, Ehde DM, Gibbons LE, Sullivan M, Bowen JD, Kraft GH. Depressive symptoms and severity of illness in multiple sclerosis: epidemiologic study of a large community sample. Am J Psychiat 2002 Nov; 159(11): 1862–8.

7 Beiske A, Svensson E, Sandanger I, Czujko B, Pedersen E, Aarseth J, et al. Depression and anxiety amongst multiple sclerosis patients. Euro J Neurol 2008; 15(3): 239–45.

8 Dahl O, Stordal E, Lydersen S, Midgard R. Anxiety and depression in multiple sclerosis. A comparative population-based study in Nord-Trøndelag County, Norway. Mult Scler 2009; 15(12): 1495.

9 Koch M, Mostert J, Heerings M, Uyttenboogaart M, De Keyser J. Fatigue, depression and disability accumulation in multiple sclerosis: a cross sectional study. Euro J Neurol 2009; 16(3): 348–52.

10 Cetin K, Johnson K, Ehde D, Kuehn C, Amtmann D, Kraft G. Antidepressant use in multiple sclerosis: epidemiologic study of a large community sample. Mult Scler 2007; 13(8): 1046.

11 Spitzer RL W, J. Instruction Manual for the Structured Clinical Interview for DSM-III (SCID) New York, NY: Biomedical Research Division, New York State Psychiatric Institute; 1985.

12 Di Legge S, Piattella MC, Pozzilli C, Pantano P, Caramia F, Pestalozza IF, et al. Longitudinal evaluation of depression and anxiety in patients with clinically isolated syndrome at high risk of developing early multiple sclerosis. Mult Scler 2003; 9(3): 302–6.

13 Glanz B, Holland, C, Rintell D, Cook, S., Himmelberger, K., Delft, K, Weiner H (editor) The Impact of Social Support on Depressive Symptoms in Patients with Early MS. Consortium of Multiple Sclerosis Centers, 2004; Toronto, ON.

14 Association AP. Diagnostic and Statistical Manual of Mental Disorders (DSM IV-TR): American Psychiatric Association, 2000.

15 Minden SL, Orav J, Reich P. Depression in multiple sclerosis. Gen Hosp Psychiat 1987 Nov; 9(6): 426–34.

16 Wallin M, Wilken J, Turner A, Williams R, Kane R. Depression and multiple sclerosis: review of a lethal combination. J Rehabil Res Devel 2006; 43(1): 45.

17 Kessler R, Gruber M, Hettema J, Hwang I, Sampson N, Yonkers K. Co-morbid major depression and generalized anxiety disorders in the National Comorbidity Survey follow-up. Psychol Med 2008; 38(3): 365–74.

18 Katon W, Ciechanowski P. Impact of major depression on chronic medical illness. J Psychosom Res 2002; 53(4): 859–64.

19 Patten SB, Beck CA, Williams JVA, Barbui C, Metz LM. Major depression in multiple sclerosis - A population-based perspective. Neurology 2003 Dec; 61(11): 1524–7.

20 Patten SB, Williams JVA, Lavorato DH, Modgill G, Jette N, Eliasziw M. Major depression as a risk factor for chronic disease incidence: longitudinal analyses in a general population cohort. Gen Hosp Psychiat 2008 Sep–Oct; 30(5): 407–13.

21 Schubert D, Foliart R. Increased depression in multiple sclerosis patients: a meta-analysis. Psychosomatics 1993; 34(2): 124–30.

22 Egede LE. Major depression in individuals with chronic medical disorders: prevalence, correlates and association with health resource utilization, lost productivity and functional disability. Gen Hosp Psychiat 2007; 29(5): 409–16.

23 Bol Y, Duits AA, Vertommen-Mertens C, E. R., Hupperts R, M. M., Romberg-Camps M, J. L., Verhey F, R. J., et al. The contribution of disease severity, depression and negative affectivity to fatigue in multiple sclerosis: A comparison with ulcerative colitis. J Psychosom Res 2010; 69(1): 43–9.

24 Patten SB, Beck CA, Kassam A, Williams JV, Barbui C, Metz LM. Long-term medical conditions and major depression: Strength of association for specific conditions in the general population. Canad J Psychiat – Revue Canad Psychiat 2005 Mar; 50(4): 195–202.

25 McGuigan C, Hutchinson M. Unrecognised symptoms of depression in a community-based population with multiple sclerosis. J Neurol 2006 Feb; 253(2): 219–23.

26 Marrie RA, Horwitz R, Cutter G, Tyry T, Campagnolo D, Vollmer T. The burden of mental comorbidity in multiple sclerosis: frequent, underdiagnosed, and under-treated. Mult Scler 2009 Mar; 15(3): 385–92.

27 Mohr DC, Dick LP, Russo D, Pinn J, Boudewyn AC, Likosky W, et al. The psychosocial impact of multiple sclerosis: exploring the patient's perspective. Health Psychol 1999 Jul; 18(4): 376–82.

28 Bakshi R. Depression in multiple sclerosis: a review. MSQR: Mult Scler Qtly Rep 2001; 20: 6–9.

29 Bakshi R, Czarnecki D, Shaikh ZA, Priore RL, Janardhan V, Kaliszky Z, et al. Brain MRI lesions and atrophy are related to depression in multiple sclerosis. Neuroreport 2000 Apr; 11(6): 1153–8.

30 Feinstein A, O'Connor P, Akbar N, Moradzadeh L, Scott CJM, Lobaugh NJ. Diffusion tensor imaging abnormalities in depressed multiple sclerosis patients. Mult Scler [Article] 2010 Feb; 16(2): 189–96.

31 Feinstein A, Roy P, Lobaugh N, Feinstein K, O'Connor P, Black S. Structural brain abnormalities in multiple sclerosis patients with major depression. Neurology [Article] 2004 Feb; 62(4): 586–90.

32 van Tol M-J, van der Wee NJA, van den Heuvel OA, Nielen MMA, Demenescu LR, Aleman A, et al. Regional brain volume in depression and anxiety disorders. Arch Gen Psychiatry 2010 Oct; 67(10): 1002–11.

33 Klapper J. Interferon beta treatment of multiple sclerosis. Neurology 1994; 44(1): 188.

34 Loftis JM, Hauser P. The phenomenology and treatment of interferon-induced depression. J Affec Disord 2004; 82(2): 175–90.

35 Jacobs L, Beck R, Simon J, Kinkel R, Brownscheidle C, Murray T, et al. CHAMPS Study Group. Intramuscular interferon beta-1a therapy initiated during a first demyelinating event in multiple sclerosis. N Engl J Med 2000; 343(13): 898–904.

36 Bakshi R, Czarnecki D, Shaikh Z, Priore R, Janardhan V, Kaliszky Z, et al. Brain MRI lesions and atrophy are related to depression in multiple sclerosis. Neuroreport 2000; 11(6): 1153.

37 Williams R, Turner A, Hatzakis Jr., M, Bowen J, Rodriquez A, Haselkorn J. Prevalence and correlates of depression among veterans with multiple sclerosis. Neurology 2005; 64(1): 75.

38 Krupp L, Alvarez L, LaRocca N. et al. Fatigue in multiple sclerosis. Arch Neurol 1988; 45: 435–7.

39 Bakshi R, Shaikh ZA, Miletich RS, Czarnecki D, Dmochowski J, Henschel K, et al. Fatigue in multiple sclerosis and its relationship to depression and neurologic disability. Mult Scler 2000 Jun; 6(3): 181–5.

40 Rabinowitz A, Fisher A, Arnett P. Neurovegetative symptoms in patients with multiple sclerosis: Fatigue, not depression. J Int Neuropsychol Soc 2006: 1–10.

41 Bamer AM, Johnson KL, Amtmann DA, Kraft GH. Beyond fatigue: Assessing variables associated with sleep problems and use of sleep medications in multiple sclerosis. Clin Epidemiol 2010 May; 00(2): 99–106.

42 Janardhan V, Bakshi R. Quality of life in patients with multiple sclerosis: the impact of fatigue and depression. J Neurol Sci 2002 Dec; 205(1): 51–8.

43 Fischer JS LN, Miller DM RP, Andrews H, D P. Recent developments in the assessment of quality of life in multiple sclerosis (MS). Mult Scler 1999; 5: 251–9.

44 Vickrey BG HR, Harooni R, Myers LW EG. A health related quality of life measure for multiple sclerosis. Qual Life Res 1995; 4: 187–206.

45 D'Alisa S, Miscio G, Baudo S, Simone A, Tesio L, Mauro A. Depression is the main determinant of quality of life in multiple sclerosis: A classification-regression (CART) study. Disabil Rehabil 2006 Mar; 28(5): 307–14.

46 Benedict RH, Wahlig E, Bakshi R, Fishman I, Munschauer F, Zivadinov R, et al. Predicting quality of life in multiple sclerosis: accounting for physical disability, fatigue, cognition, mood disorder, personality, and behavior change. J Neurol Sci 2005 Apr; 231(1–2): 29–34.

47 Glanz BI, Healy BC, Rintell DJ, Jaffin SK, Bakshi R, Weiner HL. The association between cognitive impairment and quality of life in patients with early multiple sclerosis. J Neurol Sci 2010 Mar; 290(1–2): 75–9.

48 Gilchrist AC, Creed FH. Depression, cognitive impairment and social stress in multiple-sclerosis. J Psychosom Res 1994 Apr; 38(3): 193–201.

49 Bambara JK, Turner AP, Williams RM, Haselkorn JK. Perceived social support and depression among Veterans with multiple sclerosis. Disabil Rehabil 2010 Sep.

50 Maor Y, Olmer L, Mozes B. The relation between objective and subjective impairment in cognitive function among multiple sclerosis patients–the role of depression. Mult Scler 2001 Apr; 7(2): 131–5.

51 Gronwall D. Paced auditory serial-addition task: A measure of recovery from concussion. Percept Mot Skills 1977; 44: 367–73.

52 Smith A. The symbol-digit modalities test: A neuropsychologic test for economic screening of learning and other cerebral disorders. Learn Discord 1968; 3: 83–91.

53 Rabinowitz AR, Arnett PA. A longitudinal analysis of cognitive dysfunction, coping, and depression in multiple sclerosis. Neuropsychology 2009; 23(5): 581–91.

54 Sachdev P, Smith J, Angus-Lepan H, Rodriguez P. Pseudodementia twelve years on. J Neurol Neurosurg Psychiat 1990; 53(3): 254.

55 Sperling R, Guttmann C, Hohol M, Warfield S, Jakab M, Parente M, et al. Regional magnetic resonance imaging lesion burden and cognitive function in multiple sclerosis: a longitudinal study. Arch Neurol 2001; 58(1): 115.

56 Mohr DC, Goodkin DE, Likosky W, Gatto N, Baumann KA, Rudick RA. Treatment of depression improves adherence to interferon beta-1b therapy for multiple sclerosis. Arch Neurol [Article] 1997 May; 54(5): 531–3.

57 Katon W, Von Korff M, Lin E, Lipscomb P, Russo J, Wagner E, et al. Distressed high utilizers of medical care* 1: : DSM-III-R diagnoses and treatment needs. Gen Hosp Psychiat 1990; 12(6): 355–62.

58 Schiffer RB. The Goldman Consensus statement on depression in multiple sclerosis. Mult Scler (13524585). [Article] 2005; 11(3): 328–37.

59 Schiffer RB, Wineman NM. Antidepressant pharmacotherapy of depression associated with multiple sclerosis. Am J Psychiat 1990 Nov; 147(11): 1493–7.

60 Hamilton M. A rating scale for depression. J Neurol Neurosurg Psychiat 1960; 23(1): 56.

61 Ehde DM, Kraft GH, Chwastiak L, Sullivan MD, Gibbons LE, Bombardier CH, et al. Efficacy of paroxetine in treating major depressive disorder in persons with multiple sclerosis. Gen Hosp Psychiat [Article] 2008 Jan–Feb; 30(1): 40–8.

62 Mohr DC, Hart SL, Fonareva I, Tasch ES. Treatment of depression for patients with multiple sclerosis in neurology clinics. Mult Scler (13524585). [Article] 2006; 12(2): 204–8.

63 Mohr DC, Goodkin DE. Treatment of depression in multiple sclerosis: Review and meta-analysis. Clin Psychol: Science and Practice 1999; 6(1): 1–9.

64 Mohr D. The Stress and Mood Management Program for Individuals With Multiple Sclerosis: Therapist Guide: Oxford University Press, 2010.

65 Mohr DC, Hart SL, Julian L, Catledge C, Honos-Webb L, Vella L, et al. Telephone-administered psychotherapy for depression. Arch Gen Psychiat 2005 Sep; 62(9): 1007–14.

66 Dalgas U, Stenager E, Jakobsen J, Petersen T, Hansen HJ, Knudsen C, et al. Fatigue, mood and quality of life improve in MS patients after progressive resistance training. Mult Scler 2010 Apr; 16(4): 480–90.

67 Arnstein. From chronic pain patient to peer: Benefits and risks of volunteering * 1. Pain Manag Nurs 2002; 3(3): 94.

68 Korostil M, Feinstein A. Anxiety disorders and their clinical correlates in multiple sclerosis patients. Mult Scler (13524585). [Article] 2007; 13(1): 67–72.

69 Burns MN, Siddique J, Fokuo JK, Mohr DC. Comorbid anxiety disorders and treatment of depression in people with multiple sclerosis. Rehabil Psychol 2010; 55(3): 255–62.

70 Beiske AG, Svensson E, Sandanger I, Czujko B, Pedersen ED, Aarseth JH, et al. Depression and anxiety amongst multiple sclerosis patients. Euro J Neurol 2008; 15(3): 239–45.

71 Poder K, Ghatavi K, Fisk J, Campbell T, Kisely S, Sarty I, et al. Social anxiety in a multiple sclerosis clinic population. Mult Scler 2009; 15(3): 393.

72 Janssens ACJW, Buljevac D, van Doorn PA, van der Meché FGA, Polman CH, Passchier J, et al. Prediction of anxiety and distress following diagnosis of multiple sclerosis: a two-year longitudinal study. Mult Scler (13524585). [Article] 2006; 12(6): 794–801.

73 Zorzon M, de Masi R, Nasuelli D, Ukmar M, Pozzi Mucelli R, Cazzato G, et al. Depression and anxiety in multiple sclerosis. A clinical and MRI study in 95 subjects. J Neurol 2001; 248(5): 416–21.

74 Rintell D, Minden, S., Frankel, D., Glanz, B. Patients perspectives on quality mental health care for people with multiple sclerosis. Annual Meeting of the Consortium of Multiple Sclerosis Centers; Atlanta, GA: International JMS Care 2009; PO4, p. 2.

75 Bruce J, Hancock L, Arnett P, Lynch S. Treatment adherence in multiple sclerosis: association with emotional status, personality, and cognition. J Behav Med 2010; 33(3): 219–27.

76 Mohr DC, Cox D. Multiple sclerosis: empirical literature for the clinical health psychologist. J Clin Psychol 2001; 57(4): 479–99.

77 Baldwin D, Woods R, Lawson R, Taylor D. Efficacy of drug treatments for generalised anxiety disorder: systematic review and meta-analysis. Br Med J 2011 March 11, 2011; 342.

78 Tan KR, Rudolph U, Lüscher C. Hooked on benzodiazepines: GABAA receptor subtypes and addiction. Trends Neurosci 2011; 34(4): 188–97.

79 Schiffer R, Wineman N, Weitkamp L. Association between bipolar affective disorder and multiple sclerosis. Am J Psychiat 1986; 143(1): 94.

80 Feinstein A, Feinstein K, Gray T, Oconnor P. Prevalence and neurobehavioral correlates of pathological laughing and crying in multiple sclerosis. Arch Neurol [Article] 1997 Sep; 54(9): 1116–21.

81 Ghaffar O, Chamelian L, Feinstein A. Neuroanatomy of pseudobulbar affect - A quantitative MRI study in multiple sclerosis. J Neurol 2008 Mar; 255(3): 406–12.

82 Panitch HS, Thisted RA, Smith RA, Wynn DR, Wymer JP, Achiron A, et al. Randomized, controlled trial of dextromethorphan/quinidine for pseudobulbar affect in multiple sclerosis. Ann Neurol 2006; 59(5): 780–7.

83 Feinstein A. The Clinical Neuropsychiatry of Multiple Sclerosis. Cambridge University Press, 2007.

84 Anderson R, Smith B. Deaths: leading causes for 2001. Nat Vital Stat Rep 2003; 52(9): 1–85.

85 Sadovnick AD, Eisen K, Ebers GC, Paty DW. Cause of death in patients attending multiple-sclerosis clinics. Neurology [Article] 1991 Aug; 41(8): 1193–6.

86 Feinstein A. An examination of suicidal intent in patients with multiple sclerosis. Neurology 2002; 59(5): 674.

87 Stenager E, Stenager E, Koch-Henriksen N, Brønnum-Hansen H, Hyllested K, Jensen K, et al. Suicide and multiple sclerosis: an epidemiological investigation. J Neurol Neurosurg Psychiat 1992; 55(7): 542.

88 Stenager E, Koch-Henriksen N, Stenager E. Risk factors for suicide in multiple sclerosis. Psychother Psychosom 1996; 65(2): 86–90.

89 Turner A, Williams R, Bowen J, Kivlahan D, Haselkorn J. Suicidal ideation in multiple sclerosis. Arch Phys Med Rehabil 2006; 87(8): 1073–8.

90 Singh G, Siahpush M. Increasing rural-urban gradients in US suicide mortality, 1970–1997. Am J Public Health 2002; 92(7): 1161.

91 Lambert M. Suicide risk assessment and management: focus on personality disorders. Curr Opin Psychiat 2003; 16(1): 71.

92 Maris R. Suicide. Lancet 2002; 360(9329): 319–37.

93 Rintell D, Minden, S., Glanz, B., Healy, B., Cleary, P. Improving the recognition and management of mental health problems in persons with multiple sclerosis. ACTRIMS: Americas Committee for Treatment and Research in Multiple Sclerosis; 6/5/2010; San Antonio, TX2010.

94 Mohr DC, Goodkin DE, Likosky W, Beutler L, Gatto N, Langan MK. Identification of Beck Depression Inventory items related to multiple sclerosis. J Behav Med 1997 Aug; 20(4): 407–14.

95 Kalb P. Multiple sclerosis: The questions you have, the answers you need: Demos Health; 2008.

96 Bandura A. Self-efficacy: The Exercise of Control. New York, NY US: WH Freeman/ Times Books/Henry Holt & Co, 1997.

97 Pinson DMK, Ottens AJ, Fisher TA. Women coping successfully with multiple sclerosis and the precursors of change. Qual Health Res 2009; 19(2): 181–93.

98 O'Connor EJ, McCabe MP, Firth L. The impact of neurological illness on marital relationships. J Sex Marit Ther 2008; 34(2): 115–32.

99 Berkman L. The role of social relations in health promotion. Psychosom Med 1995 May 1, 1995; 57(3): 245–54.

100 Ertel KA, Glymour MM, Berkman LF. Effects of social integration on preserving memory function in a nationally representative US elderly population. Am J Public Health 2008 July; 98(7): 1215–20.

101 Williams RM, Turner AP, Hatzakis M, Chu S, Rodriquez AA, Bowen JD, et al. Social support among veterans with multiple sclerosis. Rehabil Psychol 2004 May; 49(2): 106–13.

102 Pakenham KI, Cox S. The dimensional structure of benefit finding in multiple sclerosis and relations with positive and negative adjustment: A longitudinal study. Psychol Health 2009; 24(4): 373–93.

103 Pakenham KI. The nature of benefit finding in multiple sclerosis (MS). Psychology, Health Med [Article] 2007; 12(2): 190–6.

104 Malcomson KS, Dunwoody L, Lowe-Strong AS. Psychosocial interventions in people with multiple sclerosis. J Neurol 2007; 254(1): 1–13.

105 Diagnostic and Statistical Manual of Mental Disorders, Fourth Edition, Text revision (Copyright © 2000). American Psychiatric Association. DSM-IV TR Diagnostic Criteria for Major Depressive Disorder.

106 Diagnostic and Statistical Manual of Mental Disorders, Fourth Edition, Text revision, (Copyright © 2000). American Psychiatric Association. DSM-IV TR Diagnostic Criteria for Mood Disorder Due to a General Medical Condition.

107 Mohr DC, et al. Screening for depression among patients with multiple sclerosis: two questions may be enough. Mult Scler 2007; 13: 215–19.

108 Rintell D, Minden S, Glanz B, Healy B, Cleary P. Improving the recognition and management of mental health problems in persons with multiple sclerosis. ACTRIMS: Americas Committee for Treatment and Research in Mult Scler; 6/5/2010; San Antonio, TX2010.

CHAPTER 12
Future Therapeutic Approaches

Howard L. Weiner and Laura Edwards

Partners Multiple Sclerosis Center, Center for Neurologic Diseases, Brigham and Women's Hospital and Department of Neurology, Harvard Medical School, Boston, MA, USA

Introduction

Multiple sclerosis (MS) is a presumed autoimmune disease of the central nervous system. This has been established on the basis of pathologic analysis, genetic susceptibility genes, and the mechanism of action of treatments that have been shown to affect the disease process. The past 20 years have seen the FDA approval of several therapies primarily for the treatment of relapsing forms of MS. In addition, there are promising results with other agents, and it is expected that over the next decade additional drugs will be approved for the treatment of MS. Thus MS, which was once an untreatable disease, has now become a disease with a plethora of treatments, which creates a conundrum for both the physician and the patient. This raises a central challenge regarding the therapy of MS, namely, which drugs to use, when to use them, and how to choose drugs for individual patients. Furthermore, there is a need to develop drugs for the treatment of progressive forms of the disease. This chapter will address these issues and the challenges that confront us as we consider the future therapy of multiple sclerosis.

Therapeutic targets for the treatment of MS

Many drugs have been shown to affect the disease process, primarily the relapsing-remitting form. Although there are common mechanisms of action among them, there are also important differences. In addition, there are new targets that are being developed for the future. These targets are shown schematically in Figure 12.1. In addition to current targets that relate to inflammation, newer targets will involve neuroprotection and remyelinaiton.

Multiple Sclerosis: Diagnosis and Therapy, First Edition. Edited by Howard L. Weiner and James M. Stankiewicz. © 2012 John Wiley & Sons, Ltd.
Published 2012 by John Wiley and Sons, Ltd.

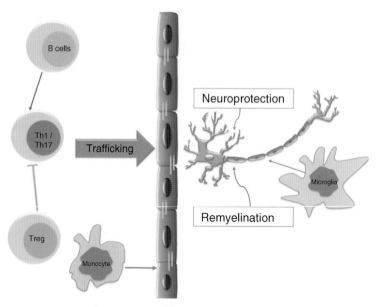

Figure 12.1 Therapeutic targets for the treatment of MS. There are multiple targets for the treatment of MS both in the periphery and in the CNS.

Suppression of Th1/Th17 responses

It has long been held that MS is driven by a disease-inducing myelin reactive T cell that is triggered in the periphery and migrates to the CNS where it initiates damage. This was the basis for trials of immunosuppressive agents early in the history of MS therapeutics, such as azathioprine and cyclophosphamide. It has long been thought that Th1 cells that produce IFNg were the primary disease-inducing T cells. Indeed, a trial of gamma interferon worsened MS and was associated with the activation of T cells [1]. Response to the immunosuppressant cyclophosphamide is linked to a decrease in the production of IL-12, a cytokine that drives Th1 responses [2], although a recent trial targeting the IL-12/23p40 chain of IL-12 did not show any benefit in MS [3]. However, gamma interferon can have protective effects, as can be seen in the EAE model of MS in which it has been shown that IFNg-deficient animals have worse EAE [4]. In addition, certain classes of regulatory T cells produce gamma interferon. More importantly, the phenotype of disease-inducing T cells has significantly changed with the recent description of Th17 cells. Th17 cells have been shown to play a major role in EAE and other autoimmune models and elevated levels of Th17 have been described in patients with MS [5]. This has raised a question of whether there may be different subtypes of MS, such as a subtype driven predominantly by Th1 cells and a subtype driven by Th17 cells. Some have suggested that response to therapy, such as the interferons, may be linked to whether the disease is driven by Th1 vs Th17 cells [6]. It is known that specific cytokines drive Th1 and Th17 responses. For example, IL-6 is important for the induction of Th17 responses and could serve as a target of therapy in the future. Tocilizamab is an anti-IL-6R antibody, which is approved for the treatment of rheumatoid arthritis. Transcription factors and pathways involved in the induction of Th17 cells are being defined, which are likely to yield new drug candidates. It is likely that the IFNg/IL-17 axis is central to the pathogenesis of relapsing forms of MS and that most currently approved drugs, and those being developed in the future, will affect this axis.

A number of drugs with positive results in phase II/III studies act as "immunosuppressants," and most likely work primarily by decreasing Th1/Th17 responses although they may have secondary effects that include the emergence of regulatory T cells (described below). These include alemtuzumab, which recognizes CD52 and is one of the most potent immunosuppressant drugs being developed for MS. One of the major side effects is the development of thyroid autoimmunity, which appears to be related to IL-21. Cladribine is a purine antagonist that decreases T cell number and affects relapse rate, gadolinium-enhancing lesions, and disability. Teriflunomide is a general immunosuppressant that has been used in rheumatology and is currently in phase III trials in MS. Other oral drugs currently in phase III trials include laquinimod and BG-12. Although their mechanism of action has not been established in MS, BG-12 may work by affecting the Nrf2 transcription factor and thus have neuroprotectant/antioxidant properties. Laquinimod appears to modulate pro-inflammatory responses and may also have effects in the CNS [7]. Nonetheless, both affect relapses and gadolinium-enhancing lesions and thus most likely also affect the Th1/Th17 axis. Decisions regarding MS therapy in the future, including drug choice, and the drug combinations to use, will be related to measuring biomarkers that are linked to pathogenic immune responses. Thus, it may be that drugs in the future will be measured in part by their ability to affect the IFNg/IL-17 axis.

Induction of regulatory T cells

Regulatory T cells (Tregs) are a major component of the immune system. Abnormalities of Tregs have been reported in animal models of autoimmunity and in human autoimmune diseases [8]. Tregs have been shown to control autoimmunity in the animal model of MS and defects in Treg function have been reported for MS patients [9]. Although a complete understanding of the mechanisms by which Tregs exert their effects is still evolving, and there are different types of Treg, a major mode of action relates to the secretion of anti-inflammatory factors such as TGF-b and IL-10. Drugs that benefit MS affect these anti-inflammatory pathways. For example, IFN-b causes the increased secretion of IL-10 [10] and cyclophosphamide, in addition to decreasing Th1/Th17 responses, increases TGF-b [2]. Glatiramer acetate (GA), the widely used first-line treatment for MS, appears to act primarily by the induction of Tregs/anti-inflammatory cytokines [11]. Although the mechanism of action of GA is not completely understood, it appears to have a major effect on monocytes and the innate immune system. GA conditions T cells towards an anti-inflammatory Treg phenotype. A major goal for the treatment of autoimmune diseases is the induction of Tregs and it is likely that Treg induction will be applied to the treatment of MS in the future. There are specific pathways for the induction of Th1/Th17 cells and transcription factors associated with Th1 cells (T-bet) Th17 cells (RORgt). The same holds true for Tregs with Foxp3 being the signature transcription factor for Tregs. The pathways involved in the induction of Th17 cells and Tregs may in some way be related as TGF-b induces Foxp3 Tregs while TGF-b plus IL-6 induces IL-17 cells [12]. Another type of Tregs, Tr1 cells, which are induced by IL-27 and beta interferon, may also work by affecting the IL-27 immune axis [13]. Extensive studies are underway to characterize the pathways for the induction of Tregs. New therapeutic targets and drugs are likely to be developed, based on the induction of Tregs. Daclizumab is an anti-IL-2 receptor antibody which appears to act by inducing an NK type 2 regulatory cell and has shown positive results in the treatment of MS in phase II trials [14].

We have found that oral administration of anti-CD3 monoclonal antibody induces Tregs in the gut, which then migrate systemically to suppress animal models of MS [15] as well as other autoimmune diseases such as diabetes, lupus, and arthritis. Positive results have been observed in initial pilot trials of oral anti-CD3, reviewed in [16]. Another approach we have been investigating to induce Tregs is the oral administration of ligands which bind to the aryl hydrocarbon receptor (AHR). AHR is a ligand-activated transcription factor that induces the Treg transcription factor Foxp3 in T cells and also conditions dendritic cells to drive Tregs, in a manner similar to the action of glatiramer acetate. One ligand of AHR is TCDD (dioxin), an environmental toxin [17]. In an attempt to develop AHR ligands for the treatment of MS we have investigated a natural AHR ligand (ITE) and found that the oral administration of the AHR ligand, ITE, induces Tregs and suppresses the animal model of EAE [18].

The gut is a major source for the induction of Tregs. The primary method by which oral tolerance occurs is the induction of Tregs [16]. Thus, it is likely that the gut will be used in future therapeutic approaches to induce Tregs for the treatment of MS. In this regard, helminths are known to induce Tregs and trials of helminths have been initiated in MS [19]. MS patients that have been infected with parasites appear to have less relapses, perhaps due to the propensity of parasites to induce Tregs [20]. In this regard we found that positive effects of cyclophosphamide are related to the eosinophilia that is induced with treatment [21]. Furthermore, the gut microbiota is a burgeoning area of immunologic investigation and the gut flora appears to have a major influence on the immune system, both in the induction of Tregs and in Th17 responses [22]. Understanding the immune system in the gut is likely to help to answer questions related to why some individuals are more susceptible to contracting MS and how environmental factors play a role in MS. It is of note that, in Japan, "Western" type MS is more prevalent than in the past, even though the genetics of the population has not changed. It is postulated that this may be related to dietary factors. Experimental studies in the animal model of MS are being reported and susceptibility to EAE and manipulation of the gut microbiota affects autoimmunity [23]. Thus, it is possible that therapeutic targets in the future may be directed at the gut microbiota. Furthermore a major effort is currently in progress to understand the pathways involved in inducing Tregs, and drugs to induce Tregs will be a new therapeutic target for the treatment of MS. Tregs most likely act by decreasing pathogenic Th1/Th17 responses. Thus biomarkers that measure the Th1/Th17 responses discussed above will be used to assess the efficacy of Treg induction. Of note, regarding Tregs, anti-TNF was of benefit in MS animal models but did not work in clinical trials where patients were in fact worse [24, 25].

Furthermore, in some patients receiving anti-TNF therapy for rheumatoid arthritis, the underlying demyelinating disease has exacerbated [26, 27]. Although it is not known why anti-TNF therapy makes MS worse, it has been reported that TNF is required for the induction of CD8 Tregs [28].

B cell depletion

An unexpected finding regarding the therapy of MS is the dramatic effect of the anti-CD20 monoclonal antibody, rituximab, in reducing relapses and gadolinium-enhancing lesions on MRI [29]. Rituximab was initially tested in MS on the basis of the theory that B cells and antibodies may play a direct role in the pathogenesis of the disease. However, the effect of rituximab occurs within months of initiation of therapy and there is no effect of rituximab on levels of antibodies. The currently held view is that the effect of rituximab is indirect and affects relapses and gadolinium-enhancing lesions by affecting T cells. B cells have strong antigen presenting properties and likely participate in the induction of pathogenic Th1/Th17 cells, although the depletion of B cells appears to remove this effect. There are different subsets of B cells, some that drive Th1/Th17 responses and others that could enhance Treg induction [30]. However, targeting of B cells may not always have a positive effect in MS. Treatment of relapsing MS patients with the anti-B cell monoclonal atacicept resulted in more relapses and brain lesions. Additional anti-B cell monoclonal antibodies are being studied, such as ocrelizumab. It is likely that drugs affecting B cells in a manner that is beneficial to MS patients will be available to physicians in the future.

Altering T cell traffic

Natalizumab is an anti-VLA 4 inhibitor that acts by blocking the movement of T cells and other cells into the brain. This was first shown in the animal model and later in human studies where the number of T cells, B cells, and monocytes in the brain decreased [31]. There is no evidence that there is an increase in Treg induction; in fact, there may be an accumulation of Th17 type cells in the bloodstream of patients treated with natalizumab [32]. FTY 720 is a sphingosine inhibitor that acts by blocking the egress of cells from the lymph nodes and may also react within the nervous system affecting the oligodendrocyte. How it affects other aspects of immune regulation are not known at this time, though it may have an effect by inducing Tregs [33]. It is clear that altering T cell traffic is beneficial in the inflammatory component of MS.

Macrophages/microglia

An important target for therapy in MS involves cells of the innate immune system. Although targeting these cells in animal models has shown their potential, these approaches have not been translated into the clinic. We have recently shown that the micro-RNA, mir-124, acts to maintain microglial cells in a quiescent state. These properties have been successfully used to treat EAE, the animal model of MS, by deactivating inflammatory macrophages in the periphery [34]. Older studies in which macrophages were targeted with silica have also demonstrated their important role in the EAE model [35]. Microglia are the primary innate immune cells in the CNS and it has recently been shown that resident or indigenous microglia are distinct from infiltrating monocytes from the periphery [36]. We have found that there may be a dysfunction of indigenous microglia in progressive forms of the EAE model that could serve as an additional target for therapy once unique structures on microglia are identified. We have also found, in the progressive EAE model, that PARP-1 activates innate cells in the CNS such as monocytes and microglia, and that targeting PARP-1 has beneficial effects in this model [37]. Another agent that appears to affect microglia is the antibiotic minocycline, which has been tested in human disease, including MS [38], with mixed results [39].

Neuroprotection

It is now recognized that toxic factors such as glutamate and nitric oxide are released in association with the infiltration of immune cells into the CNS. These factors are believed to play a role in the progression of MS and axonal damage. Clinical trials have been carried out using some of these compounds. One example is the anticonvulsant lamotrigine, which acts by blocking voltage-gated sodium channels and is neuroprotective in experimental models of inflammatory demyelinating disease. A clinical trial of lamotrigine in progressive MS showed minimal benefit [40]. In the animal model of progressive MS, we have shown that a fullerene-based compound decreases glutamate toxicity and protects axonal function [41]. One of the mechanisms by which this works relates to decreasing the CCL2 expression on astrocytes, which in turn decreases the number of CCR2+ monocytes from infiltrating the CNS. This demonstrates the interconnection of the pathways for the treatment of MS.

Remyelination

Lingo-1 is a compound that impedes the movement of nerve cells. It has been shown in animal models of MS that anti-Lingo-1 enhances nerve outgrowth and thus can be used as a treatment to enhance remyelination [42]. It is currently in clinical development. Nogo is another compound that impedes the movement of nerve cells. Anti-Lingo-1 antibody has also been used to enhance nerve outgrowth in animal models [43]. Stem cell therapy has been investigated in animal models of MS and is a potential future therapy, but much more is required before clinical application can be successful [44]. Some stem cell approaches in the animal model have actually been shown to affect the immune system, rather than direct effects on neuronal structures [45].

Antigen-specific therapy

It is generally believed that myelin antigen-specific T cells enter the brain and initiate the immune cascade drive MS. Thus, the most direct and least toxic approach for the treatment of the disease would be antigen-specific therapy in which pathogenic antigen-specific T cells are inactivated or in which antigen-specific Tregs are induced. There are many examples in animal models of successful antigen-specific therapy, including IV administration of antigen, antigen coupled to cell membranes, use of altered peptide ligands, antigen given by the oral or nasal route, DNA vaccination, and epicutaneous administration of antigen. Positive results have recently been reported for DNA vaccination [46] and epicutaneous administration of myelin antigen [47]. Given the appeal of antigen-specific therapy and the multiple avenues to affect antigen-specific T cells, it is likely that in the future nontoxic, antigen-specific therapy will become an important treatment modality in MS. We are focusing on the oral and nasal routes [16].

MS biomarkers

As discussed above, one of the major unmet needs in MS is the availability of validated blood biomarkers that can be used to establishing which drug to use and when, which drugs to use in combination, and when is it appropriate to stop therapy. The primary biomarker that currently affects therapeutic decisions is magnetic resonance imaging (MRI).

Magnetic resonance imaging

MRI has served as the primary biomarker for MS [48, 49] and although conventional imaging does not link strongly to clinical outcomes, every FDA-approved MS drug has had positive results on MRI. Advances in MRI are beginning to better define MS and its heterogeneity. It is highly significant that MRI and pathologic studies have shown gray matter atrophy in MS, which is linked to cognitive impairment [50]. In addition, cortical foci of demyelination, microglial activation, leptomeningeal inflammation, iron deposition, and neuronal loss occur in the gray matter (Figure 12.2). The degree to which current therapy attenuates gray matter destruction is not known. It is likely that the processes affecting the gray matter are highly clinically relevant and will ultimately provide new therapeutic targets. MRI has also shown diffuse involvement of the normal appearing white matter, including demyelination, inflammation, and axonal injury not seen by conventional imaging [51] but which can be visualized by magnetization transfer, diffusion-weighted, and spectroscopic imaging. These changes can precede overt gadolinium-enhancing lesions by months and result from early migration of lymphocytes into the brain.

Gadolinium-enhancing lesions on MRI have been used to test anti-inflammatory drugs and physicians routinely use the MRI measure to assess ongoing inflammatory disease and the effect of anti-inflammatory drug therapy. Gadolinium-enhancement is also used as a measure by which to enter patients into clinical trials. Nonetheless, current imaging processes that rely on gadolinium and T2 imaging are not as sensitive as they might be. For example, we have found that subtraction imaging shows new lesions that otherwise might not be identified [52].

Spinal cord dysfunction is primarily responsible for gait impairment in MS, the major disabling feature of the illness. Better spinal cord imaging should improve clinical MRI correlation [53]. Spinal cord atrophy may occur early and the clinical heterogeneity of MS and benign forms of MS may relate to atrophy and spinal cord involvement. The factors that predict benign vs nonbenign MS are poorly understood. We have found that the rate of atrophy progression is less in benign MS [54] and an MRI study using double inversion-recovery imaging to detect cortical lesions suggests the importance of gray matter sparing in predicting a benign clinical course [50]. We have developed a Magnetic Resonance Disease Severity Scale (MRDSS) that combines multiple measures to provide an index of disease severity and progression as measured by MRI [48, 49]. The addition of spinal cord imaging and gray matter involvement to the MRDSS should enhance its value as a biomarker.

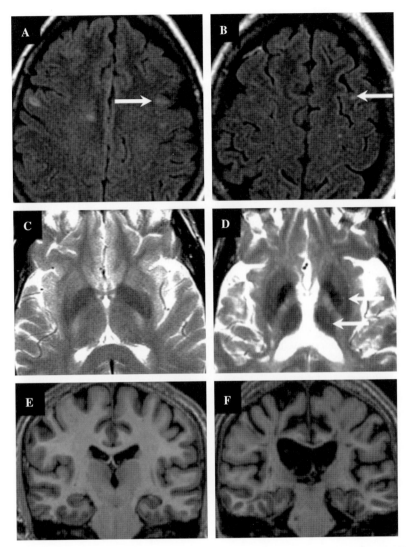

Figure 12.2 MRI-defined gray matter involvement in multiple sclerosis. A and B: FLAIR axial images of a 40-year-old woman with RRMS of 2 years duration and mild disability demonstrate cortical lesions (arrows, note hyperintensities). C: Fast spin-echo T2-weighted axial images of a 43-year-old man with RRMS of 4 years duration and mild to moderate disability demonstrates bilateral hypointensity in the thalamus and basal ganglia (arrows) most likely representing excessive iron deposition and diffuse brain atrophy indicated by the widening of the cortical sulci/fissures and ventricles. D: Age-matched normal control. E: SPGR coronal images of a 54-year-old man with secondary progressive MS of 29 years duration with moderate to severe disability demonstrate widespread gray matter atrophy of the cortical mantle and the deep gray nuclei, such as the thalamus in the patient with MS. F: Age-matched normal control. (Reproduced from Stankiewicz et al. [82] with permission from Elsevier (parts C and D); courtesy of Drs Mohit Neema and Rohit Bakshi (parts A, B, E, and F).)

Immune biomarkers

We and others have shown immune measures that are associated with disease activity and MRI activity [55–57] and RNA profiling is beginning to identify gene expression patterns associated with different forms of MS and disease progression [58, 59]. Building on the approach of Robinson [60, 61] we performed antigen microarray analysis to characterize patterns of low affinity antibody reactivity in MS serum against a panel of CNS proteins, lipid autoantigens, and heat shock proteins. Using informatic analysis for validation, we found unique autoantibody signatures that distinguished RRMS, SPMS, and PPMS from healthy controls and other neurologic or autoimmune diseases [17, 41, 62]. RRMS was characterized by autoantibodies to heat shock proteins that were not observed in PPMS or SPMS. In addition, RRMS, SPMS, and PPMS were characterized by unique patterns of reactivity to CNS antigens (Plate 12.1). We also examined sera from patients with different immunopathologic patterns of MS as determined by brain biopsy [63] and identified unique antibody patterns to lipids and CNS-derived peptides that were linked to type I and type II patterns. The demonstration of unique serum immune signatures linked to different stages and pathologic processes in MS provides a new avenue to understand disease heterogeneity, to monitor MS, and to characterize immunopathogenic mechanisms and therapeutic targets in the disease. We have also found that lipid indices we have identified on antigen arrays link to measures of gray matter atrophy on MRI, and this provides a crucial link between blood biomarkers and MRI. It is clear that the development of biomarkers that could allow more individualized therapy would have a major impact on MS management; for example, the ability to test for exposure to JC virus helps physicians to make decisions about the use of natalizumab in MS [64].

Induction vs first-line therapy

There is a debate about the best approach for treating patients at disease onset. One school argues that first-line therapy should be tried, and if there is a disease breakthrough, more aggressive therapy should be instituted. A second school argues that strong immunosuppressive therapy at the beginning, or induction therapy, is the best approach. This would prevent epitope spreading and would result in less disease over longer periods of time. Indeed, this is one of the arguments for the use of alemtuzumab. Induction therapy using mitoxantrone and cyclophosphamide has been attempted. It is likely that the categorization of patients at disease onset might identify those that would be best treated by induction therapy. Thus a patient with optic neuritis and two small lesions in the brain would be treated differently from a patient who presents with multiple-enhancing lesions and extensive disease in the spinal cord and brain.

Another challenge for the physician will be which first-line therapy to use. In the future we will have multiple medications, including the currently used injectables, new oral medications, and drugs given intravenously by infusion. At this time there is no clear way to distinguish which of these is best as a first-line therapy. It will ultimately depend on head-to-head trials, adverse event profiles, patient preferences, and disease biomarkers.

Chronic/sequential/combination/ halting therapy

We currently assume that patients should be on treatment for long periods of time, perhaps for a lifetime, although there are no studies to support such a view. Thus, in the future there may be biomarkers and guidelines for discontinuing treatment in certain groups of patients. Furthermore, different types of combination therapy based on the mechanism of action described above may be used. An issue that has not been addressed is: At what stage could a person stop medication? This raises the situation of the disease entering a quiescent stage where treatment is no longer required, and trials on stopping medication are likely to occur in the future.

Progressive disease

One of the major problems in MS is the effective treatment of progressive disease. Anti-inflammatory drugs, including beta interferon [65], rituximab [66], cyclophosphamide [67, 68], and mitoxantrone [69] have been reported to be of benefit in some patients with progressive disease. This is likely due to an inflammatory component that occurs in some patients with progressive disease that these drugs are targeting. The pathologic processes associated with disease progression are not well understood. In order to better understand the disease progression, CSF biomarkers or new types of imaging, including imaging of microglia, may be required. We have found that activation of the innate immune system is observed in the peripheral blood of patients with progressive MS, reflecting chronic inflammation in the CNS of these patients [70]. It is of note that progression does not always occur when there is damage to the nervous system as in stroke, which results in fixed deficits. We will require a better understanding of the underlying pathologic processes that drive disease progression in chronic CNS progressive illnesses such as MS, Alzheimer disease and Parkinson disease. A major question in MS is whether strong anti-inflammatory drugs given early will prevent or significantly delay the onset of progressive MS.

Curing MS

I: Immunotherapy for halting disease activity and progression

One could argue that a cure is a treatment that eradicates MS. This may be true for an infection or tumor but not for MS in which there is an inherent defect of the immune system and chronic inflammation of the brain. If, however, one treated MS at the clinical onset and prevented disease progression for the remainder of the patient's life, it would be considered a cure. There may be patients that are being "cured" with current therapy though they may have less severe forms of the disease. Interferons and glatiramer acetate are only partially effective in MS, with stronger effects observed with natalizumab and alemtuzumab [71, 72]. This raises a central question: Will aggressive and early immunotherapy prevent the secondary progressive form of the disease? With the strong anti-inflammatory effects of a drug such as alemtuzumab, this question could be addressed in the future, though widespread testing may be prohibited by side effects. Other approaches of aggressive immunotherapy at disease onset to test this hypothesis includes bone marrow transplantation, nonablative chemotherapy utilizing cyclophosphamide [73], or induction with a drug such as cyclophosphamide or mitoxantrone followed by maintenance immune modulation [74].

Because the immune damage to myelin and axons initiates secondary pathways of CNS damage, nonimmune-based therapy may be required to control disease progression. The presence of glutamate and nitric oxide leads to axon injury and demyelination which, in itself, can set up an inflammatory response on astrocytes that express CCL2 and lead to infiltration of CD11B cells.

Thus, a complex disease such as MS will require treatment(s) that have an effect on multiple pathways, including the suppression of Th1/Th17 responses, the induction of Tregs, altering the traffic of cells into the CNS, and protecting axons and myelin from degeneration initiated by inflammation that affects the innate immune system. If multiple drugs are required to achieve this effect, one must be certain that one treatment does not interfere with another. It has been reported, for example, that statins may interfere with the action of interferons [75]. It may also be that one must first suppress Th1 and Th17 responses before inducing Tregs. Because of disease heterogeneity, there will be responders and nonresponders to each "effective" therapy. Finally, the earlier treatment is initiated, the more likely it is to be effective.

Inherent to the concept of curing MS by halting progression, is the ability to demonstrate that progression has been halted in a group of patients, and to identify those factors associated with preventing the onset of progressive disease. We have initiated the CLIMB natural history study in which nearly 2000 patients with new-onset MS will be followed over a 20-year period with clinical evaluation, MRI imaging, and immune and genetic markers, to identify the factors that are associated with disease progression [76].

II: Repairing a damaged nervous system

There is evidence of repair in the CNS of those with MS, though the mechanisms involved are not well understood. Furthermore, it has been shown in animal models that reducing inflammation promotes repair even with nonspecific immunosuppressants such as cyclophosphamide [77]. Blocking molecules that inhibit axonal (Nogo) or myelin (Lingo-1) growth may promote repair, and the treatment of animal models with anti-Lingo-1, anti-Nogo, or antibodies reacting with oligodendrocytes have shown positive effects [74, 78, 79]. Furthermore, treatments that affect sodium channels may not only affect nerve conduction but may have effects in microglia activation [80]. Nonetheless, it must be emphasized that when severe neuronal and oligodendrocyte loss occurs, it is unlikely that one would be able to reverse neurologic deficits significantly. It is of note that stem cell therapy may be inhibited by CNS inflammation [81].

III: Preventing MS

If MS is triggered in the environment in susceptible individuals it may be possible to prevent MS, though one must first be able to identify those at risk. In this respect it has been found that autoantibody signatures in the serum have the potential to identify those at risk [62]. Some believe that vaccination against EBV virus or treating children at high risk of developing MS with vitamin D, may be initial approaches. Ultimately, approaches are now being considered to prevent disease in those susceptible or in the general population. This, of course, requires an understanding of those at risk and factors that could be used for disease prevention. One area that has sparked interest is the use of Vitamin D, and it is likely that Vitamin D will be studied in greater depth not only in MS but also in other diseases. EBV virus appears to be a clear disease risk factor for MS, and whether any vaccination programs related to EBV could be of benefit is not yet understood.

Conclusion

Future therapeutic approaches for the treatment of MS are likely to move away from injectable modalities toward the use of oral and periodic intravenous treatment. Biomarkers will allow the choice of one therapy over another, and in some patients induction therapy with strong immunosuppression may be used. Combination therapy is also likely to be employed. A central question for the future is whether aggressive treatment of early inflammation will prevent the progressive phase to the extent that specific drugs for progressive MS will not be required.

TOP TIPS 12.1

- Th1/Th17 cells are the main drivers of autoimmunity in relapsing forms MS.
- Immune targets change as MS becomes more progressive.
- Biomarkers will be needed to categorize different stages of MS.
- Combination therapy will be linked to different modes of action of drugs.
- Strong anti-inflammatory therapy at disease onset may prevent later progression.

References

1 Panitch HS, Hirsch RL, Schindler J, Johnson KP. Treatment of multiple sclerosis with gamma interferon: exacerbations associated with activation of the immune system. Neurology 1987 Jul; 37(7): 1097–102.

2 Comabella M, Balashov K, Issazadeh S, Smith D, Weiner HL, Khoury SJ. Elevated interleukin-12 in progressive multiple sclerosis correlates with disease activity and is normalized by pulse cyclophosphamide therapy. J Clin Invest 1998 Aug; 102(4): 671–8.

3 Segal BM, Constantinescu CS, Raychaudhuri A, Kim L, Fidelus-Gort R, Kasper LH. Repeated subcutaneous injections of IL12/23 p40 neutralising antibody, ustekinumab, in patients with relapsing-remitting multiple sclerosis: a phase II, double-blind, placebo-controlled, randomised, dose-ranging study. Lancet Neurol 2008 Sep; 7(9): 796–804.

4 Ferber IA, Brocke S, Taylor-Edwards C, Ridgway W, Dinisco C, Steinman L, et al. Mice with a disrupted IFN-gamma gene are susceptible to the induction of experimental autoimmune encephalomyelitis (EAE). J Immunol 1996 Jan; 156(1): 5–7.

5 Miossec P, Korn T, Kuchroo VK. Interleukin-17 and type 17 helper T cells. N Engl J Med 2009 Aug; 361(9): 888–98.

6 Axtell RC, de Jong BA, Boniface K, van der Voort LF, Bhat R, De Sarno P, et al. T helper type 1 and 17 cells determine efficacy of interferon-beta in multiple sclerosis and experimental encephalomyelitis. Nat Med 2010 Apr; 16(4): 406–12.

7 Gold R. Oral therapies for multiple sclerosis: a review of agents in phase III development or recently approved. CNS Drugs 2011 Jan; 25(1): 37–52.

8 Sakaguchi S. Regulatory T cells: history and perspective. Methods Mol Biol 2011; 707: 3–17.

9 Viglietta V, Baecher-Allan C, Weiner HL, Hafler DA. Loss of functional suppression by CD4+CD25+ regulatory T cells in patients with multiple sclerosis. J Exp Med 2004 Apr; 199(7): 971–9.

10 Waubant E, Gee L, Bacchetti P, Sloan R, Cotleur A, Rudick R, et al. Relationship between serum levels of IL-10, MRI activity and interferon beta-1a therapy in patients with relapsing remitting MS. J Neuroimmunol 2001 Jan; 112(1–2): 139–45.

11 Racke MK, Lovett-Racke AE. Glatiramer acetate treatment of multiple sclerosis: an immunological perspective. J Immunol 2011 Feb; 186(4): 1887–90.

12 Bettelli E, Carrier Y, Gao W, Korn T, Strom TB, Oukka M, et al. Reciprocal developmental pathways for the generation of pathogenic effector TH17 and regulatory T cells. Nature 2006 May; 441(7090): 235–8.

13 Mitsdoerffer M, Kuchroo V. New pieces in the puzzle: how does interferon-beta really work in multiple sclerosis? Ann Neurol 2009 May; 65(5): 487–8.

14 Hao J, Campagnolo D, Liu R, Piao W, Shi S, Hu B, et al. Interleukin-2/interleukin-2 antibody therapy induces target organ natural killer cells that inhibit central nervous system inflammation. Ann Neurol 2011 Apr; 69(4): 721–34.

15 Ochi H, Abraham M, Ishikawa H, Frenkel D, Yang K, Basso AS, et al. Oral CD3-specific antibody suppresses autoimmune encephalomyelitis by inducing CD4+ CD25– LAP+ T cells. Nat Med 2006 Jun; 12(6): 627–35.

16 Weiner HL, da Cunha AP, Quintana F, Wu H. Oral tolerance. Immunol Rev 2011 May; 241(1): 241–59.

17 Quintana FJ, Basso AS, Iglesias AH, Korn T, Farez MF, Bettelli E, et al. Control of T(reg) and T(H)17 cell differentiation by the aryl hydrocarbon receptor. Nature 2008 May; 453(7191): 65–71.

18 Quintana FJ, Murugaiyan G, Farez MF, Mitsdoerffer M, Tukpah AM, Burns EJ, et al. An endogenous aryl hydrocarbon receptor ligand acts on dendritic cells and T cells to suppress experimental autoimmune encephalomyelitis. Proc Natl Acad Sci U S A 2010 Nov; 107(48): 20768–73.

19 Fleming J, Isaak A, Lee J, Luzzio C, Carrithers M, Cook T, et al. Probiotic helminth administration in relapsing-remitting multiple sclerosis: a phase 1 study. Mult Scler 2011 Mar 3.

20 Correale J, Farez MF. The impact of parasite infections on the course of multiple sclerosis. J Neuroimmunol 2011 Apr; 233(1–2): 6–11.

21 Smith DR, Balashov KE, Hafler DA, Khoury SJ, Weiner HL. Immune deviation following pulse cyclophosphamide/methylprednisolone treatment of multiple sclerosis: increased interleukin-4 production and associated eosinophilia. Ann Neurol 1997 Sep; 42(3): 313–8.

22 Ivanov II, Littman DR. Modulation of immune homeostasis by commensal bacteria. Curr Opin Microbiol 2011 Feb; 14(1): 106–14.

23 Ochoa-Reparaz J, Mielcarz DW, Ditrio LE, Burroughs AR, Begum-Haque S, Dasgupta S, et al. Central nervous system demyelinating disease protection by the human commensal Bacteroides fragilis depends on polysaccharide A expression. J Immunol 2010 Oct; 185(7): 4101–8.

24 TNF neutralization in MS: results of a randomized, placebo-controlled multicenter study. The Lenercept Multiple Sclerosis Study Group and The University of British Columbia MS/MRI Analysis Group. Neurology 1999 Aug; 53(3): 457–65.

25 van Oosten BW, Barkhof F, Truyen L, Boringa JB, Bertelsmann FW, von Blomberg BM, et al. Increased MRI activity and immune activation in two multiple sclerosis patients treated with the monoclonal anti-tumor necrosis factor antibody cA2. Neurology 1996 Dec; 47(6): 1531–4.

26 Mohan N, Edwards ET, Cupps TR, Oliverio PJ, Sandberg G, Crayton H, et al. Demyelination occurring during anti-tumor necrosis factor alpha therapy for inflammatory arthritides. Arthritis Rheum 2001 Dec; 44(12): 2862–9.

27 Toussirot E, Pertuiset E, Martin A, Melac-Ducamp S, Alcalay M, Grardel B, et al. Association of rheumatoid arthritis with multiple sclerosis: report of 14 cases and discussion of its significance. J Rheumatol 2006 May; 33(5): 1027–8.

28 Ablamunits V, Bisikirska B, Herold KC. Acquisition of regulatory function by human CD8(+) T cells treated with anti-CD3 antibody requires TNF. Eur J Immunol 2010 Oct; 40(10): 2891–901.

29 Hauser SL, Waubant E, Arnold DL, Vollmer T, Antel J, Fox RJ, et al. B-cell depletion with rituximab in relapsing-remitting multiple sclerosis. N Engl J Med 2008 Feb; 358(7): 676–88.

30 Bar-Or A, Fawaz L, Fan B, Darlington PJ, Rieger A, Ghorayeb C, et al. Abnormal B-cell cytokine responses a trigger of T-cell-mediated disease in MS? Ann Neurol 2010 Apr; 67(4): 452–61.

31 Stuve O. The effects of natalizumab on the innate and adaptive immune system in the central nervous system. J Neurol Sci 2008 Nov; 274(1–2): 39–41.

32 Kivisakk P, Healy BC, Viglietta V, Quintana FJ, Hootstein MA, Weiner HL, et al. Natalizumab treatment is associated with peripheral sequestration of proinflammatory T cells. Neurology 2009 Jun; 72(22): 1922–30.

33 Ledgerwood LG, Lal G, Zhang N, Garin A, Esses SJ, Ginhoux F, et al. The sphingosine 1–phosphate receptor 1 causes tissue retention by inhibiting the entry of peripheral tissue T lymphocytes into afferent lymphatics. Nat Immunol 2008 Jan; 9(1): 42–53.

34 Ponomarev ED, Veremeyko T, Barteneva N, Krichevsky AM, Weiner HL. MicroRNA-124 promotes microglia quiescence and suppresses EAE by deactivating macrophages via the C/EBP-alpha-PU.1 pathway. Nat Med 2011 Jan; 17(1): 64–70.

35 Brosnan CF, Bornstein MB, Bloom BR. The effects of macrophage depletion on the clinical and pathologic expression of experimental allergic encephalomyelitis. J Immunol 1981 Feb; 126(2): 614–20.

36 Ransohoff RM, Cardona AE. The myeloid cells of the central nervous system parenchyma. Nature 2010 Nov; 468(7321): 253–62.

37 Farez MF, Quintana FJ, Gandhi R, Izquierdo G, Lucas M, Weiner HL. Toll-like receptor 2 and poly(ADP-ribose) polymerase 1 promote central nervous system neuroinflammation in progressive EAE. Nat Immunol 2009 Sep; 10(9): 958–64.

38 Chen X, Ma X, Jiang Y, Pi R, Liu Y, Ma L. The prospects of minocycline in multiple sclerosis. J Neuroimmunol 2011 May 10.

39 Gordon PH, Moore DH, Miller RG, Florence JM, Verheijde JL, Doorish C, et al. Efficacy of minocycline in patients with amyotrophic lateral sclerosis: a phase III randomised trial. Lancet Neurol 2007 Dec; 6(12): 1045–53.

40 Kapoor R, Furby J, Hayton T, Smith KJ, Altmann DR, Brenner R, et al. Lamotrigine for neuroprotection in secondary progressive multiple sclerosis: a randomised, double-blind, placebo-controlled, parallel-group trial. Lancet Neurol 2010 Jul; 9(7): 681–8.

41 Basso AS, Frenkel D, Quintana FJ, Costa-Pinto FA, Petrovic-Stojkovic S, Puckett L, et al. Reversal of axonal loss and disability in a mouse model of progressive multiple sclerosis. J Clin Invest 2008 Apr; 118(4): 1532–43.

42 Mi S, Miller RH, Tang W, Lee X, Hu B, Wu W, et al. Promotion of central nervous system remyelination by induced differentiation of oligodendrocyte precursor cells. Ann Neurol 2009 Mar; 65(3): 304–15.

43 Yang Y, Liu Y, Wei P, Peng H, Winger R, Hussain RZ, et al. Silencing Nogo-A promotes functional recovery in demyelinating disease. Ann Neurol 2010 Apr; 67(4): 498–507.

44 Lindvall O, Kokaia Z. Stem cells for the treatment of neurological disorders. Nature 2006 Jun; 441(7097): 1094–6.

45 Pluchino S, Quattrini A, Brambilla E, Gritti A, Salani G, Dina G, et al. Injection of adult neurospheres induces recovery in a chronic model of multiple sclerosis. Nature 2003 Apr; 422(6933): 688–94.

46 Garren H, Robinson WH, Krasulova E, Havrdova E, Nadj C, Selmaj K, et al. Phase 2 trial of a DNA vaccine encoding myelin basic protein for multiple sclerosis. Ann Neurol 2008 May; 63(5): 611–20.

47 Jurynczyk M, Walczak A, Jurewicz A, Jesionek-Kupnicka D, Szczepanik M, Selmaj K. Immune regulation of multiple sclerosis by transdermally applied myelin peptides. Ann Neurol 2010 Nov; 68(5): 593–601.

48 Bakshi R, Neema M, Healy B, et al. Predicting Clinical Progression in Multiple Sclerosis with the Magnetic Resonance Disease Severity Scale. Arch Neurol 2008 Nov; 65(11): 1449–53.

49 Bakshi R, Thompson AJ, Rocca MA, Pelletier D, Dousset V, Barkhof F, et al. MRI in multiple sclerosis: current status and future prospects. Lancet Neurol 2008 Jul; 7(7): 615–25.

50 Pirko I, Lucchinetti CF, Sriram S, et al. Gray matter involvement in multiple sclerosis. Neurology 2007 Feb; 68(9): 634–42.

51 Miller DH, Thompson AJ, Filippi M. Magnetic resonance studies of abnormalities in the normal appearing white matter and grey matter in multiple sclerosis. J Neurol 2003 Dec; 250(12): 1407–19.

52 Liguori M, Meier DS, Hildenbrand P, Healy BC, Chitnis T, Baruch NF, et al. One year activity on subtraction MRI predicts subsequent 4 year activity and progression in multiple sclerosis. J Neurol Neurosurg Psychiat 2011; 82: 1125–31.

53 Agosta F, Filippi M. MRI of spinal cord in multiple sclerosis. J Neuroimaging 2007 Apr; 17Suppl 1: 46S–9S.

54 Gauthier S, Berger AM, Liptak Z, et al. Benign MS is characterized by a lower rate of brain atrophy as compared to early MS. Arch Neurol 2008.

55 Comabella M, Balashov K, et al. Elevated interleukin-12 in progressive multiple sclerosis correlates with disease activity and is normalized by pulse cyclophosphamide therapy. J Clin Invest 1998 Aug; 102(4): 671–8.

56 Khoury SJ, Guttmann CR, Orav EJ, et al. Longitudinal MRI in multiple sclerosis: correlation between disability and lesion burden. Neurology 1994 Nov; 44(11): 2120–4.

57 Khoury SJ, Guttmann CR, Orav EJ, et al. Changes in activated T cells in the blood correlate with disease activity in multiple sclerosis. Arch Neurol 2000 Aug; 57(8): 1183–9.

58 Achiron A, Gurevich M, Friedman N, et al. Blood transcriptional signatures of multiple sclerosis: unique gene expression of disease activity. Ann Neurol 2004 Mar; 55(3): 410–7.

59 Corvol JC, Pelletier D, Henry RG, et al. Abrogation of T cell quiescence characterizes patients at high risk for multiple sclerosis after the initial neurological event. Proc Natl Acad Sci U S A 2008 Aug; 105(33): 11839–44.

60 Robinson WH, DiGennaro C, Hueber W, et al. Autoantigen microarrays for multiplex characterization of autoantibody responses. Nat Med 2002 Mar; 8(3): 295–301.

61 Kanter JL, Narayana S, Ho PP, et al. Lipid microarrays identify key mediators of autoimmune brain inflammation. Nat Med 2006 Jan; 12(1): 138–43.

62 Quintana F, Farez M, Viglietta V, et al. Antigen microarrays identify unique serum autoantibody signatures associated with different clinical forms and pathologic subtypes of multiple sclerosis. Proc Natl Acad Sci U S A 2008 Dec 2; 105(48): 18889–94.

63 Lassmann H, Bruck W, Lucchinetti CF. The immunopathology of multiple sclerosis: an overview. Brain Pathol 2007 Apr; 17(2): 210–8.

64 Gorelik L, Lerner M, Bixler S, Crossman M, Schlain B, Simon K, et al. Anti-JC virus antibodies: implications for PML risk stratification. Ann Neurol 2010 Sep; 68(3): 295–303.

65 Kappos L, Weinshenker B, Pozzilli C, Thompson AJ, Dahlke F, Beckmann K, et al. Interferon beta-1b in secondary progressive MS: a combined analysis of the two trials. Neurology 2004 Nov; 63(10): 1779–87.

66 Hawker K, O'Connor P, Freedman MS, Calabresi PA, Antel J, Simon J, et al. Rituximab in patients with primary progressive multiple sclerosis: results of a randomized double-blind placebo-controlled multicenter trial. Ann Neurol 2009 Oct; 66(4): 460–71.

67 Zephir H, de Seze J, Duhamel A, Debouverie M, Hautecoeur P, Lebrun C, et al. Treatment of progressive forms of multiple sclerosis by cyclophosphamide: a cohort study of 490 patients. J Neurol Sci 2004 Mar; 218(1–2): 73–7.

68 Elkhalifa A, Weiner H. Cyclophosphamide Treatment of MS: Current Therapeutic Approaches and Treatment Regimens. Int MS J 2010 May; 17(1): 12–8.

69 Esposito F, Radaelli M, Martinelli V, Sormani MP, Martinelli Boneschi F, Moiola L, et al. Comparative study of mitoxantrone efficacy profile in patients with relapsing-remitting and secondary progressive multiple sclerosis. Mult Scler 2010 Dec; 16(12): 1490–9.

70 Karni A, Abraham M, Monsonego A, Cai G, Freeman GJ, Hafler D, et al. Innate immunity in multiple sclerosis: myeloid dendritic cells in secondary progressive multiple sclerosis are activated and drive a proinflammatory immune response. J Immunol 2006 Sep; 177(6): 4196–202.

71 Rudick RA, Stuart WH, Calabresi PA, et al. Natalizumab plus interferon beta-1a for relapsing multiple sclerosis. N Engl J Med 2006 Mar; 354(9): 911–23.

72 Coles AJ, Compston DA, Selmaj KW, et al. Alemtuzumab vs. interferon beta-1a in early multiple sclerosis. N Engl J Med 2008 Oct; 359(17): 1786–801.

73 Krishnan C, Kaplin AI, Brodsky RA, et al. Reduction of disease activity and disability with high-dose cyclophosphamide in patients with aggressive multiple sclerosis. Arch Neurol 2008 Aug; 65(8): 1044–51.

74 Le Page E, Leray E, Taurin G, et al. Mitoxantrone as induction treatment in aggressive relapsing remitting multiple sclerosis: treatment response factors in a 5 year follow-up observational study of 100 consecutive patients. J Neurol Neurosurg Psychiat 2008 Jan; 79(1): 52–6.

75 Birnbaum G, Cree B, Altafullah I, et al. Combining beta interferon and atorvastatin may increase disease activity in multiple sclerosis. Neurology 2008 Oct; 71(18): 1390–5.

76 Gauthier SA, Glanz BI, Mandel M, et al. A model for the comprehensive investigation of a chronic autoimmune disease: the multiple sclerosis CLIMB study. Autoimmun Rev 2006 Oct; 5(8): 532–6.

77 Rodriguez M, Lindsley MD. Immunosuppression promotes CNS remyelination in chronic virus-induced demyelinating disease. Neurology 1992 Feb; 42(2): 348–57.

78 Karnezis T, Mandemakers W, McQualter JL, et al. The neurite outgrowth inhibitor Nogo A is involved in autoimmune-mediated demyelination. Nat Neurosci 2004 Jul; 7(7): 736–44.

79 Warrington AE, Asakura K, Bieber AJ, et al. Human monoclonal antibodies reactive to oligodendrocytes promote remyelination in a model of multiple sclerosis. Proc Natl Acad Sci USA 2000 Jun; 97(12): 6820–5.

80 Craner MJ, Damarjian TG, Liu S, et al. Sodium channels contribute to microglia/macrophage activation and function in EAE and MS. Glia 2005 Jan; 49(2): 220–9.

81 Pluchino S, Muzio L, Imitola J, et al. Persistent inflammation alters the function of the endogenous brain stem cell compartment. Brain 2008 Oct; 131 (Pt 10): 2564–78.

82 Stankiewicz J, Panter SS, Neema M, et al. Iron in chronic brain disorders: imaging and neurotherapeutic implications. Neurotherapeutics 2007; 4: 371–86.

Index

Multiple Sclerosis: Diagnosis and Therapy, First Edition. Edited by Howard L. Weiner and
James M. Stankiewicz. © 2012 John Wiley & Sons, Ltd.
Published 2012 by John Wiley and Sons, Ltd.